Plant-Based Bioactive Natural Products

Plant-Based Bioactive Natural Products

Insights into Molecular Mechanisms of Action

Editor

Hari Prasad Devkota

MDPI • Basel • Beijing • Wuhan • Barcelona • Belgrade • Manchester • Tokyo • Cluj • Tianjin

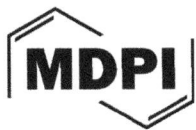

Editor
Hari Prasad Devkota
Graduate School of
Pharmaceutical Sciences,
Kumamoto University
Japan

Editorial Office
MDPI
St. Alban-Anlage 66
4052 Basel, Switzerland

This is a reprint of articles from the Special Issue published online in the open access journal *Applied Sciences* (ISSN 2076-3417) (available at: https://www.mdpi.com/journal/applsci/special_issues/Bioactive_Natural_Products).

For citation purposes, cite each article independently as indicated on the article page online and as indicated below:

LastName, A.A.; LastName, B.B.; LastName, C.C. Article Title. *Journal Name* **Year**, *Volume Number*, Page Range.

ISBN 978-3-0365-2412-2 (Hbk)
ISBN 978-3-0365-2413-9 (PDF)

© 2021 by the authors. Articles in this book are Open Access and distributed under the Creative Commons Attribution (CC BY) license, which allows users to download, copy and build upon published articles, as long as the author and publisher are properly credited, which ensures maximum dissemination and a wider impact of our publications.

The book as a whole is distributed by MDPI under the terms and conditions of the Creative Commons license CC BY-NC-ND.

Contents

About the Editor . . . . **vii**

Hari Prasad Devkota
Plant-Based Bioactive Natural Products: Insights into Molecular Mechanisms of Action
Reprinted from: *Appl. Sci.* **2021**, *11*, 10220, doi:10.3390/app112110220 1

Lucía López-Salas, Isabel Borrás-Linares, David Quintin, Presentación García-Gomez, Rafael Giménez-Martínez, Antonio Segura-Carretero and Jesús Lozano-Sánchez
Artichoke By-Products as Natural Source of Phenolic Food Ingredient
Reprinted from: *Appl. Sci.* **2021**, *11*, 3788, doi:10.3390/app11093788 5

Marisa Colone, Filippo Maggi, Rianasoambolanoro Rakotosaona and Annarita Stringaro
Vepris macrophylla Essential Oil Produces Notable Antiproliferative Activity and Morphological Alterations in Human Breast Adenocarcinoma Cells
Reprinted from: *Appl. Sci.* **2021**, *11*, 4369, doi:10.3390/app11104369 19

Hae Jin Lee, Dae Young Lee, Hae Lim Kim and Seung Hwan Yang
Scrophularia buergeriana Extract Improves Memory Impairment via Inhibition of the Apoptosis Pathway in the Mouse Hippocampus
Reprinted from: *Appl. Sci.* **2020**, *10*, 7987, doi:10.3390/app10227987 31

Hae-Jin Lee, Hae-Lim Kim, Dae-Young Lee, Dong-Ryung Lee, Bong-Keun Choi and Seung-Hwan Yang
Scrophularia buergeriana Extract (Brainon) Improves Scopolamine-Induced Neuronal Impairment and Cholinergic Dysfunction in Mice through CREB-BDNF Signaling Pathway
Reprinted from: *Appl. Sci.* **2021**, *11*, 4286, doi:10.3390/app11094286 45

Hae Lim Kim, Hae Jin Lee, Dong-Ryung Lee, Bong-Keun Choi and Seung Hwan Yang
Anti-Osteoarthritic Effects of *Terminalia Chebula* Fruit Extract (AyuFlex®) in Interleukin-1β-Induced Human Chondrocytes and in Rat Models of Monosodium Iodoacetate (MIA)-Induced Osteoarthritis
Reprinted from: *Appl. Sci.* **2020**, *10*, 8698, doi:10.3390/app10238698 57

Moon Young Jun, Rajendra Karki, Keshav Raj Paudel, Nisha Panth, Hari Prasad Devkota and Dong-Wook Kim
Liensinine Prevents Vascular Inflammation by Attenuating Inflammatory Mediators and Modulating VSMC Function
Reprinted from: *Appl. Sci.* **2021**, *11*, 386, doi:10.3390/app11010386 75

Lorina I. Badger-Emeka, Promise Madu Emeka and Hairul Islam M. Ibrahim
A Molecular Insight into the Synergistic Mechanism of *Nigella sativa* (Black Cumin) with β-Lactam Antibiotics against Clinical Isolates of Methicillin-Resistant *Staphylococcus aureus*
Reprinted from: *Appl. Sci.* **2021**, *11*, 3206, doi:10.3390/app11073206 87

Farhat Ullah, Muhammad Ayaz, Abdul Sadiq, Farman Ullah, Ishtiaq Hussain, Muhammad Shahid, Zhanibek Yessimbekov, Anjana Adhikari-Devkota and Hari Prasad Devkota
Potential Role of Plant Extracts and Phytochemicals Against Foodborne Pathogens
Reprinted from: *Appl. Sci.* **2020**, *10*, 4597, doi:10.3390/app10134597 105

Rosa Tundis, Maria C. Tenuta, Monica R. Loizzo, Marco Bonesi, Federica Finetti, Lorenza Trabalzini and Brigitte Deguin
Vaccinium Species (Ericaceae): From Chemical Composition to Bio-Functional Activities
Reprinted from: *Appl. Sci.* **2021**, *11*, 5655, doi:10.3390/app11125655 . . . . **141**

About the Editor

Hari Prasad Devkota completed his Bachelor of Pharmaceutical Sciences (B. Pharm.) from Pokhara University, Nepal in 2005. After working at the same institute as a Teaching Associate till 2007, he received Japanese Government (MEXT) Scholarship and entered the Graduate School of Pharmaceutical Sciences, Kumamoto University, Japan in 2007, and completed his Master's and PhD in Pharmaceutical Sciences in 2010 and 2013, respectively. He was working as Postdoctoral Fellow in Kumamoto University (2013–2014) with the support from Takeda Science Foundation (TSF), Japan. Since 2014, he has been working as Assistant Professor at Kumamoto University. His main research interests are plant-based bioactive natural products, functional foods and ethnopharmacology. To date, he has authored more than 130 publications including original research articles, review articles, books and book chapters. He is actively involved in the research on medicinal plants from Asia and Africa for their ethnopharmacological surveys, chemical constituents and pharmacological activities.

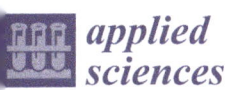

Editorial

Plant-Based Bioactive Natural Products: Insights into Molecular Mechanisms of Action

Hari Prasad Devkota

Graduate School of Pharmaceutical Sciences, Kumamoto University, 5-1 Oe-honmachi, Chuo-ku, Kumamoto 862-0973, Japan; devkotah@kumamoto-u.ac.jp

Keywords: natural products; bioactive compounds; medicinal plants; bioactivity; mechanism of action; traditional medicines

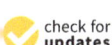

Citation: Devkota, H.P. Plant-Based Bioactive Natural Products: Insights into Molecular Mechanisms of Action. *Appl. Sci.* 2021, 11, 10220. https://doi.org/10.3390/app112110220

Received: 21 October 2021
Accepted: 26 October 2021
Published: 1 November 2021

Publisher's Note: MDPI stays neutral with regard to jurisdictional claims in published maps and institutional affiliations.

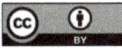

Copyright: © 2021 by the author. Licensee MDPI, Basel, Switzerland. This article is an open access article distributed under the terms and conditions of the Creative Commons Attribution (CC BY) license (https://creativecommons.org/licenses/by/4.0/).

Medicinal plants have been used for the maintenance of human health since ancient times in the form of food, spices, and traditional medicines [1–3]. Traditional plant-based medicines serve as the primary healthcare systems in various countries even in recent times [4,5]. Additionally, medicinal plants have also served as the one of the main sources for the discovery of new therapeutic agents [3,6].

At present, various plant extracts and their isolated phytochemicals are screened and evaluated for their diverse pharmacological activities related to both communicable and non-communicable diseases. However, comparatively little focus is given to the detailed mechanism of action of these agents on the molecular level. Molecular mechanism-based studies are essential for the development of evidence-based traditional medicines as well as for the development of isolated natural products as the lead candidates for novel drug discovery.

This main focus of this Special Issue "Plant-based Bioactive Natural Products: Insights into Molecular Mechanisms of Action" is to cover the recent advances in science related to the molecular mechanisms of action of natural products. A total of nine articles were published under this Special Issue including seven original research articles and two review articles.

Food by-products have been receiving great attention in recent years for their valorization to obtain bioactive natural products that can contribute to sustainable development and circular economy [7–9]. In this issue, López-Salas et al. [10] reported the potential of artichoke by-products as a rich source of phenolic compounds. The authors optimized the extraction condition for polyphenols using an advanced extraction technique, pressurized liquid extraction (PLE), with ethanol–water mixture as solvent. Compounds were identified by using high-performance liquid chromatography (HPLC) coupled to electrospray time-of-flight mass spectrometry (HPLC-ESI-TOF/MS) analysis.

Colone et al. [11] reported the potent antiproliferative activity of essential oil (EO) obtained from the leaves of *Vepris macrophylla* against human breast adenocarcinoma cell line SKBR3.

Lee et al. [12] reported the memory improving activity of 70% ethanol extract of roots of *Scrophularia buergeriana* in model mice with beta-amyloid-induced memory loss. The extract improved the memory impairment by reducing neurotoxicity and regulating oxidative stress and inhibiting the apoptosis pathway. The authors further analyzed the memory improving activity of the extract in scopolamine-induced neuronal impairment in mice [13]. The extract was reported to inhibit the acetylcholinesterase activity and to exert memory-improving effects through the phosphorylated cAMP response element-binding (CREB) and brain-derived neurotrophic factor (BDNF) pathway.

Fruits of *Terminalia chebula* are used as crude drugs in many traditional medicine systems around the world due to potent antioxidant, hepatoprotective and anti-diabetic activities [14]. Kim et al. [15] reported the anti-osteoarthritic activity of aqueous extracts of *Terminalia chebula* fruit in interleukin-1β-induced human chondrocytes and monosodium iodoacetate-induced osteoarthritis in model rats.

Jun et al. [16] reported the vascular inflammation preventive activity of liensinine, a bisbenzylisoquinoline alkaloid found in *Nelumbo nucifera*. Liensinine showed potent in vitro antioxidative and anti-inflammatory activity by attenuating inflammatory mediators in human vascular smooth muscle cells (VSMC).

Badger-Emeka et al. [17] reported the synergistic activity of cold pressed oil of *Nigella sativa* with various β-lactam antibiotics against clinical isolates of methicillin-resistant *Staphylococcus aureus* (MRSA).

Ullah et al. [18] reported a comprehensive review on the role of plant extracts and their isolated phytochemicals against food-borne pathogens, one of the major causative agents of food-borne illness worldwide.

Tundis et al. [19] reported an extensive review on the traditional uses, bioactive chemical constituents and biological properties of various species of *Vaccinium* genus. The authors also highlighted their potential uses in functional food and cosmetic markets.

This Special Issue has provided some new experimental data on bioactive natural products and their detailed mechanisms of action for biological activities. Similarly, review articles have provided state-of-the-art information on the related topics. I would like to thank all the authors for submitting their manuscripts and the reviewers and editors for their contribution to this Special Issue. Furthermore, I am also grateful to the handling editors and staff of *Applied Sciences* for their support during the preparation and finalization of this Special Issue.

Funding: This research received no external funding.

Conflicts of Interest: The author declares no conflict of interest.

References

1. Kunwar, R.M.; Bussmann, R.W. Ethnobotany in the Nepal Himalaya. *J. Ethnobiol. Ethnomed.* **2008**, *4*, 24. [CrossRef] [PubMed]
2. Khanal, A.; Devkota, H.P.; Kaundinnyayana, S.; Gyawali, P.; Ananda, R.; Adhikari, R. Culinary herbs and spices in Nepal: A review of their traditional uses, chemical constituents, and pharmacological activities. *Ethnobot. Res. Appl.* **2021**, *21*, 40.
3. Atanasov, A.G.; Waltenberger, B.; Pferschy-Wenzig, E.M.; Linder, T.; Wawrosch, C.; Uhrin, P.; Temml, V.; Wang, L.; Schwaiger, S.; Heiss, E.H.; et al. Discovery and resupply of pharmacologically active plant-derived natural products: A review. *Biotechnol. Adv.* **2015**, *33*, 1582–1614. [CrossRef] [PubMed]
4. Cordell, G.A.; Colvard, M.D. Some thoughts on the future of ethnopharmacology. *J. Ethnopharmacol.* **2005**, *100*, 5–14. [CrossRef]
5. Yuan, H.; Ma, Q.; Ye, L.; Piao, G. The traditional medicine and modern medicine from natural products. *Molecules* **2016**, *21*, 559. [CrossRef]
6. David, B.; Wolfender, J.L.; Dias, D.A. The pharmaceutical industry and natural products: Historical status and new trends. *Phytochem. Rev.* **2015**, *14*, 299–315. [CrossRef]
7. Durazzo, A.; Lucarini, M.; Santini, A. Plants and Diabetes: Description, Role, Comprehension and Exploitation. *Int. J. Mol. Sci.* **2021**, *22*, 3938. [CrossRef]
8. Vermeir, I.; Weijters, B.; De Houwer, J.; Geuens, M.; Slabbinck, H.; Spruyt, A.; Van Kerckhove, A.; Van Lippevelde, W.; De Steur, H.; Verbeke, W. Environmentally Sustainable Food Consumption: A Review and Research Agenda From a Goal-Directed Perspective. *Front. Psychol.* **2020**, *11*, 1603. [CrossRef] [PubMed]
9. Torres-León, C.; Ramírez-Guzman, N.; Londoño-Hernandez, L.; Martinez-Medina, G.A.; Díaz-Herrera, R.; Navarro-Macias, V.; Alvarez-Pérez, O.B.; Picazo, B.; Villarreal-Vázquez, M.; Ascacio-Valdes, J.; et al. Food Waste and Byproducts: An Opportunity to Minimize Malnutrition and Hunger in Developing Countries. *Front. Sustain. Food Syst.* **2018**, *2*, 52. [CrossRef]
10. López-Salas, L.; Borrás-Linares, I.; Quintin, D.; García-Gomez, P.; Giménez-Martínez, R.; Segura-Carretero, A.; Lozano-Sánchez, J. Artichoke By-Products as Natural Source of Phenolic Food Ingredient. *Appl. Sci.* **2021**, *11*, 3788. [CrossRef]
11. Colone, M.; Maggi, F.; Rakotosaona, R.; Stringaro, A. Vepris macrophylla Essential Oil Produces Notable Antiproliferative Activity and Morphological Alterations in Human Breast Adenocarcinoma Cells. *Appl. Sci.* **2021**, *11*, 4369. [CrossRef]
12. Lee, H.J.; Lee, D.Y.; Kim, H.L.; Yang, S.H. *Scrophularia buergeriana* Extract Improves Memory Impairment via Inhibition of the Apoptosis Pathway in the Mouse Hippocampus. *Appl. Sci.* **2020**, *10*, 7987. [CrossRef]
13. Lee, H.-J.; Kim, H.-L.; Lee, D.-Y.; Lee, D.-R.; Choi, B.-K.; Yang, S.-H. *Scrophularia buergeriana* Extract (Brainon) Improves Scopolamine-Induced Neuronal Impairment and Cholinergic Dysfunction in Mice through CREB-BDNF Signaling Pathway. *Appl. Sci.* **2021**, *11*, 4286. [CrossRef]

14. Nigam, M.; Mishra, A.P.; Adhikari-Devkota, A.; Dirar, A.I.; Hassan, M.M.; Adhikari, A.; Belwal, T.; Devkota, H.P. Fruits of *Terminalia chebula* Retz.: A review on traditional uses, bioactive chemical constituents and pharmacological activities. *Phyther. Res.* **2020**, *34*, 2518–2533. [CrossRef] [PubMed]
15. Kim, H.L.; Lee, H.J.; Lee, D.-R.; Choi, B.-K.; Yang, S.H. Anti-Osteoarthritic Effects of *Terminalia Chebula* Fruit Extract (AyuFlex®) in Interleukin-1β-Induced Human Chondrocytes and in Rat Models of Monosodium Iodoacetate (MIA)-Induced Osteoarthritis. *Appl. Sci.* **2020**, *10*, 8698. [CrossRef]
16. Jun, M.Y.; Karki, R.; Paudel, K.R.; Panth, N.; Devkota, H.P.; Kim, D.-W. Liensinine Prevents Vascular Inflammation by Attenuating Inflammatory Mediators and Modulating VSMC Function. *Appl. Sci.* **2021**, *11*, 386. [CrossRef]
17. Badger-Emeka, L.I.; Emeka, P.M.; Ibrahim, H.I.M. A Molecular Insight into the Synergistic Mechanism of *Nigella sativa* (Black Cumin) with β-Lactam Antibiotics against Clinical Isolates of Methicillin-Resistant *Staphylococcus aureus*. *Appl. Sci.* **2021**, *11*, 3206. [CrossRef]
18. Ullah, F.; Ayaz, M.; Sadiq, A.; Ullah, F.; Hussain, I.; Shahid, M.; Yessimbekov, Z.; Adhikari-Devkota, A.; Devkota, H.P. Potential Role of Plant Extracts and Phytochemicals Against Foodborne Pathogens. *Appl. Sci.* **2020**, *10*, 4597. [CrossRef]
19. Tundis, R.; Tenuta, M.C.; Loizzo, M.R.; Bonesi, M.; Finetti, F.; Trabalzini, L.; Deguin, B. *Vaccinium* Species (Ericaceae): From Chemical Composition to Bio-Functional Activities. *Appl. Sci.* **2021**, *11*, 5655. [CrossRef]

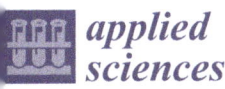

Article

Artichoke By-Products as Natural Source of Phenolic Food Ingredient

Lucía López-Salas [1], Isabel Borrás-Linares [2,*], David Quintin [3], Presentación García-Gomez [3], Rafael Giménez-Martínez [1], Antonio Segura-Carretero [2,4,†] and Jesús Lozano-Sánchez [1,2,†]

1. Department of Food Science and Nutrition, Campus Universitario s/n, University of Granada, 18071 Granada, Spain; lslucia@correo.ugr.es (L.L.-S.); rafaelg@ugr.es (R.G.-M.); jesusls@ugr.es (J.L.-S.)
2. Functional Food Research and Development Centre (CIDAF), Health Sciencie Technological Park, Avda. Del Conocimiento S/N, 18016 Granada, Spain; ansegura@cidaf.es
3. Centro Tecnológico Nacional de la Conserva y Alimentación, Concordia, s/n, 30500 Molina de Segura, Spain; dquintin@ctnc.es (D.Q.); sese@ctnc.es (P.G.-G.)
4. Department of Analytical Chemistry, Faculty of Sciences, University of Granada, 18071 Granada, Spain
* Correspondence: iborras@cidaf.es; Tel.: +34-958-637-083
† These authors are joint senior authors on this work.

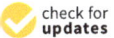

Citation: López-Salas, L.; Borrás-Linares, I.; Quintin, D.; García-Gomez, P.; Giménez-Martínez, R.; Segura-Carretero, A.; Lozano-Sánchez, J. Artichoke By-Products as Natural Source of Phenolic Food Ingredient. *Appl. Sci.* **2021**, *11*, 3788. https://doi.org/10.3390/app11093788

Academic Editors: Luca Mazzoni and Hari Prasad Devkota

Received: 13 March 2021
Accepted: 19 April 2021
Published: 22 April 2021

Publisher's Note: MDPI stays neutral with regard to jurisdictional claims in published maps and institutional affiliations.

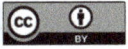

Copyright: © 2021 by the authors. Licensee MDPI, Basel, Switzerland. This article is an open access article distributed under the terms and conditions of the Creative Commons Attribution (CC BY) license (https:// creativecommons.org/licenses/by/ 4.0/).

Abstract: Nowadays, the transformation activity of the food industry results in the generation of a huge amount of daily discarded vegetables wastes. One of those undervalued by-products are produced during the post-harvesting and processing process of artichokes. In the present research, the potential of artichokes' bracts and stalks have been evaluated as a natural source of phenolic compounds which could be used as bioactive food ingredients, among others. In this study, the bioactive composition of those wastes has been evaluated using recent advances in extraction and analytical technologies, concretely, pressurized liquid extraction (PLE) followed by high-performance liquid chromatography (HPLC) coupled to electrospray time-of flight mass spectrometry (ESI-TOF/MS) analysis. To achieve this goal, first, the extraction process was evaluated by a comparative study using GRAS (Generally Recognized As Safe) solvents (mixtures of ethanol and water) at different temperatures (40–200 °C). The second step was to deeply characterize the composition of individual polyphenols by HPLC-ESI-TOF/MS in order to establish a comparison among the different PLE conditions applied to extract the phenolic fraction. The analysis revealed a wide variety of phenolic-composition, mainly phenolic acids and flavonoids. The results also highlighted that high percentages of ethanol and medium-high temperatures pointed out to be useful PLE conditions for recovering this kind of phytochemicals, which could be used in different applications, such as functional food ingredients, cosmetics, or nutraceuticals.

Keywords: artichoke by-products; phenolic compounds; HPLC-ESI-TOF-MS; PLE; GRAS

1. Introduction

Nowadays, consumption of fruit and vegetable is very widespread as they provide health benefits. These benefits are partly due to the phenolic compounds that products contain. Phenolic compounds are plant secondary metabolites, with a structure composed of an aromatic ring linked to one or more hydroxyl substitutes. They are synthesized in the normal plant growth and reproduction and, also, during stress conditions such as high temperatures, hydric stress, ultraviolet radiation, or parasites [1]. These phytochemicals are bioactive molecules with antioxidant, antithrombotic, anti-inflammatory, and antidiabetic properties, among others [2–4]. Among phenolic compounds, simple phenols and polyphenols can be distinguished. The first group includes phenolic acids (benzoic and cinnamic acids) and benzoquinones, while flavonoids, stilbenes, lignans, tannins, and other polymerized compounds are part of polyphenols group.

The current need of a sustainable food chain demands an implementation of a circular economy approach in the processing industries. The major focus of this approach is to revalorize the discarding parts of vegetables due to their great contents in bioactive compounds. This trend is supported by the potential of these food wastes, which could be used for the production of valued products. In fact, peels, seeds, stems, or vegetable pulps are considered raw materials to obtain bioactive ingredients with multiple applications, mainly for the production of food ingredients, cosmetics, or nutraceuticals. Furthermore, bioactive compounds of vegetable wastes have demonstrated antioxidant and antimicrobial actions in developed food additives used for conservative purposes. Its formulation in nutraceuticals with different presentations, such as syrups, capsules, pills or tablets, is very common [5,6]. These applications are possible due to the content in phytochemicals of these vegetable wastes with potent bioactive activities, such as phenolic compounds.

Artichoke (*Cynara scolymus* L.) is an herbaceous perennial plant belonging to *Cynara* genus and Asteraceae family. Commonly known as globe artichoke, it is traditionally consumed in the Mediterranean diet in different popular preparations. It can be consumed fresh, canned, roasted, or baked, among others. Therefore, this vegetable is extensively cultivated in Mediterranean countries such as Italy, France, Spain, Egypt, and Morocco. Their cultivation is considered an important activity of the agro-economy of these countries [7,8], indeed, the Mediterranean region has an annual production of about 770,000 tons. The edible portion of this plant includes the receptacle of immature flowers and the inner bracts, named "capitula" or heads. During the artichoke processing, the residues, principally external leaves or stems, represent approximately 60–80% of the total harvested plant material, which is translated in more than 460,000 tons of wastes generated annually. Nevertheless, these by-products possess a great content of bioactive phenolic compounds, inulin, fibers, and minerals [9–13]. This information highlighted the significance of the evaluation of artichoke wastes for the extraction of bioactive compounds.

The artichoke is one of the most consumed plants of its genus due to its high nutritional value, being rich in water, minerals, vitamins, and carotenoids. Despite its content in these interesting compounds, it is the presence of bioactive compounds that has aroused greater interest, especially phenolic compounds [14,15]. The interest in their phytochemicals has been linked to various pharmacological activities exerted on humans. Thus, hepatoprotective, antioxidant, hypocholesterolemic, anticarcinogenic, antibacterial, or diuretic effects have been described for artichoke. Therefore, the artichoke has been used for medicinal purposes since antiquity, being considered a functional food [9,10,16,17].

Consequently, the re-valorization of food by-products as a bioactive source material has experienced a great growth due to the economic and environmental benefits that it produces. In the case of artichoke, recent studies based their research on external bracts, leaves and floral stems by-products, which are considered the principal discarding parts of the artichoke processing because they are not suitable for human consumption [18].

The main objective of this article was to explore the potential of artichoke by-products generated in the food industry as a green and efficient source of phytochemicals with many applications. For this purpose, the present research optimized the extraction of the phenolic profile from artichoke bracts and stems, which were obtained as industrial by-products, through an advanced extraction system and characterized the composition of the obtained extracts by a powerful analytical platform. Thus, pressurized liquid extraction (PLE) using water and ethanol as GRAS extraction solvents was chosen due to its great potential to extract phenolic compounds in green and efficient processes from vegetable matrices. Similarly, reversed-phase high-performance liquid chromatography coupled to electrospray time-of-flight mass spectrometry (HPLC-ESI-TOF-MS) was selected for the analytical characterization of the PLE extracts due to its great potential.

2. Materials and Methods

2.1. Reagents

The chemicals employed during the development of this study have analytical reagent grade. Purified water used for extraction and analytical experiments was obtained from a Milli-Q system from Millipore (Bedford, MA, USA). Moreover, ethanol used to obtain artichoke PLE extracts was purchased from VWR Chemicals (Radnor, PA, USA), whereas sand and cellulose filters were from Fisher Chemicals (Waltham, MA, USA). The mobile phases used for the analysis were prepared with formic acid and LC-MS-grade methanol provided from Sigma–Aldrich (Steinheim, Germany) and Fisher Chemicals (Waltham, MA, USA), respectively.

2.2. Plant Material

By-products such as bracts and stems were obtained from the industrial processing of artichokes. The post-harvest processing of artichokes consists in a minimally blanching step carried out in the same day of harvesting before peeling. This processing was performed with water for 20 min at 98 °C. After blanching, the artichokes were pealed and the bracts and stems were separated from the artichoke hearts. These by-products were frozen at −45 °C and lyophilized for 24 h in a freeze-dryer (Vertis SP Scientific, Thermo Fisher (Madrid, Spain).

2.3. Pressurized Liquid Extraction

PLE extracts from artichoke by-products were obtained with an accelerated solvent extractor (ASE 350, Dionex, Sunnyvale, CA, USA) applying different combinations of temperature and solvent composition (mixtures of ethanol and water in different proportions) previously applied to food by-products. These conditions were selected to cover a wide range of dielectric constant (from 19 to 59.1) [19,20].

Briefly, PLE static extractions were performed during 20 min under a pressure of 1500 psi. Thus, the tested ranges of instrumental parameters were as follow: 0–100% of aqueous ethanol mixtures as extraction solvent and 40 to 200 °C as extraction temperature.

The experiments were performed with extraction cells of 33 mL filled with a homogenous mixture composed of 4 g of artichoke sample plus 8 g of sand. This sample-sand ratio (1:2, w:w) allows to perform the experiments avoiding technical problems (fundamentally blockage of the lines of the PLE instrument) with the maximum amount of sample. The solvents used in each PLE experiment were previously sonicated for 15 min in order to eliminate the oxygen dissolved in the mixture, which could provoke a degradation of compounds susceptible of oxidation.

The PLE process begins with a cell heat-up step previous to the extraction in order to attain the pertinent extraction temperature. The duration of this phase is dependent of the temperature set-point and established by the instrument (lasting from 5 to 9 min). Then, the extraction step was carried out applying the corresponding conditions according to Table 1.

Table 1. Experimental pressurized liquid extraction (PLE) conditions.

Experimental Condition	Temperature and Percentage of Ethanol in the Extraction Solvent	Dielectric Constant
PLE 1	120 °C; EtOH 100%	19.0
PLE 2	176 °C; EtOH 85%	21.6
PLE 3	200 °C; EtOH 50%	26.0
PLE 4	63 °C; EtOH 85%	31.0
PLE 5	176 °C; EtOH 15%	33.4
PLE 6	120 °C; EtOH 50%	34.7
PLE 7	40 °C; EtOH 50%	48.0
PLE 8	120 °C; EtOH 0%	50.4
PLE 9	63 °C; EtOH 15%	59.1

The obtained extracts were immediately cooled at room temperature in an ice-bath. The supernatants were separated after a centrifugation step of 15 min at 4 °C applying

12,499 as relative centrifugal force (RCF). Then, they were completely evaporated under vacuum at 35 °C in a Savan SC250EXP Speed-Vac (Thermo Scientific, Leicestershire, UK). The dry extracts were stored refrigerated (−20 °C) avoiding light exposure until further use.

2.4. HPLC-ESI-TOF-MS Analysis

The analysis of the artichoke by-products PLE extracts was carried out by high-performance liquid chromatography (HPLC) with a diode array detector (DAD) coupled to time-of-flight mass spectrometry with an electrospray interface (ESI-TOF-MS). The instrument was an Agilent 1200-RRLC system (Agilent Technologies, Palo Alto, CA, USA) equipped with a vacuum degasser, a binary pump, an auto-sampler, a thermostatically controlled column compartment, and a DAD detector. Mass detection was performed using a micrOTOF II analyzer from Bruker Daltonik (Bremen, Germany). The extracts were dissolved in aqueous ethanol (50:50, v/v) at 5 mg/mL and analyzed in triplicate. Before the HPLC injection, the samples were filtered through a 0.45 µm syringe filters of regenerated cellulose to avoid solid particles.

The separation occurs in an Agilent Zorbax Eclipse Plus C18 column (150 mm × 4.6 mm id, 1.8 µm). The mobile phases consist of water with 0.1% formic acid (A) and methanol (B) at a flow rate of 0.8 mL/min. The analytical method used an elution gradient according to the following linear multi-step profile: 0 min, 5% B; 3 min, 50% B; 25 min, 75% B; 35 min, 100% B, 40 min, and 5% B plus 5 min of stabilization at initial conditions before the next analysis. The analyses were carried out at 25 °C injecting 10 µL of sample in each run.

Detection was performed within a mass range of 50–1000 m/z operating in negative ionization mode. In order to achieve a stable ionization, the flow rate from the HPLC was split before the connection to the ESI interface (Agilent Technologies) until 125 µL/min. Ultrapure nitrogen was used as drying and nebulizing gas with flows of 9.0 L min^{-1} and 2.0 bar, respectively. The operating parameters applied for the ionization and ion transfer were: capillary voltage of +4.5 kV; drying gas temperature, 190 °C; capillary exit, −150 V; skimmer 1, −50 V; hexapole 1, −23 V; RF hexapole, 100 Vpp; and skimmer 2, −22.5 V.

In order to recalibrate the mass spectra acquired during the analysis to achieve accurate mass measurements with a precision better than 5 ppm, 10 mM sodium formate solution was used as calibrant. This mixture is automatically injected at the beginning of each run by means of a 74900-00-05 Cole Palmer syringe pump (Vernon Hills, IL, USA) directly connected to the ESI interface, equipped with a Hamilton syringe (Reno, NV, USA). All data acquisition and processing operations were controlled with HyStar 3.2 and Data Analysis 4.0 software, respectively (Bruker Daltonics GmbH, Bremen, Germany). The software provides a list of possible elemental formulas using the Generate-Molecular Formula Editor. This information provided by the analytical platform was used for identification purposes together with the one reported in databases and bibliography.

2.5. Statistical Analysis

Data were statistically treated using Origin (Version Origin Pro 8.5, Northampton, MA, USA). For these data, set one-way analysis of variance (ANOVA, Tukey's test) at a 95% confidence level ($p \leq 0.05$) was performed to point out the differences in semi-quantitative bioactive compounds contents found between PLE artichoke samples with statistical significance.

3. Results

3.1. Identification of Phytochemical Compounds of Artichoke By-Products by HPLC-ESI-TOF-MS

The compounds were identified by the data provided by the HPLC-ESI-TOF-MS instrument. Thus, for all the peaks detected in the chromatogram, a list of possible molecular formulas was obtained with DataAnalysis 4.0 software. The identification was achieved comparing with the data previously reported in databases and literature for artichoke composition.

The bibliography search consulted for the tentative identification of the detected compounds was composed by studies carried out on artichoke. Therefore, one of the studies reported the inflorescence of artichoke, which were lyophilized and extracted by ultrasound-assisted extraction (UAE) using 80% methanol as solvent [21]. Other authors evaluated the phenolic profile of the edible parts of artichokes (receptacle and internal bracts) using a conventional procedure and mixture of solvents, concretely sonication in methanol/water (70:30, v/v) [10,22]. Finally, another study was based on the study of the chemical composition of artichoke by-products (leaves, floral stems, and bracts) applying maceration with 80% methanol–water mixture able to obtain extracts enriched in polar compounds [18].

Figure 1 shows a representative base peak chromatogram (BPC) of artichoke by-products PLE extract obtained by HPLC-ESI-TOF-MS analyzed in negative polarity. Moreover, Figure 2 includes the extracted ion chromatograms and mass spectra of the major phenolic compounds characterized in those extracts. Furthermore, Table 2 summarizes the main peaks detected according to their elution order, including the information provided by the MS spectrometer: experimental and theoretical *m/z*, error (ppm), molecular formula, proposed compound, and the PLE condition in which each of them was detected. As can be observed, a total of 23 compounds were detected, being 19 of them tentatively identified. Despite the information provided by the analyzer and the effort made for their identification, unfortunately four compounds remain unknown (listed as UK in Table 2). The proposed compounds were tentatively identified as phenolic acids, flavones, and derivatives (flavonoids), saponins, lipids, and other polar compounds. In the following sections, the tentatively identification of these compounds has been described according to these chemical sub-classes.

Table 2. Phenolic and other polar compounds characterized in *Cynara scolymus* L. PLE extracts analyzed by HPLC-time-of-flight mass spectrometry with an electrospray interface (ESI-TOF/MS).

Peak	RT (min)	Proposed Compound	Theoretical m/z	Experimental m/z	Molecular Formula	Error (ppm)	PLE Experiment
1	2.14	Quinic acid	191.0561	191.0567	$C_7H_{12}O_6$	−3.2	*
2	6.14	Chlorogenic acid	353.0878	353.0883	$C_{16}H_{18}O_9$	−1.5	*
3	6.51	UK 1	375.0663	375.067	$C_{25}H_{12}O_4$	−5.4	1,2,4,5,6,7,9
4	6.62	Rosamarinic acid	359.0772	359.0735	$C_{18}H_{16}O_8$	10.5	1,4,5,6,7,8,9
5	7.36	Cynarin isomer 1	515.1195	515.1211	$C_{25}H_{24}O_{12}$	−4.5	*
6	7.65	Luteolin-rutinoside	593.1512	593.1514	$C_{27}H_{30}O_{15}$	−0.3	*
7	7.95	Luteolin-glucoside	447.0933	447.0919	$C_{21}H_{20}O_{11}$	−4	*
8	8.08	Cynarin isomer 2	515.1195	515.1207	$C_{25}H_{24}O_{12}$	−2.2	*
9	8.58	Apigenin-rutinoside	577.1563	577.1571	$C_{27}H_{30}O_{14}$	−1.4	*
10	8.98	Apigenin-glucoside	431.0984	431.0965	$C_{21}H_{20}O_{10}$	−3.1	*
11	10.27	UK 2	345.0405	345.0374	$C_{20}H_{10}O_6$	9	*
12	11.62	UK 3	207.0663	207.0657	$C_{11}H_{12}O_4$	2.7	1,2,3,5,6
13	13.40	Luteolin	285.0405	285.0412	$C_{15}H_{10}O_6$	−2.5	1,3,4,5,6,7,8,9
14	15.95	Apigenin	269.0455	269.0459	$C_{15}H_{10}O_5$	−6.8	*
15	20.65	Trihydroxy-octadecenoic acid	329.2333	329.2331	$C_{18}H_{34}O_5$	0.6	*
16	22.51	Dihydroxy-hexadecanoic acid	287.2228	287.2229	$C_{16}H_{32}O_4$	−0.3	1,3,4,5,6,7,8,9
17	23.15	Methylapigenin	283.0612	283.0607	$C_{16}H_{12}O_5$	1.7	1,2,3,4,6
18	26.62	Cynarasaponin A/H isomer	925.4802	925.476	$C_{47}H_{74}O_{18}$	4.6	1,6,7,9

Table 2. *Cont.*

Peak	RT (min)	Proposed Compound	Theoretical m/z	Experimental m/z	Molecular Formula	Error (ppm)	PLE Experiment
19	26.92	Cynarasaponin A/H isomer	925.4802	925.478	$C_{47}H_{74}O_{18}$	2.4	1,6,7,9
20	30.05	UK 4	205.1598	205.1606	$C_{14}H_{22}O$	−3.8	2,3,4,5,6,7,8,9
21	31.10	Hydroxy-octadecatrienoic acid	293.2122	293.2111	$C_{18}H_{30}O_3$	3.9	1,2,4,6,7,9
22	31.27	Hydroxy-octadecadienoic acid	295.2279	295.2286	$C_{18}H_{32}O_3$	−2.6	*
23	33.19	Linolenic acid	277.2173	277.2170	$C_{18}H_{30}O_2$	1.1	*

(*) Indicate that these compounds were identified in all the PLE extracts. For those compounds that were not identified in all the extracts, the number of the PLE experiment in which they were detected was annotated. UK, unknown.

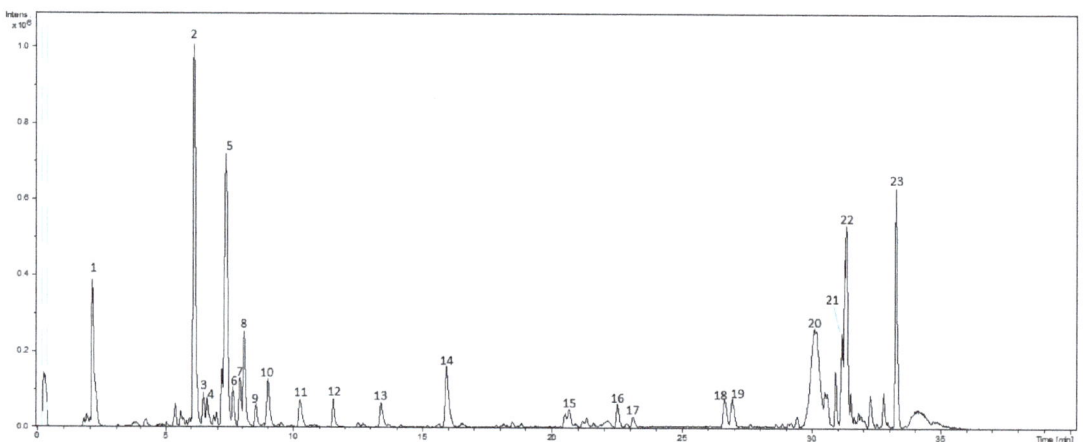

Figure 1. Base peak chromatogram (BPC) of representative pressurized liquid extraction (PLE) extracts of *Cynara scolymus* L. by-products.

3.1.1. Phenolic Acids

Peak 2, with a precursor ion at *m/z* 353.0878 was identified as chlorogenic acid [21], whereas peak 4, with *m/z* 359.0772 and a molecular formula $C_{18}H_{16}O_8$, was proposed as rosamarinic acid [22]. Moreover, peaks 5 and 8, which displayed a *m/z* 515.1195 and retention times of 7.36 and 8.08 min, respectively, were identified as cynarin isomers, also named "dicaffeoylquinic acid isomers" [21,22].

3.1.2. Flavonoids

With regard to flavonoids and its several sub-classes, only flavones and their derivatives were detected in artichokes by-products. Thereby, peak 6, with *m/z* at 593.1512, was tentatively identified as luteolin-rutinoside [18], while peak 7 with *m/z* at 447.0933 was proposed as luteolin-glucoside (cymaroside) according to bibliographic data [10,21]. Furthermore, the compound eluting at 8.58 min (peak 9) and displaying *m/z* 577.1563 was considered as apigenin-rutinoside (isorhoifolin) [21]. In the same way, peak 10, detected at 8.98 min and *m/z* 431.0984, was tentatively assigned to apigenin-glucoside according to the comparison of the molecular formula provided by the detector and literature data [21]. Similarly, peak 13 at *m/z* 285.0405 and molecular formula $C_{15}H_{10}O_6$ along with peak 14 at 15.44 min and *m/z* 269.0455 were proposed according to the literature as luteolin [10,21] and apigenin [10,21], respectively. Finally, peak 17 with *m/z* 283.0612 was tentatively assigned to methylapigenin [22].

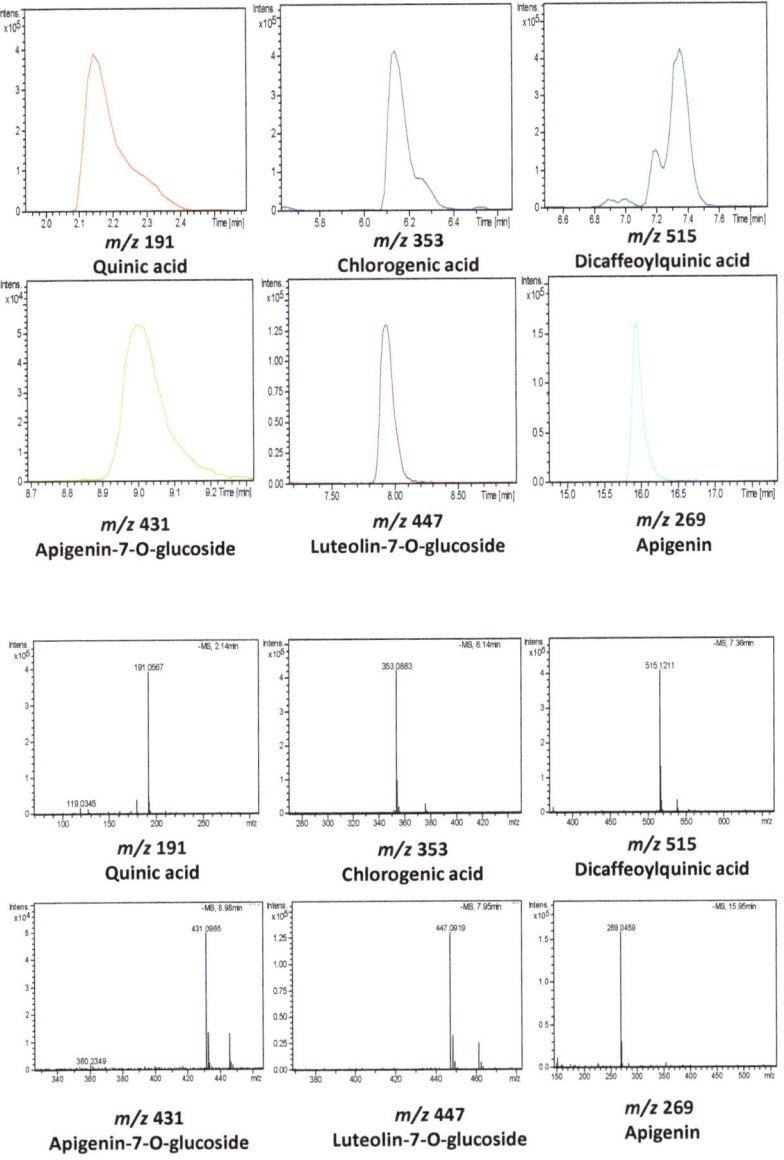

Figure 2. Extracted ion chromatograms (EIC) and mass spectra of some phenolic compounds characterized by HPLC-time-of-flight mass spectrometry with an electrospray interface (ESI-TOF/MS) in artichoke by-products.

3.1.3. Saponins, Lipids, and Other Polar Compounds

Peak 1, with *m/z* at 191.0561, was proposed as quinic acid, a carboxylic acid commonly found in artichoke [21].

On the other hand, compounds belonging to saponins family correspond to peaks 18 and 19. They displayed a *m/z* 925.4802 and retention times of 26.62 and 26.92 min, respectively. Both were identified as isomers of cynarasaponin A or H [21].

Lastly, several lipids were also found in these artichoke samples. Thence, hydroxy-octadecatrienoic acid (peak 21) is a lipid previously identified in artichoke [21]. Trihydroxy-octadecenoic acid (peak 15), hydroxy-octadecadienoic acid (peak 22), and linolenic acid (peak 23) were also detected in the present analysis. All these lipids have been previously identified in other vegetable PLE extracts, such as *Morus nigra* [23] and *Prunus avium* [24]. Similarly, dihydroxyhexadecanoic acid (peak 16) was identified in the present study as well as in *Symphytum officinale* L. samples [25]. Although these plant matrices belong to different species, both molecular formula and *m/z* generated by the software match with data reported in the bibliography.

3.2. Extraction Yield and Extraction Efficiency

In this study, different PLE conditions were evaluated and compared in terms of yield and recovery of individual phenolic compounds from artichoke by-products. The extraction yield was expressed as weight of collected extract per dry plant material (w/w, in grams) used in the extraction procedure. The extraction efficiency of individual compounds was estimated by a semi-quantitative approach, measuring the peak areas of the compounds identified in the chromatogram as expressed as mean ± standard deviation of three consecutive injections. Table 3 includes the extraction yield and phenolic extraction efficiency for the *C. scolymus* L. PLE extracts.

Table 3. Extraction yield and phenolic compounds recovery for *C. scolymus* L. obtained in each PLE condition. Yield (%), individual phenolic compounds (peak area × E + 4). Value = mean ± standard deviation.

Experimental Condition	Dielectric Constant	Extraction Conditions	Yield	Total Phenolic Acids	Total Flavonoids	Total Phenolic Compounds
PLE 1	19.0	120 °C; EtOH 100%	7.4 ± 0.3	787 ± 25	488 ± 13	1274 ± 37
PLE 2	21.6	176 °C; EtOH 85%	50 ± 1	190 ± 10	94.1 ± 0.3	284 ± 10
PLE 3	26	200 °C; EtOH 50%	57 ± 2	285 ± 10	157 ± 1	442 ± 10
PLE 4	31.0	63 °C; EtOH 85%	10.5 ± 0.8	728 ± 24	365 ± 8	1092 ± 33
PLE 5	33.4	176 °C; EtOH 15%	45 ± 2	134 ± 4	43.9 ± 0.4	178 ± 4
PLE 6	34.7	120 °C; EtOH 50%	40 ± 2	343 ± 5	145 ± 2	489 ± 4
PLE 7	48.0	40 °C; EtOH 50%	19 ± 1	594 ± 16	253 ± 16	848 ± 17
PLE 8	50.4	120 °C; EtOH 0%	37 ± 2	302 ± 8	66 ± 1	368 ± 7
PLE 9	59.1	63 °C; EtOH 15%	25 ± 2	291 ± 18	75 ± 4	365 ± 22

Concerning the extraction yield, the obtained results in the different PLE experiments are highly inconstant. Similar variations were observed in other PLE extracts from plants such as black mulberry or sweet cherry stems, ranging from 11% to 48% or from 3% to 49%, respectively [23,25]. In general, it could be observed that the application of elevated temperatures (above 170 °C) resulted in higher extraction yields. Indeed, PLE 3 (200 °C, EtOH 50%), PLE 2 (176 °C, EtOH 85%), and PLE 5 (176 °C, EtOH 15%) were the extraction conditions with the highest yield values (57 ± 2%, 50 ± 1%, and 45 ± 2%, respectively). This fact could be explained by the increase in solvent diffusivity with increasing temperature, which enhances the extraction of several components from vegetable matrices [26]. In contrast to this observation, it could not establish a relationship between the percentage of ethanol and extraction yield.

Focusing on the individual recovery of phenolic compounds of each PLE condition, a relationship between the extraction parameters (temperature and percentage of ethanol) and the enhancement extraction of particular compounds could be revealed.

In this sense, regarding phenolic compounds, as described above, both sub-classes of polyphenols (phenolic acids and flavonoids) identified in the samples were extracted under all the PLE experiments. The individual areas of all compounds identified in PLE extracts were also analyzed to evaluate significant differences among the different PLE conditions. Figure 3 draws the peak area (mean value ± standard deviation) of the individual compounds detected in each artichoke PLE extract as well as the total phenolic acids and flavonoids (see Table S1).

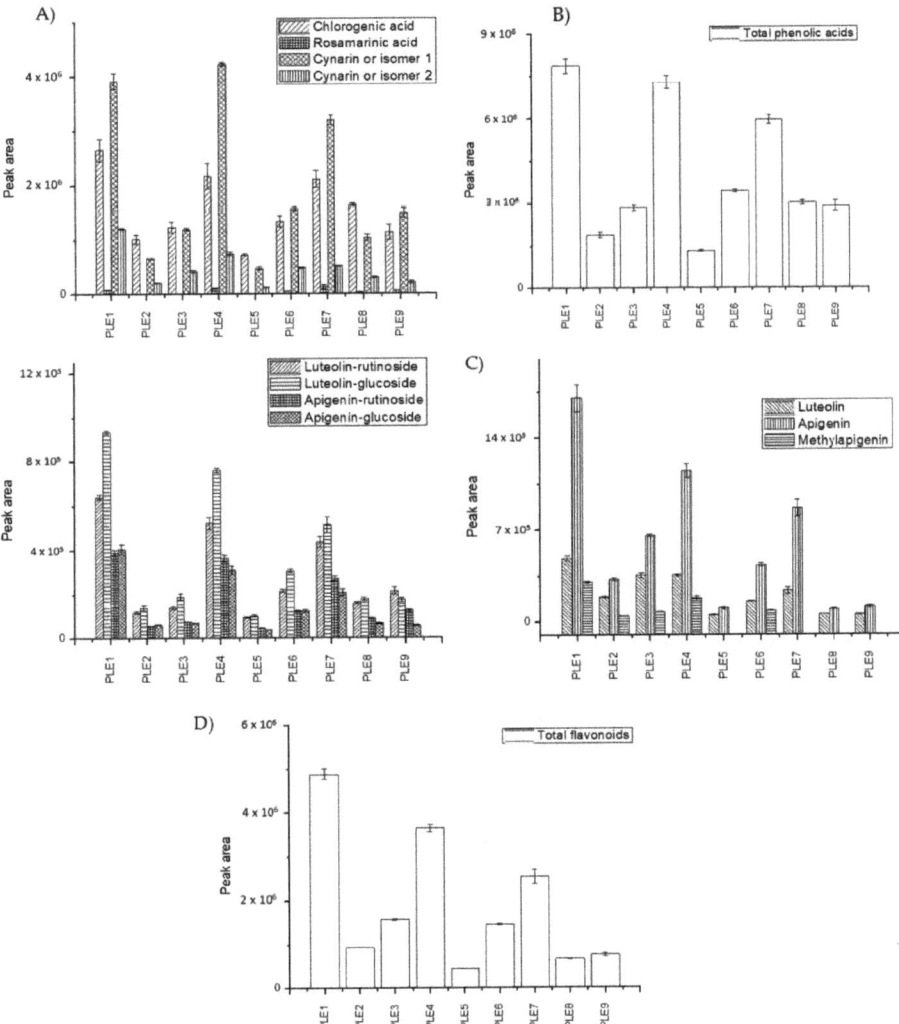

Figure 3. Abundance of phenolic compounds characterized in each *C. scolymus* PLE extracts by HPLC-ESI-TOF-MS: (**A**) individual phenolic acids, (**B**) total phenolic acids, (**C**) individual flavonoids, and (**D**) total flavonoids.

In regards to the total abundance of phenolic acids in the *C. scolymus* PLE extracts, it could be observed that PLE 1 (120 °C, EtOH 100%), PLE 4 (63 °C, EtOH 85%), and PLE 7

(40 °C, EtOH 50%) conditions showed the best recovery for this chemical sub-class. On the contrary, PLE 5 (176 °C, EtOH 15%) and PLE 2 (176 °C, EtOH 85%) present the worst extraction recoveries for this kind of substances. In light of these data, it can be concluded that higher percentages of ethanol in aqueous mixtures and moderate to high extraction temperature enhances the extraction of these compounds. On the contrary, very high temperatures, such as in PLE 5 and PLE 2, seem to act to the detriment of the extraction of phenolic acids.

Additionally, the individual behavior of phenolic acids was also monitored. Chlorogenic acid was extracted in greater abundance by PLE 1 condition (with the highest percentage of ethanol, 100%), followed by PLE 4 (63 °C, EtOH 85%) and PLE 7 (40 °C, EtOH 50%) experiments, which presented similar abundances. In the case of rosamarinic acid, the best extraction conditions were PLE 7 and PLE 4. Both experiments were performed with low-intermediate temperatures and medium-high percentages of ethanol. In fact, higher temperatures such as the applied in PLE 5 (176 °C, EtOH 15%) recovered this compound in very low amount or could not extract rosamarinic acid from artichoke by-products, as in PLE 2 (176 °C, EtOH 85%) and PLE 3 (200 °C, EtOH 50%). Finally, within the family of phenolic acids, cynarin isomers showed different behavior over the tested extraction conditions. PLE 1 run (120 °C, EtOH 100%) reported a high value of cynarin isomer 1 peak area, while cynarin isomer 2 was not recovered in abundance. The same phenomena could be described for PLE 4 (63 °C, EtOH 85%) and PLE 7 (40 °C, EtOH 50%).

On the other hand, the analysis of the total abundance of flavonoids in the artichoke extracts indicated that PLE 1 (120 °C, EtOH 100%) was the best condition, followed by PLE 4 (63 °C, EtOH 85%) and PLE 7 (40 °C, EtOH 50%). All these runs applied intermediate conditions within the range of temperature and percentage of ethanol as solvent combinations. On the contrary, the conditions PLE 2 (176 °C, EtOH 85%), PLE 5 (176 °C, EtOH 15%), PLE 8 (120 °C, EtOH 0%), and PLE 9 (63 °C, EtOH 15%) reported a lower abundance with respect to the other PLE extracts.

Analyzing individual flavonoids, the highest abundance of glycoside structures was obtained under the conditions PLE 1 (120 °C, EtOH 100%) and PLE 4 (63 °C, EtOH 85%). On further consideration, aglycon flavonoids as luteolin and apigenin showed the same trend, being better extracted by the PLE 1 condition. The abundance of simple flavonoids, luteolin and apigenin, was not increased as extraction temperatures raised. This fact suggests that high temperatures did not generate the hydrolysis of glycoside forms over the extraction process (luteolin-glucoside, apigenin-glucoside, luteolin-rutinoside, and apigenin-rutinoside).

Taking into account all these results, a comparison of the extraction yield and phenolic compounds recovery in each experimental PLE run showed important differences. Although the high temperatures would improve the diffusivity of the solvent and break component–matrix interactions, which increase the solubility of the analytes and consequently enhance the extraction yields [27], it does not necessarily mean a greater recovery of phenolic compounds. This fact seems to occur with artichoke by-products, which could be related to different factors. Indeed, an excessive increase in temperature is demonstrated to negatively affect the extraction of thermolabile compounds, such as phenolic compounds [26].

In addition to the possible thermal degradation of compounds, different combinations of solvent composition and temperature provide changes in the dielectric constant value, which is crucial for the extraction recovery of the phytochemicals from natural sources. In this way, special attention has to be paid to PLE 1 condition (120 °C, 100% EtOH) with a dielectric constant value of 19. Despite this condition reported the lowest yield, the recovery of phenolic compounds was higher compared to other PLE conditions. This phenomenon has also been reported in other plant matrices extracted by PLE at the same conditions (100% EtOH and 120 °C) [23].

Thereby, PLE 1 condition provided 2.6, 7.6, and 3.4 times higher recovery of phenolic acids, flavonoids, and total phenolic compounds than PLE 8 (120 °C, EtOH 0%, dielectric constant 50.4), respectively. Analyzing individual phenolic compounds identified in both PLE conditions, significant differences could be observed concerning the abundance of all of them (see Table S2). A similar trend was observed when the yield and recovery of phytochemical compounds of PLE 6 (120 °C, EtOH 50%, dielectric constant 34.7) were compared to those obtained for PLE 1 (120 °C, EtOH 100%, dielectric constant 19.0). Thus, the yield obtained for PLE 6 is 5.4 times higher than for PLE 1. Nevertheless, PLE 1 condition showed 2.6 times higher phenolic recovery than PLE 6.

Nonetheless, tt is important to remark that at dielectric constant values higher than 19, minor differences were observed on the yield and recovery of phenolic compounds among the experimental conditions. Indeed, PLE 8 (dielectric constant value, 50.4) obtained an extraction yield 1.1 times higher than PLE 6 (dielectric constant value, 34.7). Moreover, PLE 6 had 1.1, 2.2, and 1.3 times higher recovery of phenolic acids, flavonoids, and total phenolic compounds than PLE 8, respectively, significant differences among all the characterized phenolic compounds were found for PLE 8 and PLE 6, except for chlorogenic and rosamarinic acids (Table S2).

Therefore, similar differences on the yield and phytochemical recovery were also observed for PLE conditions where the same temperature was applied in combination with different percentages of ethanol, which consequently provides different values of dielectric constants. Some examples are: (a) temperature of 63 °C combined with 15% of ethanol (PLE 9, dielectric constant value 59.1) or 85% of ethanol (PLE 4, dielectric constant 31) and (b) extractions at 176 °C using 15% EtOH (PLE 5, dielectric constant 33.4) or 85% EtOH (PLE 2, dielectric constant 21.6). These results pointed out that at the same working temperature, the recovery of phenolic compounds is improved when the solvent composition (% EtOH) provides the lowest value of dielectric constant.

Nevertheless, despite this focus in the targeted extraction of individual compounds provided by concrete PLE parameters, the total extraction yield should be considered if the main purpose is to obtain the maximum quantity of extract with a particular compound.

4. Conclusions

In the present work, the efficiency of PLE extraction for the recovery of phytochemicals from artichoke by-products was studied. The proposed extraction system by PLE obtained 9 extracts under different extraction conditions delimited by the technical limits of the PLE extractor. The analytical characterization of these extracts allowed the detection of 23 compounds, most of them were phenolic and other polar bioactive compounds previously identified in artichoke samples. The individual phenolic compounds recovery through the different PLE extraction conditions was estimated by considering the peak area of each compound in the chromatogram (three replicates), which permits a comparison of the same compound between extracts. This information could establish the best extraction condition for each compound or family. The best PLE parameters, for both phenolic acids and flavonoids, consist in high percentages of ethanol and medium-high temperatures. In addition, it should be pointed into light that at the same temperature, the recovery of individual phenolic compounds is improved when the solvent composition provides the lowest value of dielectric constant.

Supplementary Materials: The following are available online at https://www.mdpi.com/article/10.3390/app11093788/s1, Table S1: Peak areas of the identified compounds in *C. scolymus* pressurized liquid extraction (PLE), extracts expressed as mean ± standard deviation of the three analyses replicates. Table S2: Statistical data of the PLE extraction conditions for individual phenolic compounds.

Author Contributions: Conceptualization, J.L.-S. and I.B.-L.; methodology, J.L.-S. and R.G.-M.; software, L.L.-S.; validation, J.L.-S., I.B.-L. and A.S.-C.; formal analysis, L.L.-S.; investigation, L.L.-S., P.G.-G. and D.Q.; data curation, L.L.-S.; writing—original draft preparation, L.L.-S.; writing—review and editing, J.L.-S. and I.B.-L.; visualization, R.G.-M.; supervision, J.L.-S., A.S.-C. and R.G.-M. All authors have read and agreed to the published version of the manuscript.

Funding: This research received no external funding.

Institutional Review Board Statement: Not applicable.

Informed Consent Statement: Not applicable.

Data Availability Statement: All the data generated by this research have been included in the article. For any assistance it is possible to contact with the corresponding author.

Conflicts of Interest: The authors declare no conflict of interest.

References

1. Shirahigue, L.D.; Ceccato-Antonini, S.R. Agro-industrial wastes as sources of bioactive compounds for food and fermentation industries. *Cienc. Rural* **2020**, *50*, 50. [CrossRef]
2. Muñoz-Jauregui, A.M.; Ramos-Escudero, F. Componentes fenólicos de la dieta y sus propiedades biomedicinales—Phenolics compounds of the diet and his biomedicinal properties. *Horiz. Méd.* **2007**, *7*, 23–38.
3. Bataglion, G.A.; Da Silva, F.M.A.; Eberlin, M.N.; Koolen, H.H.F. Determination of the phenolic composition from Brazilian tropical fruits by UHPLC-MS/MS. *Food Chem.* **2015**, *180*, 280–287. [CrossRef]
4. Bataglion, G.A.; Da Silva, F.M.A.; Eberlin, M.N.; Koolen, H.H.F. Simultaneous quantification of phenolic compounds in buriti fruit (*Mauritia flexuosa* L.f.) by ultra-high performance liquid chromatography coupled to tandem mass spectrometry. *Food Res. Int.* **2014**, *66*, 396–400. [CrossRef]
5. Mármol, I.; Quero, J.; Jiménez-Moreno, N.; Rodríguez-Yoldi, M.J.; Ancín-Azpilicueta, C. A systematic review of the potential uses of pine bark in food industry and health care. *Trends Food Sci. Technol.* **2019**, *88*, 558–566. [CrossRef]
6. Cruzado, M.; Cedrón, J. Nutracéuticos, alimentos funcionales y su producción. *Rev. Química PUCP* **2012**, *2*, 33–36.
7. Sonnante, G.; Pignone, D.; Hammer, K. The Domestication of Artichoke and Cardoon: From Roman Times to the Genomic Age. *Ann. Bot.* **2007**, *100*, 1095–1100. [CrossRef] [PubMed]
8. Abu-Reidah, I.M.; Arraez-Roman, D.; Segura-Carretero, A.; Fernandez-Gutierrez, A. Extensive characterisation of bioactive phenolic constituents from globe artichoke (*Cynara scolymus* L.) by HPLC-DAD-ESI-QTOF-MS. *Food Chem.* **2013**, *141*, 2269–2277. [CrossRef]
9. Lattanzio, V.; Kroon, P.A.; Linsalata, V.; Cardinali, A. Globe artichoke: A functional food and source of nutraceutical ingredients. *J. Funct. Foods* **2009**, *1*, 131–144. [CrossRef]
10. El-Mesallamy, A.M.D.; Abdel-Hamid, N.; Srour, L.; Hussein, S.A.M. Identification of polyphenolic compounds and hepatoprotective activity of artichoke (*Cynara scolymus* L.) edible part extracts in rats. *Egypt. J. Chem.* **2020**, *63*, 2273–2285.
11. Sanchez-Rabaneda, F.; Jauregui, O.; Lamuela-Raventos, R.M. Identification of phenolic compounds in artichoke waste by high-performance liquid chromatography—Tandem mass spectrometry. *J. Chromatogr. A* **2003**, *1008*, 57–72. [CrossRef]
12. Pandino, G.; Lombardo, S.; Mauromicale, G. Globe artichoke leaves and floral stems as a source of bioactive compounds. *Ind. Crop. Prod.* **2013**, *44*, 44–49. [CrossRef]
13. Orlovskaya, T.V.; Luneva, I.L.; Chelombit'Ko, V.A. Chemical composition of *Cynara scolymus* leaves. *Chem. Nat. Compd.* **2007**, *43*, 239–240. [CrossRef]
14. Shallan, M.A.; Ali, M.A.; Meshrf, W.A.; Marrez, D.A. In vitro antimicrobial, antioxidant and anticancer activities of globe artichoke (*Cynara cardunculus* var. *scolymus* L.) bracts and receptacles ethanolic extract. *Biocatal. Agric. Biotechnol.* **2020**, *29*, 101774. [CrossRef]
15. Kukić, J.; Popović, V.; Petrović, S.; Mucaji, P.; Ćirić, A.; Stojković, D.; Soković, M. Antioxidant and antimicrobial activity of *Cynara cardunculus* extracts. *Food Chem.* **2008**, *107*, 861–868. [CrossRef]
16. Aguilera, Y.; Martin-Cabrejas, M.A.; Gonzalez de Mejia, E. Phenolic compounds in fruits and beverages consumed as part of the Mediterranean diet: Their role in prevention of chronic diseases. *Phytochem. Rev.* **2016**, *15*, 405–423. [CrossRef]
17. Shen, Q.; Dai, Z.; Lu, Y. Rapid determination of caffeoylquinic acid derivatives in *Cynara scolymus* L. by ultra-fast liquid chromatography/tandem mass spectrometry based on a fused core C18 column. *J. Sep. Sci.* **2010**, *33*, 3152–3158. [CrossRef]
18. Rejeb, I.B.; Dhen, N.; Gargouri, M.; Boulila, A. Chemical Composition, Antioxidant Potential and Enzymes Inhibitory Properties of Globe Artichoke By-Products. *Chem. Biodivers.* **2020**, *17*, e2000073. [CrossRef]
19. Lozano-Sánchez, J.; Castro-Puyana, M.; Mendiola, J.A.; Segura-Carretero, A.; Cifuentes, A.; Ibáñez, E. Recovering bioactive compounds from olive oil filter cake by advanced extraction techniques. *Int. J. Mol. Sci.* **2014**, *15*, 16270–16283. [CrossRef]
20. Gonçalves, E.C.B.A.; Lozano-Sanchez, J.; Gomes, S.; Ferreira, M.S.L.; Cameron, L.C.; Segura-Carretero, A. Byproduct Generated During the Elaboration Process of Isotonic Beverage as a Natural Source of Bioactive Compounds. *J. Food Sci.* **2018**, *83*, 2478–2488. [CrossRef]
21. Yang, M.; Ma, Y.; Wang, Z.; Khan, A.; Zhou, W.; Zhao, T.; Cao, J.; Cheng, G.; Cai, S. Phenolic constituents, antioxidant and cytoprotective activities of crude extract and fractions from cultivated artichoke inflorescence. *Ind. Crop. Prod.* **2020**, *143*, 111433. [CrossRef]
22. Palermo, M.; Colla, G.; Barbieri, G.; Fogliano, V. Polyphenol metabolite profile of artichoke is modulated by agronomical practices and cooking method. *J. Agric. Food Chem.* **2013**, *61*, 7960–7968. [CrossRef]
23. Nastić, N.; Borrás-Linares, I.; Lozano-Sánchez, J.; Švarc-Gajić, J.; Segura-Carretero, A. Optimization of the extraction of phytochemicals from black mulberry (*Morus nigra* L.) leaves. *J. Ind. Eng. Chem.* **2018**, *68*, 282–292. [CrossRef]

24. Nastić, N.; Lozano-Sánchez, J.; Borrás-Linares, I.; Švarc-Gajić, J.; Segura-Carretero, A. New technological approaches for recovering bioactive food constituents from sweet cherry (*Prunus avium* L.) stems. *Phytochem. Anal.* **2020**, *31*, 119–130. [CrossRef]
25. Nastić, N.; Borrás-Linares, I.; Lozano-Sánchez, J.; Švarc-Gajić, J.; Segura-Carretero, A. Comparative Assessment of Phytochemical Profiles of Comfrey (*Symphytum officinale* L.) Root Extracts Obtained by Different Extraction Techniques. *Molecules* **2020**, *25*, 837. [CrossRef]
26. Figueroa, J.G.; Borrás-Linares, I.; Lozano-Sánchez, J.; Quirantes-Piné, R.; Segura-Carretero, A. Optimization of drying process and pressurized liquid extraction for recovery of bioactive compounds from avocado peel by-product. *Electrophoresis* **2018**, *39*, 1908–1916. [CrossRef]
27. Vazquez-Roig, P.; Picó, Y. Pressurized liquid extraction of organic contaminants in environmental and food samples. *Trends Anal. Chem.* **2015**, *71*, 55–64. [CrossRef]

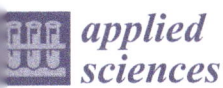

Article

Vepris macrophylla Essential Oil Produces Notable Antiproliferative Activity and Morphological Alterations in Human Breast Adenocarcinoma Cells

Marisa Colone [1], Filippo Maggi [2], Rianasoambolanoro Rakotosaona [3,4] and Annarita Stringaro [1,*]

1. National Center for Drug Research and Evaluation, Italian National Institute of Health, Viale Regina Elena 299, 00161 Rome, Italy; marisa.colone@iss.it
2. School of Pharmacy, University of Camerino, Via Sant'Agostino 1, 62032 Camerino, Italy; filippo.maggi@unicam.it
3. Centre National d'Application de Recherches Pharmaceutiques, Ambodivoanjo Ambohijatovo, Rue RP Rahajarizafy Analamahitsy, BP 702, Antananarivo 101, Madagascar; rravalison@gmail.com
4. Ecole Supérieure Polytechnique d'Antananarivo, University of Antananarivo, BP 1500, Antananarivo 101, Madagascar
* Correspondence: annarita.stringaro@iss.it

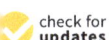

Citation: Colone, M.; Maggi, F.; Rakotosaona, R.; Stringaro, A. *Vepris macrophylla* Essential Oil Produces Notable Antiproliferative Activity and Morphological Alterations in Human Breast Adenocarcinoma Cells. *Appl. Sci.* **2021**, *11*, 4369. https://doi.org/10.3390/app11104369

Academic Editor: Hari Prasad Devkota

Received: 2 April 2021
Accepted: 7 May 2021
Published: 12 May 2021

Publisher's Note: MDPI stays neutral with regard to jurisdictional claims in published maps and institutional affiliations.

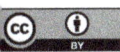

Copyright: © 2021 by the authors. Licensee MDPI, Basel, Switzerland. This article is an open access article distributed under the terms and conditions of the Creative Commons Attribution (CC BY) license (https://creativecommons.org/licenses/by/4.0/).

Abstract: Medicinal plants contain numerous bioactive molecules that synergistically provide therapeutic benefits. We have devoted our attention to various EOs without toxicity to normal cells, studying their activities against human cancer cells. In particular, we have studied the cytotoxicity of *Vepris macrophylla* (Baker) I. Verd. EO. *V. macrophylla* is an evergreen tree of Madagascar where is much appreciated as a source of traditional remedies. Its major volatile components are citral, i.e., a mixture of neral and geranial, citronellol and myrcene. The antiproliferative activities of *V. macrophylla* EO were studied against human breast adenocarcinoma cell line SKBR3. Cellular metabolism was analyzed by MTT assay at different concentrations of EO and at different times of incubation (24, 48 and 72 h). Moreover, morphological and ultrastructural analyses were performed to study its antiproliferative effects against human adenocarcinoma cells, demonstrating the ability of *V. macrophylla* EO, stored inside numerous intracellular vesicles, to damage both plasma membranes and disorganize the cytoskeleton protein as actin filaments.

Keywords: *Vepris macropylla*; essential oil; citral; antiproliferative activity; fluorescence and scanning electron microscopy; human breast cancer cell line

1. Introduction

Breast cancer is a major public health problem, representing the highest incidence rate of death for women [1,2]. The interest in products of natural origin from plants with different pharmacological activities that can be used in chemotherapy is increasingly broad. Many natural compounds have shown anticancer activities [3]. The most famous antineoplastic drug, paclitaxel, used for the treatment of breast cancer, was isolated from the bark of *Taxus brevifolia* Nutt. [4]. Furthermore, among the natural products, there are aloe-emodin, which is isolated from the root of *Rheum palmatum* L. and the leaves of aloe vera. Numerous in vitro studies have demonstrated that aloe-emodin is able to reduce the viability and proliferation of different human cancer cell lines, inducing apoptotic cell death and inhibiting adhesion and the migration process [5,6]. Another compound is curcumin, the active ingredient of turmeric, which is a polyphenolic compound with a broad range of medicinal properties, such as antibreast-cancer activity. Curcumin is able to enhance the effects of chemotherapeutic agents such as paclitaxel [3]. A natural stilbene and non-flavonoid polyphenol, resveratrol is present in grapes, peanuts and red wine. This natural product possesses anti-inflammatory, antioxidant, cardioprotective and anticancer properties [7]. Moreover, a synergistic effect has been reported by the combination of genistein and doxorubicin [8]. Additionally, rosemary (*Rosmarinus officinalis* L.) extract can increase the activity of the anti-breast-cancer agents tamoxifen, trastuzumab, and paclitaxel [9]. Currently, one of the most interesting approaches in the fight against this tumor comprises new therapeutic strategies using natural products in combination with synthetic drugs in order to increase the therapeutic index of the drug and reduce the many undesirable side effects caused by the doses used in typical chemotherapy protocols. After chemotherapy or radiotherapy, a number of adverse effects in patients occur [10]. A natural flavonoid, quercetin has anti-inflammatory and antioxidative effects. After high dose chemotherapy, quercetin, administered in capsules of 250 mg (twice daily for four weeks), can reduce oral mucositis events in patients with blood malignancy [11]. A combination of curcumin and α-tocopherol regulates rat liver enzymes via inhibition of oxidative stress, revealing protection against cisplatin-induced hepatotoxicity [12]. Naringenin, a natural flavanone isolated from *Thymus vulgaris* L., has growth inhibitory and chemosensitization effects on human breast and colorectal cancer [13]. Naringenin can reduce the nephrotoxicity induced by daunorubicin treatment in rats [14]. Several drugs derived from natural products have already received clinical approval, and many are currently undergoing in clinical trials. To date, the Food and Drug Administration (FDA) has approved the administration of resveratrol and quercetin [15].

Essential oils (EOs) are products obtained from vegetable raw material [16]. They are complex, multicomponent systems composed of volatile small molecular weight components, mainly terpenes and non-terpene components. EOs have been used for a long time by various traditional medicine systems as antiseptic agents [17]. Nowadays, scientific evidence is available showing that certain EOs have antimicrobial, antimycotic, antiviral, antioxidant, immunomodulant and anticancer properties [18,19]. Some of these characteristics are related to their functions in plants. *Vepris macrophylla* (Baker) I. Verd. (Rutaceae) is a tree endemic to Madagascar, where it is known by many names, such as itampody, ampodiberavina, mampodifotsy, mampody (evoking its euphoric properties) (Figure 1) [20]. Indeed, the roots of *V. macrophylla* are traditionally used to manufacture euphoric alcoholic beverages. In Malagasy ethnomedicine, each part of the plant has a specific use. The root bark, grated and macerated in water, is administered as a drink to treat nervous depression or apathetic states. Fruits are used to prepare steam baths during convalescence periods following infectious diseases. The leaves are used to regulate the coronary blood flow. [21–25]. The EO obtained from *V. macrophylla* leaves showed antimicrobial activities for the treatment of infectious diseases [26]. Furthermore, it was effective against phytopathogenic fungi such as *Phytophthora cryptogea* and *Fusarium avenaceum* [27].

In our previous study, the *V. macrophylla* EO showed notable effects on human tumor cells, notably breast adenocarcinoma and colon carcinoma cell lines, highlighting its cytotoxicity [26]. These results pushed us to further explore the effects of this EO on tumor cells. Thus, in the present study, we evaluated the antiproliferative activity of *V. macrophylla* EO, at different times and concentrations, on human breast cell line SKBR3.

Furthermore, the ultrastructural morphological alterations of SKBR3 cells were evaluated by fluorescence and scanning electron microscopy analyses.

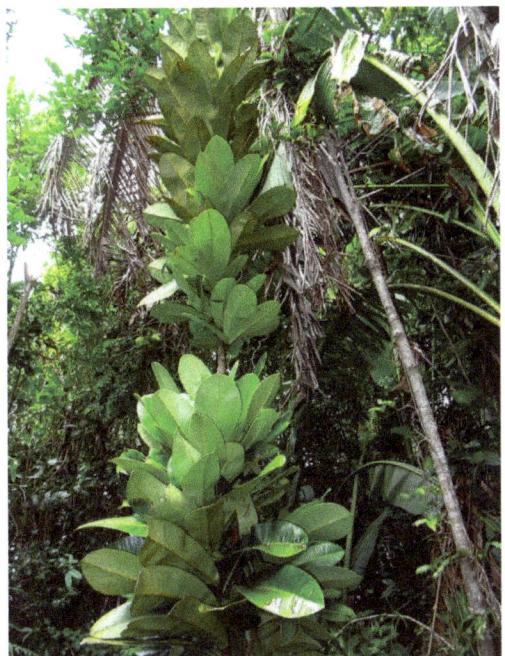

Figure 1. Vepris macrophylla tree.

2. Materials and Methods

2.1. Plant Material and Essential Oil (EO) Extraction and Composition

The EO was obtained by hydrodistillation of *V. macrophylla* leaves, collected in the east coast of Madagascar (Sahamamy/Analalava), using a portable alembic as reported in Maggi et al. [26]. Following GC and GC-MS analysis the following major components were detected in the EO chemical profile: geranial (33.2%), neral (23.1%), citronellol (14.5%), and myrcene (8.3%).

2.2. Cell Culture

SKBR3 cell line from human breast cancer was obtained from American Type Culture Collection (ATCC, Rockville, MD, USA) and was grown in Dulbecco's Modified Eagle's Medium (DMEM) medium with 10% fetal bovine serum (HyClone™ FBS (U.S.A. origin), Characterized), 1% nonessential amino acids, 1% L-glutamine, 100 IU per mL penicillin, 100 IU per mL streptomycin, in a humidified atmosphere at 37 °C with 5% CO_2.

2.3. Cell Viability Assay

MTT assay was utilized to evaluate cell viability. Briefly, cells were seeded for 24 h in a 96-well plate (NunclNunclonTM, NuncGmbH & Co., Wiesbaden, Germany) with a density of 1.2×10^4 cells/well. Then were treated with *V. macrophylla* EO at concentration of 1.25; 2.5; 5 and 10 µg/mL for 24, 48 and 72 h. After the incubation period, 0.5 mg/mL of MTT (Sigma, Deisenhofen, Germany) was added to each well for 2 h at 37 °C and the cells were dissolved with 200 µL/well of dimethylsulfoxide (Merck, Darmstadt, Germany). The absorbance of formazan was read at 570 nm on a scanning microtiter spectrophotometer plate reader. The results were calculated as the percentage of viability in relation to the untreated cells standardized to 100%. They are the mean ± SD of three separate experiments done in triplicate.

2.4. Immunfluorescence Microscopy

SKBR3 cells were grown for 24 h on 12 mm diameter coverslips and treated with *V. macrophylla* EO for an incubation time of 24 and 48 h. Cells were then fixed with 4% paraformaldehyde for 30 min and were permeabilized with 0.5% Triton X-100 (Sigma Chemicals Co., St. Louis, MO, USA) for 5 min. For actin detection, cells were stained with FITC-phalloidin (Sigma) at room temperature for 30 min. For nuclei detection, cells were stained with Hoechst 33258 (Sigma-Aldrich, St. Louis, MO, USA; #861405) at 37 °C for 15 min. After the washing with PBS coverslips were mounted with glycerol-phosphate and images were acquired with a Nikon Microphot fluorescence microscope (Nikon Instruments, Melville, NY, USA) equipped with a Zeiss CCD camera (Carl Zeiss, Oberkochen, Germany).

2.5. Scanning Electron Microscopy (SEM)

SEM analysis allowed the study of cell surface modifications induced by *V. macrophylla* EO. Samples were grown for 24 h on glass coverslips and treated for 24, 48 and 72 h with *V. macrophylla* EO with a concentration of 0.01; 0.1; 1.25 and 2.5 µg/mL. Then cells were fixed in 2.5% glutaraldehyde in 0.2 M Na-cacodylate buffer for 2 h and postfixed with 1% (w/w) OsO_4 for 1 h. Subsequently, cells were dehydrated using an ethanol gradient. After the passage in 100% ethanol, the samples were submitted to drying with CO_2 (Critical point dryer CPD 030, Bal-Tec AG, Lichtenstein) and gold coated by sputtering (SCD 050 Blazers device, Bal-Tec). Samples were observed with a scanning electron microscope FE-SEM Quanta Inspect F (FEI—Thermo Fisher Scientific; Eindhoven—The Netherlands).

2.6. Statistical Analysis

All data were repeated in at least three different experiments, and results are expressed as the mean ± standard deviation. Statistical differences were determined using a one-way ANOVA test and values with $p < 0.05$ being considered significant.

3. Results

3.1. Evaluation of Citotoxicity of V. macrophylla EO

MTT assay was used to study cell viability and consequently the proliferative capacity of SKBR3 adenocarcinoma cells after treatment with *V. macrophylla* EO. This assay allows to evaluate the toxicity of a substance, through the comparison of cell viability indices obtained from treated cells compared to control. Figure 2 shows the results of the MTT assay obtained from treatments at 24, 48 and 72 h at different concentrations of *V. macrophylla* EO (1.25; 2.5; 5 and 10 µg/mL) on human breast adenocarcinoma cells SKBR3.

The results showed that *V. macrophylla* EO was able to reduce cell proliferation below 60%, even at the lowest concentrations (1.25 µg/mL) after 24 h of treatment. This trend was also observed at longer times (48 and 72 h) for all other concentrations (2.5; 5; and 10 µg/mL).

3.2. Immunoflorescence Microscopy Observations

In the course of experimental analyses, we performed investigations by fluorescence microscopy that allowed us to evaluate the morphological alterations of cells after treatment with *V. macrophylla* EO at different times and concentrations.

After treatment with *V. macrophylla* EO, the SKBR3 cells were labeled both with Hoechst 33258, which is used to highlight morphological-ultrastructural alterations in the nucleus, and with FITC-phalloidin, to highlight changes in the cell cytoskeleton and actin filaments, induced by different treatments with EO (Figure 3). The micrographs obtained by fluorescence microscopy showed that at 1.25 and 2.5 µg/mL concentrations, the lowest concentrations of EO, after 24 h of treatment, the nuclei still possessed a morphology similar to those of the control cells, while the actin filaments of the cytoskeleton revealed a significant rearrangement of their ultrastructures. Moreover, in some cells, there were numerous vesicular structures, probably containing the same EO (Figure 4a,b, see arrowheads). Images of cells treated with the same concentration of EO for an incubation time of 48 h revealed a reduction of nuclei diameters of the cells. Moreover, the morphologies of the actin filament appeared altered, and numerous green fluorescence points were identified exclusively around the nucleus (Figure 4c,d). This result reveals that *V. macrophylla* EO is able to disorganize the actin filament network (see also Figure 3).

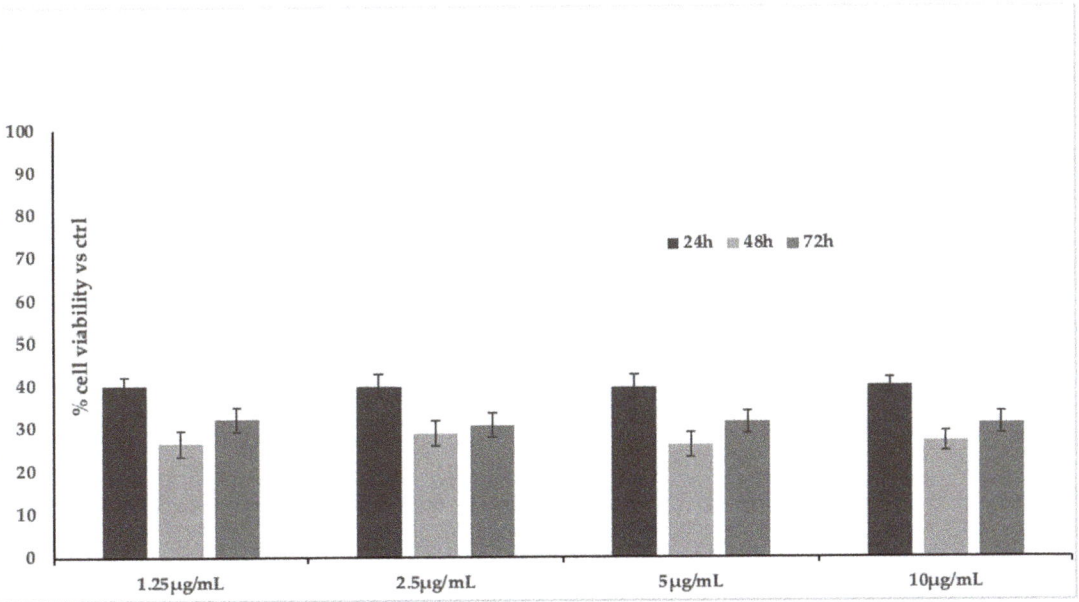

Figure 2. Evaluation of SKBR3 cell viability treated for 24, 48 and 72 h with different concentrations of EO obtained from *Vepris macrophylla* leaves. Cell viability was calculated considering the control value and standardized to 100%. Data represent mean ds (n = 3).

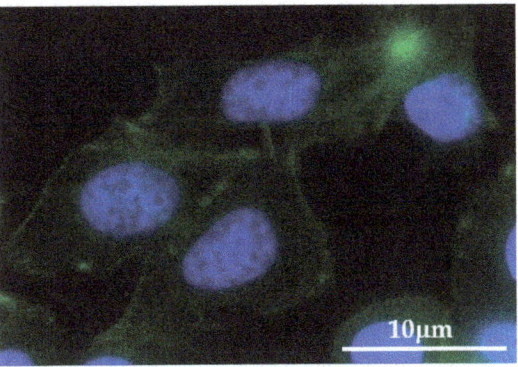

Figure 3. Images after double-cell staining with FITC-phalloidin (green) and Hoechst 33258 (blue) in SKBR3 control cells.

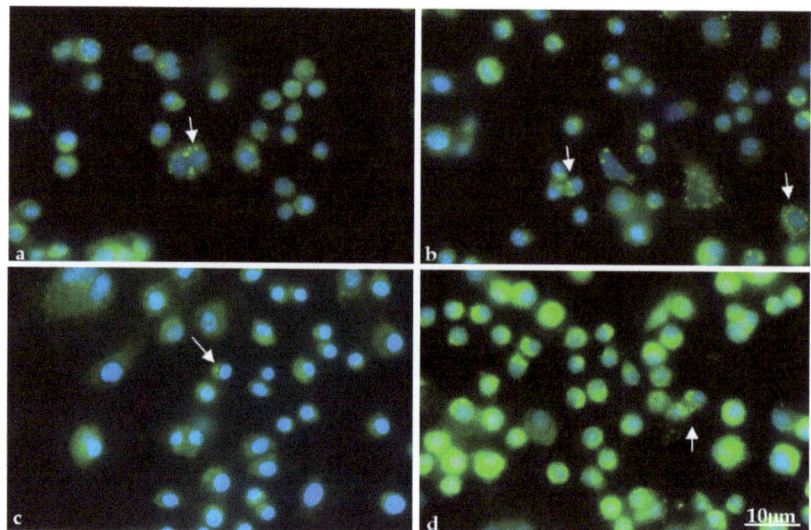

Figure 4. Immunofluorescence micrographs shown the morphological alterations on SKBR3 cells induced by *Vepris macrophylla* EO after treatment with 1.25 (**a,c**) and 2.5 µg/mL (**b,d**) concentrations at two incubation times 24 h (**a,b**) and 48 h (**c,d**). Arrowheads indicate probably vesicles filled with EO.

Immunofluorescence observations of SKBR3 cells treated with 5 and 10 µg/mL, at 48 h, were in agreement with results obtained by MTT assay (see Figure 2), showing both the same morphological alterations and numerous vesicles inside the cytoplasm of cancer cells (Figure 5a,b, arrowheads).

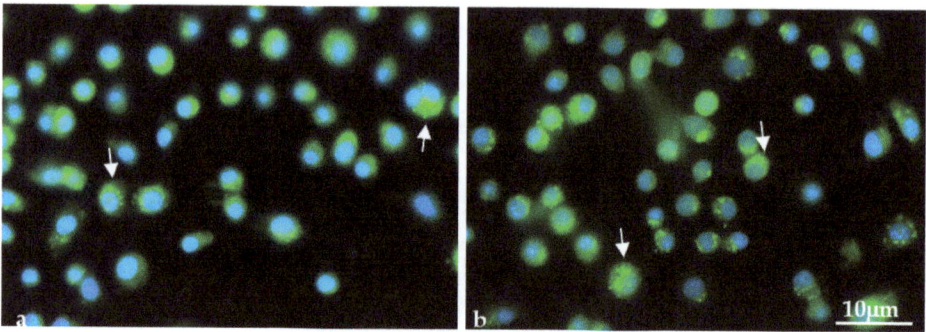

Figure 5. Morphological alterations of SKBR3 cells after treatment with 5 (**a**) and 10 (**b**) µg/mL of *Vepris macrophylla* EO at 48 h. Arrowheads indicate probably vesicles filled with EO.

3.3. SEM Analysis

SEM observations of SKBR3 control cells at 24, 48 and 72 h showed numerous microvilli and random "ruffles" on the cell surface (Figure 6).

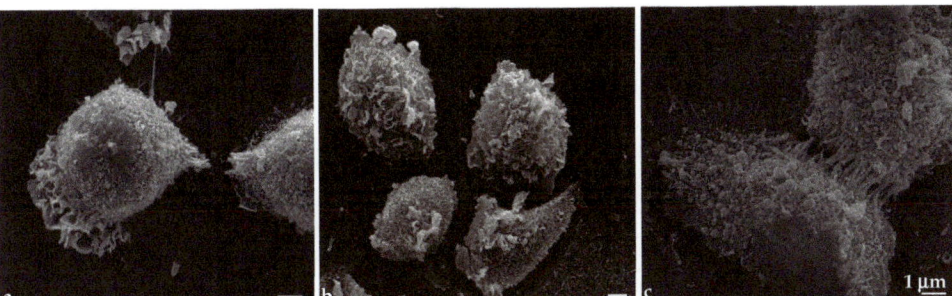

Figure 6. SEM images of SKBR3 control cells at 24, 48 and 72 h (a–c respectively).

After treatment with EO at different concentrations, cancer cells appeared very damaged. Figures 7–9 show important ultrastructural alterations of SKBR3 cells. The morphological alterations are clearly visible after only 24 h of treatment (Figure 7) with four different concentrations of EO (0.01; 0.1; 1.25 and 2.5 µg/mL, respectively). Moreover, at higher concentrations (1.25 and 2.5 µg/mL), SKBR3 cells appeared flat and adherent to the substrate, probably due the effect on cytoskeletal actin disorganization, as also shown by fluorescence microscopy analysis (Figure 4). When cells were treated with the lowest concentrations of EO (0.01 and 0.1 µg/mL), at 48 h, the plasma membranes were entirely destroyed (Figure 8a,b). Cells showed plasma membrane alterations like those observed 24 h after treatment with the highest concentration (2.5 µg/mL) of EO. Figure 8d shows cells treated with 2.5 µg/mL for 48 h, in which the plasma membranes are completely damaged. Finally, as a dose-dependent effect, after 72 h, these morphological alterations were clearly visible in all SKBR3 cells treated with V. macrophylla EO (Figure 9a–c).

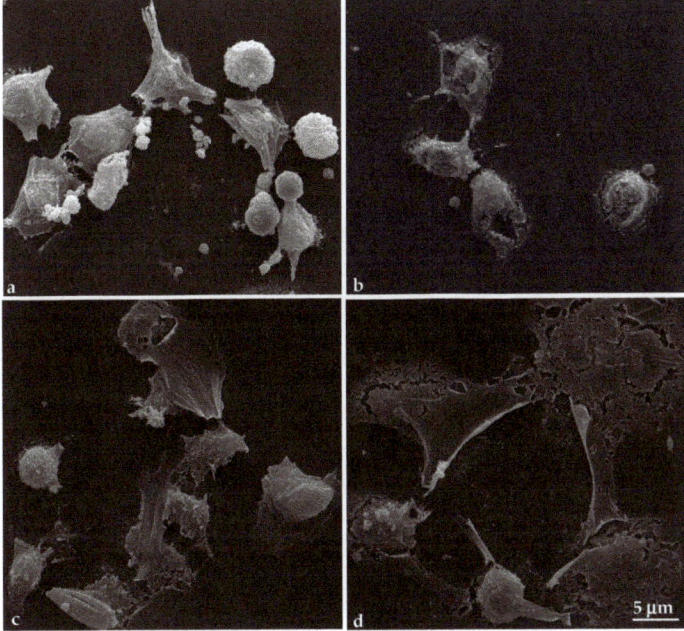

Figure 7. SEM micrographs of SKBR3 cells after 24 h of V. macrophylla EO incubation (0.01 (a), 0.1 (b), 1.25 (c) and 2.5 (d) µg/mL, respectively).

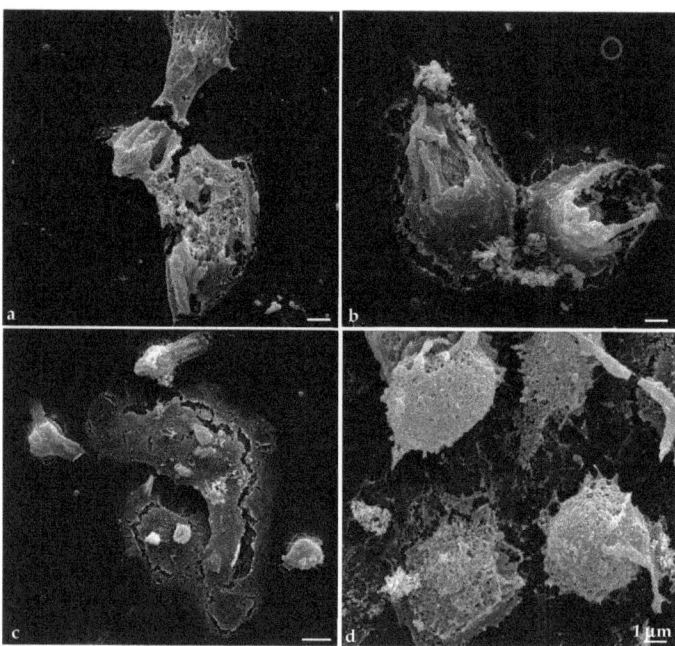

Figure 8. SEM micrographs of SKBR3 cells after 48 h of *V. macrophylla* EO incubation (0.01 (**a**), 0.1 (**b**), 1.25 (**c**) and 2.5 (**d**) µg/mL, respectively).

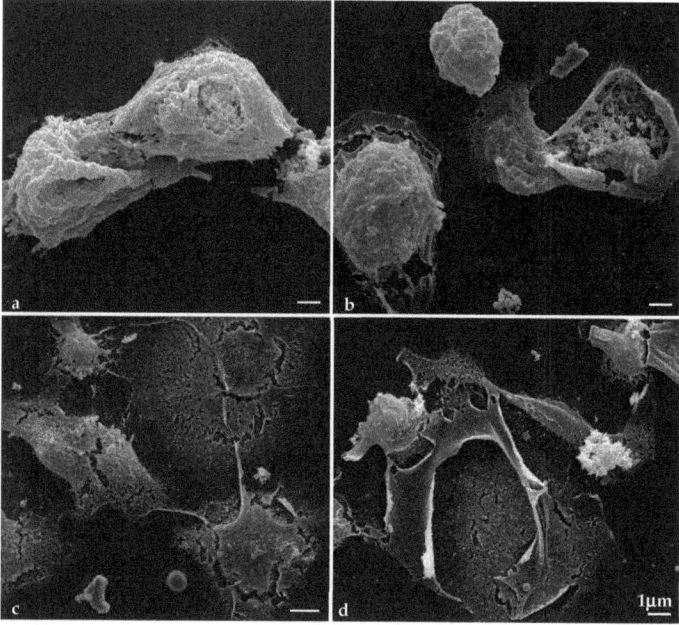

Figure 9. Micrographs of SKBR3 cells after 72 h of *V. macrophylla* EO incubation (0.01 (**a**), 0.1 (**b**), 1.25 (**c**) and 2.5 (**d**) µg/mL, respectively).

Figure 10 shows immunofluorescence and SEM images of the SKBR3 cells with some vesicles on and inside the cytoplasm (arrowheads). These structures, containing the stored EO of *V. macrophylla*, could slow the release of EOs, enhancing both the antiproliferative activity and alteration of cancer cell adhesion on the substrates by actin filaments.

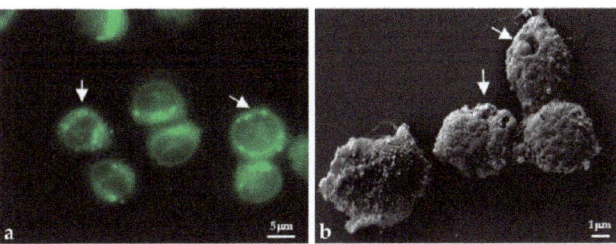

Figure 10. SKBR3 treated with *Vepris macrophylla* EO at 24 h with 1.25 µg/mL (**a**) fluorescence microscopy and (**b**) scanning electron microscopy micrographs. Arrowheads indicate probably vesicles filled with EO.

4. Discussion

EOs and some of their components exert antitumor activities against numerous cancer models, such as colon [28], lung and liver [29], by affecting multiple pathways [30–33]. Di Martile et al. [34] summarized studies showing the properties of EOs to induce in vitro and in vivo cell death in melanoma models. They also indicated the use of EOs in clinical trials with the reduction of the side effects in cancer patients. Moreover, frankincense, pine needle and geranium EOs are also able to suppress tumor progression through the regulation of the AMPK/mTOR pathway in breast cancer [35]. Several EOs also have chemopreventive properties [34]. In eukaryotic cells, EOs can cause depolarization of mitochondrial membranes and decrease their fluidity. In this way, EOs are able to induce severe damage in the mitochondria, leading to cell death. Bhakkiyalakshmi et al. demonstrated that carvacrol, a phenolic monoterpenoid, is able to cause cell death as apoptosis. This process is associated with the production of free radicals that cause the rapid consumption of the intracellular pool of antioxidants [36]. Another study by Arunasree et al. evaluated the mechanism of action of carvacrol in the MDA-MB-231 cell line. This monoterpenoid induced cell death via cytochrome C release after mitochondria permeabilization [37]. Moreover, we also demonstrated the antitumoral activity of Tea Tree Oil (TTO), with an apoptotic effect on melanoma cell lines [38]. In general, the cytotoxic effects of EOs in toto, or those of some of their components, such as monoterpenoids [39], are due to their lipophilicity, which allows them to cross membranes and destroy them [40,41].

Herein, the damage caused by *V. macrophylla* EO to the cell membranes of SKBR3 cells can be attributed to its main component, citral, which is a mixture of the two monoterpenes, neral and geranial. Citral is generally recognized as safe (GRAS) by the FDA, and is commonly used as a flavoring agent in the EU. On the other hand, this compound is endowed with antimicrotubule [42] and chemopreventive properties [43]. Several studies have shown that citral is able to cause cell death to tumor cells and severely damage cytoskeletal structures. On the other hand, other components occurring in the *V. macrophylla* EO, including both major and minor constituents, may be involved in the overall synergistic effect normally displayed by the EO [26]. Moreover, as demonstrated by other authors [44], our results show that *V. macrophylla* EO significantly changes the cytoskeletal organization of SKBR3 cancer cells, suppressing actin cytoskeletal rearrangement and destroying the cell membrane thanks in part to its monoterpenoid activities. Furthermore, this EO significantly decreased the proliferation and migration of human SKBR3 cells in a concentration and time-dependent manner.

5. Conclusions

In the present study, we examined the in vitro antitumoral activities of *V. macrophylla* EO on the SKBR3 human adenocarcinoma cell line. The results demonstrated that this EO is able to induce numerous ultrastructural alterations thanks its ability to both disorganize the cytoskeleton and damage the plasma membrane. Thus, these results suggest a potential use of *V. macrophylla* EO and its main components as a chemosensitizer in clinical practice. Future studies should clarify the mechanism of action and biochemical process activated by this EO. Other studies will be performed using fluorescence microscopy to study all cytoskeletal proteins in order to assess whether these complexes will be used to reduce the degree of invasiveness of human cancer cells by increasing their ability to adhere to the substrate.

Author Contributions: Conceptualization: F.M. and A.S.; Figures preparation: M.C. and A.S.; Writing—original draft preparation: F.M., M.C. and A.S.; Analysis of essential oils composition: R.R and F.M.; Data analysis: F.M., M.C. and A.S. All authors have read and agreed to the published version of the manuscript.

Funding: This research was partially funded by Istituto Superiore di Sanità, ISS (Ministry of Health-ISS funding) and by University of Camerino.

Informed Consent Statement: This study did not involve human.

Data Availability Statement: All the data are available.

Acknowledgments: We thank Stefania Muran for experimental support in ISS laboratory.

Conflicts of Interest: No conflict of interest are present Fondo di Ateneo per la Ricerca (FAR 2014/2015) in this study.

References

1. Ferlay, J.; Héry, C.; Autier, P.; Sankaranarayanan, R. Global Burden of Breast Cancer. In *Breast Cancer Epidemiology*; Li, C., Ed.; Springer: New York, NY, USA, 2010; pp. 1–19. [CrossRef]
2. Liu, L.; Kawashima, M.; Toi, M. Breast cancer in global health: Beyond diversity and inequality. *Int. J. Surg. Global Health* **2020**, *3*, e32. [CrossRef]
3. Samistha, M.; Rajn, D. Natural products for the management and prevention of breast cancer. *Evid. Based Complement. Alternat. Med.* **2018**. [CrossRef]
4. Amaral, R.G.; Albuquerque dos Santos, S.; Nalone Andrade, L.; Severino, P.; Andrade Carvalho, A. Natural Products as Treatment against Cancer: A Historical and Current vision. *Clin. Oncol.* **2019**, *4*, 1562.
5. Chen, R.; Zhang, J.; Hu, Y.; Wang, S.; Chen, M.; Wang, Y. Potential antineoplastic effects of Aloe-emodin: A comprehensive review. *Am. J Chin. Med.* **2014**, *42*, 275–288. [CrossRef] [PubMed]
6. Dong, X.; Zeng, Y.; Liu, Y.; You, L.; Yin, X.; Fu, J.; Ni, J. Aloe-emodin: A review of its pharmacology, toxicity, and pharmacokinetics. *Phytother. Res.* **2020**, *34*, 270–281. [CrossRef] [PubMed]
7. Ko, J.H.; Sethi, G.; Um, J.Y.; Shanmugam, M.K.; Arfuso, F.; Kumar, A.P.; Bishayee, A.; Ahn, K.S. The Role of Resveratrol in Cancer Therapy. *Int. J. Mol. Sci.* **2017**, *18*, 2589. [CrossRef]
8. Xue, J.P.; Wang, G.; Zhao, Z.B.; Wang, Q.; Shi, Y. Synergistic cytotoxic effect of genistein and doxorubicin on drug-resistant human breast cancer MCF-7/Adr cells. *Oncol. Rep.* **2014**, *32*, 1647–1653. [CrossRef]
9. González-Vallinas, M.; Molina, S.; Vicente, G.; Sánchez-Martínez, R.; Vargas, T.; García-Risco, M.R.; Fornari, T.; Reglero, G.; Ramírez de Molina, A. Modulation of estrogen and epidermal growth factor receptors by rosemary extract in breast cancer cells. *Electrophoresis* **2014**, *35*, 1719–1727. [CrossRef]
10. Zhang, Q.Y.; Wang, F.X.; Jia, K.K.; Kong, L.D. Natural Product Interventions for Chemotherapy and Radiotherapy-Induced Side Effects. *Front. Pharmacol.* **2018**, *9*, 1253. [CrossRef]
11. Kooshyar, M.M.; Mozafari, P.M.; Amirchaghmaghi, M.; Pakfetrat, A.; Karoos, P.; Mohasel, M.R.; Orafai, H.; Azarian, A.A. A Randomized Placebo-Controlled Double Blind Clinical Trial of Quercetin in the Prevention and Treatment of Chemotherapy-Induced Oral Mucositis. *J. Clin. Diagn. Res.* **2017**, *11*, ZC46–ZC50. [CrossRef]
12. Palipoch, S.; Punsawad, C.; Koomhin, P.; Suwannalert, P. Hepatoprotective effect of curcumin and alpha-tocopherol against cisplatin-induced oxidative stress. *BMC Complement. Altern. Med.* **2014**, *14*, 111. [CrossRef] [PubMed]
13. Abaza, M.S.; Orabi, K.Y.; Al-Quattan, E.; Al-Attiyah, R.J. Growth inhibitory and chemo-sensitization effects of naringenin, a natural flavanone purified from *Thymus vulgaris*, on human breast and colorectal cancer. *Cancer Cell Int.* **2015**, *15*, 46. [CrossRef]

14. Karuppagounder, V.; Arumugam, S.; Thandavarayan, R.A.; Pitchaimani, V.; Sreedhar, R.; Afrin, R.; Harima, M.; Suzuki, H.; Suzuki, K.; Nakamura, M.; et al. Naringenin ameliorates daunorubicin induced nephrotoxicity by mitigating AT1R, ERK1/2-NFκB p65 mediated inflammation. *Int. Immunopharmacol.* **2015**, *28*, 154–159. [CrossRef] [PubMed]
15. Montané, X.; Kowalczyk, O.; Reig-Vano, B.; Bajek, A.; Roszkowski, K.; Tomczyk, R.; Pawliszak, W.; Giamberini, M.; Mocek-Płóciniak, A.; Tylkowski, B. Current Perspectives of the Applications of Polyphenols and Flavonoids in Cancer Therapy. *Molecules* **2020**, *25*, 3342. [CrossRef]
16. Celia, C.; Trapasso, E.; Locatelli, M.; Navarra, M.; Ventura, C.A.; Wolfram, J.; Carafa, M.; Morittu, V.M.; Britti, D.; Di Marzio, L.; et al. Anticancer activity of liposomal bergamot essential oil (BEO) on human neuroblastoma cells. *Colloids Surf. B Biointerfaces.* **2013**, *112*, 548–553. [CrossRef]
17. Ríos, J.L.; Recio, M.C. Medicinal plants and antimicrobial activity. *J. Ethnopharmacol.* **2005**, *100*, 80–84. [CrossRef]
18. Edris, A.E. Pharmaceutical and therapeutic potentials of essential oils and their individual volatile constituents: A review. *Phytother. Res.* **2007**, *21*, 308–323. [CrossRef]
19. Blowman, K.; Magalhães, M.; Lemos, M.F.L.; Cabral, C.; Pires, I.M. Anticancer Properties of Essential Oils and Other Natural Products. *Evid. Based. Complement. Alternat. Med.* **2018**, *2018*, 3149362. [CrossRef] [PubMed]
20. Novy, J.W. Medicinal plants of the eastern region of Madagascar. *J. Ethnopharmacol.* **1997**, *55*, 119–126. [CrossRef] [PubMed]
21. Garcia, G.; Charmillon, J.M.; Roux, E.; Sutour, S.; Rakotozafy, J.B.; Désiré, O.; Paoli, M.; Tomi, F.; Rabehaja, J.R. Chemical composition of leaf and bark essential oils of *Vepris unifoliata* from Madagascar. *JEOR* **2017**, *3*, 214–220.
22. Billet, D.; Favre-Bonvin, J. Constituents de l'huile essentielle de *Vepris madagascarica* Essential oil composition of *Vepris madagascarica*. *Phytochemistry* **1973**, *2*, 1194–1197. [CrossRef]
23. Rabehaja, D.J.R.; Ihandriharison, H.; Ramanoelina, P.A.R.; Ratsimamanga-Urveg, S.; Bighelli, A.; Casanova, J.; Tomi, F. Leaf oil from *Vepris madagascarica* (Rutaceae), source of (E)- anethole. *Nat. Prod. Commun.* **2013**, *8*, 1165–1166. [CrossRef] [PubMed]
24. Poitou, F. Chemical composition of *Vepris elliotii* essential oil. *J. Essent. Oil Res.* **1995**, *7*, 447–449. [CrossRef]
25. Boiteau, P.; Boiteau, M.; Allorge-Boiteau, L. *Dictionnaire des Noms Malgaches des Ve´ge´taux*; Editions Alzieu: Grenoble, France, 1999.
26. Maggi, F.; Randriana, R.F.; Rasoanaivo, P.; Nicoletti, M.; Quassinti, L.; Bramucci, M.; Lupidi, G.; Petrelli, D.; Vitali, L.A.; Papa, F.; et al. Chemical composition and in vitro biological activities of the essential oil of *Veprys macrophylla* (Baker) I. Verd. Endemic to Madagascar. *Chem. Biodivers.* **2013**, *10*, 1–12. [CrossRef]
27. Giamperi, L.; Bucchini, A.E.A.; Ricci, D.; Tirillini, B.; Nicoletti, M.; Rakotosaona, R.; Maggi, F. *Vepris macrophylla* (Baker) I. Verd Essential Oil: An Antifungal Agent against Phytopathogenic Fungi. *Int. J. Mol. Sci.* **2020**, *21*, 2776. [CrossRef]
28. Polo, M.P.; Crespo, R.; de Bravo, M.G. Geraniol and simvastatin show a synergistic effect on a human hepatocarcinoma cell line. *Cell Biochem. Funct.* **2011**, *29*, 452–458. [CrossRef]
29. Slamenová, D.; Horváthová, E.; Sramková, M.; Marsálková, L. DNA-protective effects of two components of essential plant oils carvacrol and thymol on mammalian cells cultured in vitro. *Neoplasma* **2007**, *54*, 108–112.
30. Sitarek, P.; Rijo, P.; Garcia, C.; Skała, E.; Kalemba, D.; Białas, A.J.; Szemraj, J.; Pytel, D.; Toma, M.; Wysokińska, H.; et al. Antibacterial, Anti-Inflammatory, Antioxidant, and Antiproliferative Properties of Essential Oils from Hairy and Normal Roots of *Leonurus sibiricus* L. and Their Chemical Composition. *Oxid. Med. Cell Longev.* **2017**, *2017*, 7384061. [CrossRef]
31. Bhalla, Y.; Gupta, V.K.; Jaitak, V. Anticancer activity of essential oils: A review. *J. Sci. Food Agric.* **2013**, *93*, 3643–3653. [CrossRef] [PubMed]
32. Fitsiou, E.; Anestopoulos, I.; Chlichlia, K.; Galanis, A.; Kourkoutas, I.; Panayiotidis, M.I.; Pappa, A. Antioxidant and Antiproliferative Properties of the Essential Oils of *Satureja thymbra* and *Satureja parnassica* and their Major Constituents. *Anticancer Res.* **2016**, *36*, 5757–5763. [CrossRef]
33. Saleh, A.M.; Al-Qudah, M.A.; Nasr, A.; Rizvi, S.A.; Borai, A.; Daghistani, M. Comprehensive Analysis of the Chemical Composition and *In Vitro* Cytotoxic Mechanisms of *Pallines Spinosa* Flower and Leaf Essential Oils Against Breast Cancer Cells. *Cell Physiol. Biochem.* **2017**, *42*, 2043–2065. [CrossRef] [PubMed]
34. Di Martile, M.; Garzoli, S.; Ragno, R.; Del Bufalo, D. Essential Oils and Their Main Chemical Components: The Past 20 Years of Preclinical Studies in Melanoma. *Cancers* **2020**, *12*, 2650. [CrossRef] [PubMed]
35. <named-content content-type="background:white">Ren, P.; Ren, X.; Cheng, L.; Xu, L. Frankincense, pine needle and geranium essential oils suppress tumor progression through the regulation of the AMPK/mTOR pathway in breast cancer. *Oncol. Rep.* **2018**, *39*, 129–137. [CrossRef]
36. Bhakkiyalakshmi, E.; Suganya, N.; Sireesh, D.; Krishnamurthi, K.; Devi, S.S.; Rajaguru, P.; Ramkumar, K.M. Carvacrol induces mitochondria-mediated apoptosis in HL-60 promyelocytic and Jurkat T lymphoma cells. *Eur. J. Pharmacol.* **2016**, *772*, 92–98. [CrossRef] [PubMed]
37. Arunasree, K.M. Anti-proliferative effects of carvacrol on a human metastatic breast cancer cell line, MDA-MB 231. *Phytomedicine* **2010**, *17*, 581–588. [CrossRef] [PubMed]
38. Calcabrini, A.; Stringaro, A.; Toccacieli, L.; Meschini, S.; Marra, M.; Colone, M.; Salvatore, G.; Mondello, F.; Arancia, G.; Molinari, A. Terpinen-4-ol, the main component of *Melaleuca alternifolia* (tea tree) oil inhibits the in vitro growth of human melanoma cells. *J. Investig. Dermatol.* **2004**, *122*, 349–360. [CrossRef]
39. Grayson, D.H. Monoterpenoids. *Nat. Prod. Rep.* **1998**, *15*, 435–439. [CrossRef]

40. Bozzuto, G.; Colone, M.; Toccacieli, L.; Stringaro, A.; Molinari, A. Tea tree oil might combat melanoma. *Planta Med.* **2011**, *77*, 54–56. [CrossRef]
41. Giordani, C.; Molinari, A.; Toccacieli, L.; Calcabrini, A.; Stringaro, A.; Chistolini, P.; Arancia, G.; Diociaiuti, M. Interaction of tea tree oil with model and cellular membranes. *J. Med. Chem.* **2006**, *49*, 4581–4588. [CrossRef] [PubMed]
42. Chaouki, W.; Leger, D.Y.; Liagre, B.; Beneytout, J.L.; Hmamouchi, M. Citral inhibits cell proliferation and induces apoptosis and cell cycle arrest in MCF-7 cells. *Fundam. Clin. Pharmacol.* **2009**, *23*, 549–556. [CrossRef]
43. Ben-Yehoshua, S.; Ofir, R. Effects of Citral against Cancer, and against Pathogens of Humans and Fruits. *Acta. Hortic.* **2010**, *877*, 1465–1471. [CrossRef]
44. Cho, S.; Lee, E.; Kim, S.; Lee, H. Essential oil of *Pinus koraiensis* inhibits cell proliferation and migration via inhibition of p21-activated kinase 1 pathway in HCT116 colorectal cancer cells. *BMC Complement. Altern. Med.* **2014**, *14*, 275. [CrossRef] [PubMed]

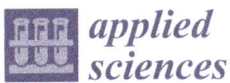

Article

Scrophularia buergeriana Extract Improves Memory Impairment via Inhibition of the Apoptosis Pathway in the Mouse Hippocampus

Hae Jin Lee [1], Dae Young Lee [2], Hae Lim Kim [1] and Seung Hwan Yang [1],*

[1] Department of Biotechnology, Chonnam National University, Yeosu 59626, Korea; haecutejin@naver.com (H.J.L.); ics1357@naver.com (H.L.K.)
[2] Department of Herbal Crop Research, National Institute of Horticultural and Herbal Science, RDA, Eumsung 27709, Korea; dylee0809@korea.kr
* Correspondence: ymichigan@jnu.ac.kr; Tel.: +82-61-659-7306

Received: 23 October 2020; Accepted: 9 November 2020; Published: 11 November 2020

Abstract: *Scrophularia buergeriana* (SB) Miq. (Scrophulariaceae) has been used to help cure swelling and fever and has reported antioxidant and neuro-protective effects. However, few mechanism–based studies have evaluated the memory improving effects in a beta-amyloid induced memory loss model. As a result of *Scrophularia buergeriana* extract (SBE) administration (30 and 100 mg/kg) for 28 days significantly recovered beta-amyloid-induced amnesia in the passive avoidance test and improved the impairment of spatial memory in the Morris Water Maze (MWM) task. Furthermore, SBE up-regulated superoxide dismutase-1 (SOD)-1, SOD-2, glutathione peroxidase-1, and B-cell lymphoma (Bcl)-2 protein expression levels. Additionally, SBE downregulated Bcl-2-associated X protein, cleaved caspase-9, cleaved poly (adenosine diphosphate-ribose) polymerase, and Aβ protein expression levels and inhibited the phosphorylation of the tau protein of Aβ-treated mice hippocampus. These results demonstrate that SBE improved memory impairment by reducing beta-amyloid induced neurotoxicity and regulated oxidative stress, anti-apoptotic pathways.

Keywords: srophularia buergeriana; cognitive impairment; amyloid beta; tau phosphorylation; oxidative stress; anti-apoptotic

1. Introduction

Alzheimer's disease (AD) is one type of dementia and a progressive neuro-degenerative disease featured by deposits of extracellular amyloid β (Aβ) peptide and flame-shaped neurofibrillary tangles of hyper-phosphorylated tau protein, inducing neurotoxicity accompanied by cognitive impairment and memory loss [1–4].

The Aβ plaque is composed of Aβ 1–40 and 1–42, major forms of Aβ found in the brains of AD patients. The Aβ 1–42 protein is more neurotoxic and induces more oxidative damage than Aβ 1–40 [5]. An important factor in AD development is considered to be Aβ accumulation, since oxidative stress is followed by Aβ cytotoxicity [1,6]. The overproduction of reactive oxygen species (ROS) induced Aβ accumulation and oxidative stress damages cellular components resulting in structural damage, functional disorder, and cell apoptosis [7].

Cells have an antioxidant defense system protecting them from ROS attacks using various enzymes, such as superoxide dismutase (SOD), glutathione peroxidases (GPx), glutathione reductases (GR) [8]. SOD is known as the first detoxification enzyme and the most powerful endogenous antioxidant in the cell. It acts as a catalyst and converse of the superoxide (O^{2-}) radical into ordinary oxygen (O_2) and hydrogen peroxide (H_2O_2), leaving the harmful superoxide anion less dangerous. SOD requires a metal cofactor, such as copper (Cu), zinc (Zn) and manganese (Mn), for activity as a metalloenzyme [9]. Cu/Zn-SOD (SOD1), which is located in chromosome 21 and encoded in the SOD1 gene located on chromosome 21 and predominantly occurs in the cytosolic compartment. Mn-SOD (SOD2), which is located in chromosome 6 and encoded in the SOD2 gene on chromosome 6, located in the mitochondrial matrix. The reduction of SOD-1 triggers oxidative cellular DNA damage, and SOD-2 protects mitochondrial DNA against damage due to oxidative stress [10]. GPx plays an import role in protecting cells from oxidative damage by converting hydrogen peroxide (H_2O_2) to H_2O with glutathione (GSH) as a substrate, after the oxidation of GSH to Glutathione disulfide (GSSG). GR is known to maintain the reduced GSH level in redox cycle. Furthermore, it resists oxidative stress and maintains a reducing environment inside the cell [11,12].

In addition, Aβ-mediated oxidative stress causes the hyper-phosphorylation of tau protein and affects neurofibrillary tangle formation. The accumulation of neurofibrillary tangles directly correlates with neuro-degeneration and cell death and is closely related to the severity of dementia [13,14].

Apoptosis is mediated by two major pathways, which are divided into extrinsic and intrinsic pathways. Death receptors release several mitochondrial intermembrane proteins by passing death signaling to mitochondria in the intrinsic pathway [15]. A common mitochondria-related apoptotic pathway in neurons is regulated principally by the pro-apoptotic Bcl-2 protein family member, Bax. On receipt of the death signal, Bax is translocated to the mitochondria and interacts with the Bcl-2 family to control the progression of apoptosis [16,17]. Bax activates down-stream effector caspases such as caspase-9 and caspase-poly (ADP) ribose polymerase (PARP) in vitro, and in vivo by stimulating cytochrome c release. Notably, Bcl-2 inhibits Bax-induced apoptosis [15,18,19].

Scrophularia buergeriana (SB) Miq. (Scrophulariaceae), called Hyun-Sam in Korea, is used to help cure fever, swelling, constipation, pharyngitis, neuritis, and laryngitis as traditional medicine. SB dried root contains various components such as E-harpagoside (CAS: 19210-12-9), 8-*O*-E-*p*-methoxycinnamoyl harpagide (MCA-Hg), E-p-methoxycinnamic acid (p-MCA, CAS: 830-09-1), cinnamic acid (CAS: 140-10-3), and angoroside C (CAS: 115909-22-3), which displays neuro protective activities [11]. In a previous study, the SB extract (SBE) demonstrated cognition-enhancing activity in a scopolamine-induced short-term memory loss mice model [12]. However, investigation evaluating the effects of SBE in a beta-amyloid induced memory loss model is lacking.

Therefore, we administered 30 or 100 mg/kg SBE based on the previous study and evaluated the effect of SBE on β-amyloid accumulation and tau phosphorylation. Furthermore, we investigated the neuro-protective effects against Aβ caused neurotoxicity through antioxidant and anti-apoptotic mechanisms in the Aβ 1–42 injected mice.

2. Materials and Methods

2.1. Sample Preparation

SBE was obtained from Nutrapharmtec co., Ltd., (Seongnam, Korea). SB dried roots were extracted for 2–4 h at 70–90 °C with 70% ethyl alcohol and filter processed, concentrated, and dried. The extraction process was performed with reference to previously described studies [11,12]. For the in vivo study, the standardized SBE was dissolved in 0.5% carboxy-methylcellulose (CMC).

2.2. Experimental Animals

Male C57BL/6N mice (8 weeks old; Orient. Co. Ltd., Gyeonggi, Korea) were used after 7 days adaptation period (20–26 °C; 12 h light cycle from 08:00 to 20:00; food, Doo Yeol Biotech, water ad libitum). All studies were conducted according to the animal experiment ethical committee (permission number: 2018-07-008) of ChemOn Inc (Yong in, Korea). The animals were cared based on the guidelines provided by this committee. We monitored changes in body weight, food and water intake once a week. To enhance the well-being of the animals, we provided hygienic and ensured proper breeding and care to prevent disease.

2.3. Aβ 1–42 Injection and Drug Administration

The experimental animals were grouped as follows: normal control group, Aβ 1–42 treated group, and co-treated groups with Aβ 1–42 and the SBE (30 or 100 mg/kg/day). SBE was dissolved in 0.5% CMC and orally administered for 4 weeks (Day 28). The passive avoidance test and Morris water maze (MWM) were performed for 3 (Days 15–17) and 7 (Days 22–28) days. The Aβ peptide was dissolved in sterile 0.1 M phosphate-buffered saline (pH 7.4) and pre-incubated at 37 °C for 7 days. Zoletil® (Virbac, Carros, France) and xylazine (Bayer, Leverkusen, Germany) (4:1, *v/v*) were used for mice to anesthetize and Aβ 1–42 was injected (5 μL/2.5 min, i.c.v.) using stereotaxic apparatus coordinates (Anterior/Posterior (AP), −1.0 mm; Mediolateral/Lateral (ML), +1.0 mm; Dorsal/Ventral (DV), −2.5 mm).

2.4. Passive Avoidance Test

The passive avoidance test equipment (Twin County Med Associates, Hudson, NY, USA) was used to perform passive avoidance experiments. This apparatus is divided into light and dark compartments with a guillotine door in the middle. The bottom is gridded to administer an electric shock. The tests were carried out for 3 days at the same time every day at 24 h intervals. For adaptation training, the animals were placed in the shaded area for 2 min, and then placed back in the illuminated area. When the animal moved into the shaded area, it was immediately placed in the illuminated compartment (day 15). Twenty-four hours later (day 16), two training sessions were performed every 2 min. After 60 s of adaptation, the animals were allowed to move between the two compartments freely for 120 s. However, on moving to the shaded area, the guillotine door was closed and a 0.20 mA scrambled shock was applied for 2 s. The animals that failed to move were excluded from and 8 mice per group participated in the experiments. On the last day of testing, (day 17), the animal was located on the illuminated area and the guillotine door was opened. The time taken to move to the shaded area was measured.

2.5. Morris Water Maze (MWM) Test

The MWM test was performed 22 days after the Aβ 1–42 peptide injection. The platform was placed in one of the four designated release points in the water pool, allowing the animal a search time of 60 s. The mice that found the platform were left on it for 30 s, but the mice that failed to find the platform within 60 s were placed on the platform and allowed to rest for about 30 s. All mice tested twice a day, and the position of the platform was randomly changed in the water pool. Using this method, we measured the time taken to locate the platform by repeating the test for 7 consecutive days (training: 2 days, behavioral test: 4 days, probe trial: 1 day). On the last 7 days (Day 28), a probe trial was conducted. Here, 1 h after vehicle or drug administration, the platform was taken out of the pool, and the number of times the mice passed the platform was measured for 60 s on Day 28. The entire experiment plan is exhibited in Figure 1.

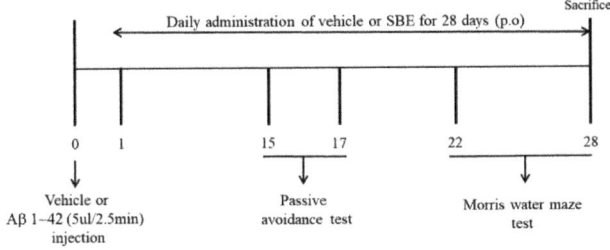

Figure 1. Experimental plan of this study.

2.6. Preparation of Tissue Samples

The mice were anesthetized and sacrificed after behavioral tasks for biochemical studies. The hippocampus was separated from the brain tissue and then immediately stored at −80 °C until further assessment.

2.7. Glutathione Reductase (GR) Activity

GR enzyme activity was determined using the Glutathione Reductase Assay Kit (Abcam, Cambridge, UK). Hippocampal tissues were homogenized in cold assay buffer, and centrifuged at 10,000× g for 15 min at 4 °C. The separated supernatant from hippocampus was taken and kept at −80 °C until further analysis. This assay is based on the reduction of glutathione by nicotinamide adenine dinucleotide phosphate (NADP)H in the presence of GR. GR activity can be detected by measuring the change in absorbance at 405 nm.

2.8. Western Blotting

Hippocampal tissues were homogenized with RIPA buffer and 1% protease inhibitor cocktail (Roche, Mannheim, Germany) and the lysate was centrifuged at 10,000× g for 15 min at 4 °C. The separated supernatant from hippocampus was taken, and protein concentrations were measured using a BCA protein assay kit (Thermo, Waltham, MA, USA). The proteins were separated using 8% or 12% SDS-PAGE and were then moved to polyvinylidene difluoride membranes (Millipore Corp., Bedford, MA, USA). The membranes were initially incubated to block with 5% non-fat skimmed milk in Tris-buffered saline containing 0.1% Tween-20 for 30 min. Next, they were incubated with specific primary antibodies against SOD-1, SOD-2, GPx-1, Aβ (1:1000; Santa Cruz Biotechnology, Santa Cruz, CA, USA), Bax, Bcl-2, cleaved Caspase-9, cleaved PARP, phospho-tau, tau, and β-actin (1:1000; Cell Signaling Technology, Inc., Danvers, MA, USA) for 1 h at 23 °C. The membranes were then incubated in the corresponding horseradish peroxidase-conjugated anti-rabbit, anti-mouse immunoglobulin G (1:10000; GenDEPOT, Barker, TX, USA) for 1 h at 23 °C. The membrane was detected using the ECL system (Atto, Tokyo, Japan). The intensity of the bands on the membrane was detected by Image-Pro Plus software (6.0 Version; Media Cybernetics, Silver Spring, MD, USA)

2.9. Statistical Analysis

The experimental results are expressed as standard error of the mean (SEM) and were assessed using the SPSS program (version 22.0, SPSS Inc., Chicago, IL, USA). Difference value of between treatment groups were analyzed by Student's *t*-test and one-way analysis of variance (ANOVA), and performed following multiple comparisons correction using Dunnett's post-hoc test using Origin 7.0 software (OriginLab, Northampton, MA, USA). $p < 0.05$ indicates that there is a statistical difference, and $p < 0.01$ was considered statistically highly significant between mean values.

3. Results

3.1. Effects of the Scrophularia Buergeriana Extract (SBE) on the Passive Avoidance Test in Aβ 1–42 Treated Mice

To determine the effect of SBE on memory deficits, we conducted the passive avoidance test in the Aβ-induced mouse model. Aβ-injected mice demonstrated a remarkable reduction in the time to move from the illuminated compartment to the shaded area compared to normal mice ($p < 0.01$), implying that the learning capacity was lowered. However, the step-through latency was dose-dependently increased in mice administered with SBE 30 mg/kg ($p < 0.05$) and 100 mg/kg ($p < 0.01$) (Figure 2) compared to Aβ-injected mice.

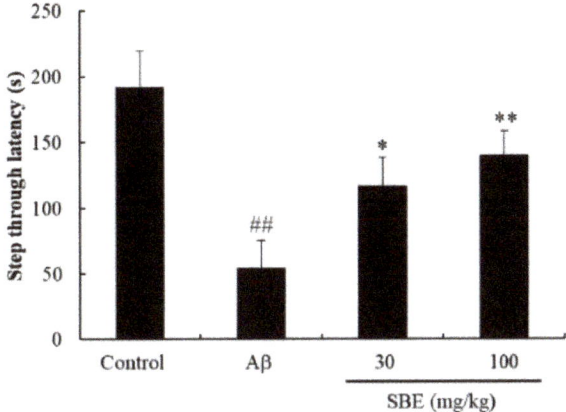

Figure 2. Effects of *Scrophularia buergeriana* extract (SBE) on the step-through latency of passive avoidance performance in Aβ 1–42 treated mice. The data are expressed as means ± standard error of the mean (SEM) of independent experiments ($n = 8$). ## $p < 0.01$ vs. Control group; * $p < 0.05$ and ** $p < 0.01$ vs. Aβ (1–42) group.

3.2. Effects of the SBE on the MWM Test in Aβ 1–42 Induced Memory Deficit Mice

To investigate the memory-enhancing effect of SBE, we next performed the MWM test in C57BL/6 mice. Normal mice quickly located the platform during four consecutive behavioral tests. The Aβ-injected group exhibited a significantly delayed escape latency compared to the normal group from days 25–27. However, mice treated with SBE 30 mg/kg and 100 mg/kg demonstrated a shortened escape latency from days 25–27 (Figure 3A). Furthermore, we observed that Aβ-injected mice demonstrated significantly increased swim distances to find the platform compared to the normal control mice (Figure 3B). We confirmed that SBE 30 mg/kg ($p < 0.05$) and 100 mg/kg ($p < 0.01$) on day 27 decreased the distance traveled to locate the platform. In the probe trials (Figure 3C), the Aβ-treated mice reported a decreased number of crossings over the previous platform position against as the control mice. The number of crossings was recovered by treatment with SBE 30 mg/kg ($p < 0.05$) and 100 mg/kg ($p < 0.01$) compared to the Aβ-injected mice and the recovery was significant. Therefore, we confirmed that SBE enhanced spatial recognition in the MWM test.

3.3. Effects of the SBE on Glutathione Reductase (GR) Activity in the Hippocampus

To evaluate the effects of SBE on GR activity of Aβ treatment mice, GR activity was measured in the hippocampal tissue. GR activity was significantly reduced in mice treated with Aβ compared with the normal group. However, mice treated with SBE 30 mg/kg ($p < 0.05$) and 100 mg/kg ($p < 0.05$) significantly increased hippocampal GR activity compared to the Aβ-treated group. Furthermore, the efficacy of SBE was comparable to the normal group mice (Figure 4).

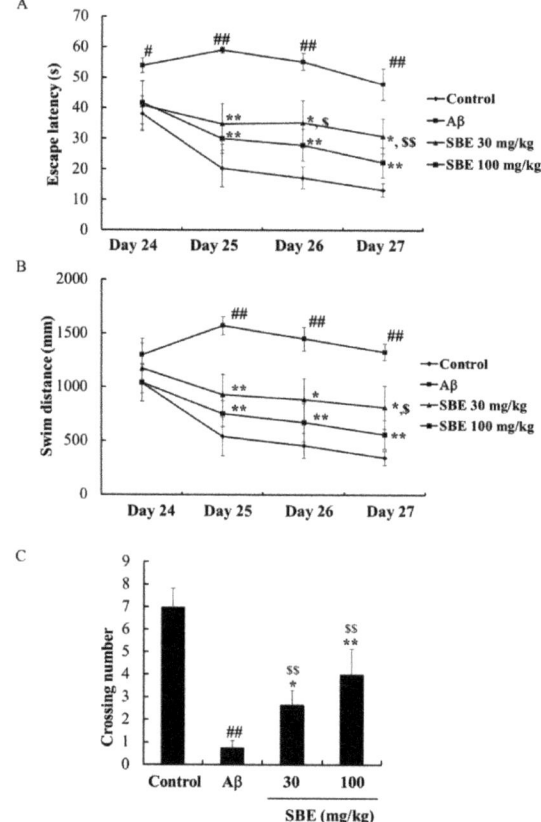

Figure 3. Effects of SBE on Aβ 1–42 induced memory impairment in the Morris water maze (MWM). (**A**) The escape latency and (**B**) Swim distance was recorded across 4 days (Day 24–Day 27). (**C**) The number of crossings in a probe trial performed on Day 28. The data are expressed as means ± SEM of independent experiments ($n = 8$). # $p < 0.05$ and ## $p < 0.01$ vs. Control group; $ < 0.05 and $$ < 0.01 vs. Control group; * $p < 0.05$ and ** $p < 0.01$ vs. Aβ (1–42) group.

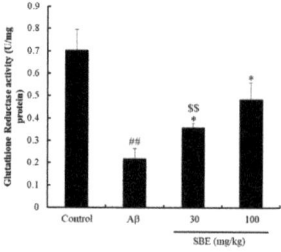

Figure 4. Effects of SBE on glutathione reductase (GR) activity in the mouse hippocampus. The hippocampus was lysed, and the supernatant was used to measurement GR activity. The results were calculated as a unit of nicotinamide adenine dinucleotide phosphate (NADPH) oxidized per protein and expressed as means ± SEM of independent experiments ($n = 3$). ## $p < 0.01$ vs. Control group; $$ < 0.01 vs. Control group; * $p < 0.05$ vs. Aβ (1–42) group.

3.4. Effects of the SBE on the Antioxidant Enzymes in Hippocampus of Aβ 1–42 Treated Mice

To investigate the effects of SBE on antioxidant enzymes in the hippocampus of Aβ treated mice, the protein levels of SOD1, SOD2, and GPx-1 were evaluated. The protein levels of SOD1, SOD2, and GPx-1 were markedly decreased in mice treated with Aβ against the control group. Furthermore, treatment with SBE 30 mg/kg increased GPx-1 protein expression by 1.3-fold. In addition, SOD1, SOD2, and GPx-1 protein levels were further increased in mice administered SBE 100 mg/kg by 4.2-, 1.7- and 2.9-fold, respectively, compared to the Aβ-treated group (Figure 5).

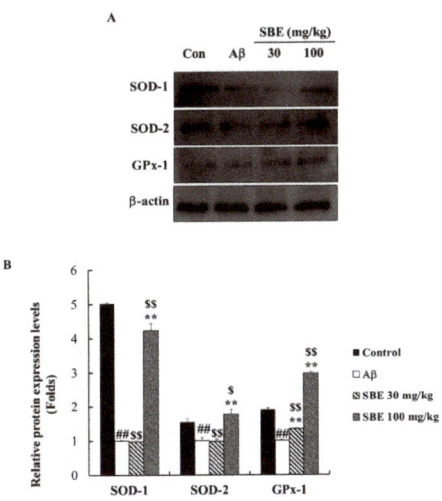

Figure 5. Effects of SBE on antioxidant protein expression levels in the hippocampus of memory-impaired mice. (**A**) The expression of superoxide dismutase 1 (SOD1), SOD2, and glutathione peroxidase-1 (GPx-1) were detected by Western blotting analysis. (**B**) The protein bands were quantified and calculated using the relevant software. Protein expression levels were normalized on β-actin level. The data are expressed as means ± SEM of independent experiments ($n = 3$). ## $p < 0.01$ vs. Control group; $ < 0.05 and $$ < 0.01 vs. Control group; ** $p < 0.01$ vs. Aβ (1–42) group.

3.5. Effects of the SBE on Apoptosis in the Hippocampus of Aβ 1–42 Treated Mice

To demonstrate the protective effect of SBE on Aβ-induced apoptosis, the protein expression levels of Bax, Bcl-2, caspase-9, and cleaved PARP were analyzed in the hippocampal tissue. Aβ treatment significantly increased the protein levels of Bax, cleaved Caspase-9, and cleaved PARP. Conversely, the Bcl-2 protein levels decreased in the Aβ-treated group. Bcl-2/Bax are known as important proteins related to apoptosis in the mitochondria. The Bax protein level was dose-dependently reduced with SBE treatment by 31% and 51%, and SBE 100 mg/kg ($p < 0.01$) significantly increased the levels of Bcl-2 and Bcl-2/Bax by 1.41- and 2.87-fold, respectively, compared to the Aβ-treated group in Figure 6. SBE 30 mg/kg and 100 mg/kg significantly reduced the levels of cleaved caspase-9 by 61%, and 76%, respectively, and reduced cleaved PARP by 33% and, 74%, respectively, compared to the Aβ treatment group. Therefore, we confirmed that SBE exhibited a prominent neuro-protective effect.

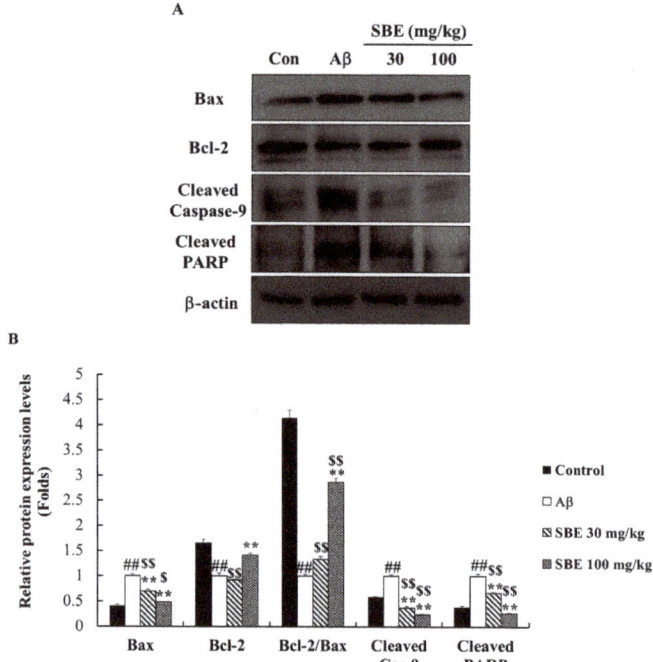

Figure 6. Effects of SBE on apoptotic protein expression levels in the hippocampus of memory-impaired mice. (**A**) The expression of Bcl-2-associated X protein (Bax), B-cell lymphoma 2 (Bcl-2), cleaved caspase-9 and cleaved poly (adenosine diphosphate (ADP)-ribose) polymerase (PARP) was detected by Western blotting analysis. (**B**) The protein bands were quantified and calculated using the software. Protein expression levels were normalized on β-actin level. The data are expressed as means ± SEM of independent experiments (n = 3). ## p < 0.01 vs. Control group; $ < 0.05 and $$ < 0.01 vs. Control group; ** p < 0.01 vs. Aβ (1–42) group.

3.6. Effects of the SBE on Aβ Accumulation and Hyper-Phosphorylation of Tau Proteins in Hippocampus of Aβ 1–42 Treated Mice

The pathological hallmarks of AD include Aβ accumulation and tau hyper-phosphorylation. The hyper-phosphorylation of the tau protein, can contribute to neuronal degeneration. Using western blot analysis, we confirmed that the Aβ injection promoted Aβ accumulation in the mouse hippocampus (Figure 7). The administration of SBE 30 mg/kg (p < 0.01) and 100 mg/kg (p < 0.01) significantly reduced Aβ accumulation in the hippocampus against as the Aβ injection group by 22% and 53%, respectively (Figure 7B). Based on the protective effect of SBE on Aβ accumulation, we confirmed the effect of SBE on tau phosphorylation in Aβ treated mice. Aβ treatment increased the tau protein phosphorylation compared to the normal group, and treatment with SBE 30 mg/kg and 100 mg/kg significantly attenuated Aβ induced hyper-phosphorylation of tau by 69% and 71%, respectively, compared to the Aβ treatment group.

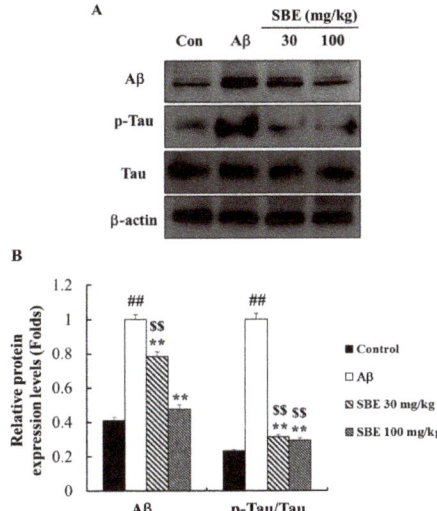

Figure 7. Effects of SBE on amyloid-beta protein expression levels and phosphorylation of tau protein levels in the hippocampus of memory-impaired mice. (**A**) The expression of amyloid-beta (Aβ) and phospho (p)-tau was detected by Western blotting analysis. (**B**) The protein bands were quantified and calculated using the software. Phosphorylation levels of the tau protein were normalized to those of tau, and Aβ protein expression level was normalized on β-actin level. The data are expressed as means ± SEM of independent experiments ($n = 3$). ## $p < 0.01$ vs. Control group; \$\$ < 0.01 vs. Control group; ** $p < 0.01$ vs. Aβ (1–42) group.

4. Discussion

Previously, we reported that SBE extracts demonstrate potent anti-amnesic activity and anti-apoptotic effects in a scopolamine-induced memory impairment mouse model and in the SH-SY5Y cell line [11,12]. In vitro studies have shown that SBE treatment inhibited cell death induced by glutamate. Furthermore, the in vivo study indicates that acute and prolonged treatment with SBE demonstrates the highest anti-oxidant activity in the scopolamine-induced memory impairment model. However, research on amyloid-beta, which affects in the development of AD, is insufficient. The first report aimed to identify the neuro-protective activities, including amyloid-beta accumulation prevention effects and related mechanisms of chronic SBE administration in the Aβ 1–42-induced cognitive deficit mice model.

AD is a progressive, neurodegenerative disorder that causes damage to the brain and is characterized by cognitive decline, and irreversible memory loss. Amyloid-beta peptides, and hyper-phosphorylated tau protein comprising neurofibrillary tangles have been considered critical factors of pathological hallmarks of AD [10]. Indeed, Aβ levels were higher in the brain of AD patients than normal aged brain samples, indicating clinical signs such as spatial memory loss [20,21].

To assess cognitive deficits, passive avoidance and MWM tasks were performed to investigate learning and memory skills. The passive avoidance task is used to confirm the memory function by measuring the escape time from the space. The MWM task is the most widely used laboratory behavioral test to assess hippocampal-dependent cognitive deficits and learning functions in mice and rats [20,22,23]. Injection of Aβ 1–42 resulted in severe cognitive impairments and memory loss in the passive avoidance test and MWM, as well as neurodegeneration. However, SBE treatment dose-dependently increased the step-through latency in the passive avoidance task and decreased escape latency and swim distance significantly for 4 days of MWM trials. This implied that SBE administration improves cognitive performance and ameliorates memory deficits, although not as completely as the normal model that did not cause memory loss.

In the previous study, we have demonstrated that neuronal cell death and cognitive deficiency due to oxidative stress are related to Aβ accumulation in the brain. [24]. Aβ is a known neuro-toxic peptide that promotes oxidative stress and lipid peroxidation in the intermembrane and also causes ROS generation by serving as a source of ROS [5,6,25]. The accumulation of Aβ may result in an increased production of ROS, subsequently leading to neuronal death through apoptotic pathways [25,26]. To prevent ROS generation and regulate the steady-state O^2 concentration, cells have anti-oxidant defense systems such as SODs, GR and GPx-1 enzymes [11,12,27]. Aβ 1–42 injection attenuated hippocampal antioxidant enzyme activities and protein expression levels, the same as in previous studies [28,29]. Nevertheless, we observed that the administration of SBE (30, 100 mg/kg) could significantly enhance GR activity and SODs, GPx-1 protein levels in the Aβ 1–42-treated mouse hippocampus.

The mitochondria are much more sensitive to oxidative stress and Aβ-mediated oxidative stress increased mitochondrial dysfunction leading to apoptotic cell death. The accumulated Aβ triggers neuronal death in the hippocampus by releasing caspase activators [24,29,30]. Aβ-induced apoptosis is regulated by mediators such as caspases, Bcl-2, and Bax [10]. The proportion of Bax and Bcl-2 affects whether a cell undergoes or escapes apoptosis. The caspase pathway promotes apoptosis and releases apoptosis-promoting factors when the Bax/Bcl-2 ratio is increased [20]. In our study, SBE treatment significantly lowered Bax, cleaved caspase-9, and cleaved PARP protein expression levels and upregulated Bcl-2 protein expression levels at the same time in mice hippocampal tissue.

Aβ injections increased the accumulation of Aβ and induced hyper-phosphorylation of the tau protein in the brain. The brains of AD patients demonstrate abnormally phosphorylated tau, 4–8-fold higher than normal brains [31]. In this study, the Aβ-injection increased the phosphorylated tau protein expression levels about 4–5 times as against the normal control. We observed that the Aβ and phosphorylated tau protein expression levels dose-dependently decreased in response to treatment with SBE compared to the normal group.

However, this pre-clinical study has some limitations and we will confirm the anti-inflammatory effects of SBE in a mouse model induced neuroinflammation and memory loss in a further study. Further studies are also needed for immunohistochemical analysis and the effect of SBE in clinical trials.

Collectively, our results indicate that SBE treatment improved memory impairment through reduction of Aβ accumulation and the regulation of oxidative stress, anti-apoptotic pathways, and tau protein hyper-phosphorylation in the Aβ 1–42 memory impairment-induced hippocampal tissue.

5. Conclusions

This study demonstrated that SBE possesses antioxidant and neuroprotective effects against a β-amyloid induced memory loss model. Amyloid beta generates oxidative stress as an early event in AD and causes tau phosphorylation, mitochondria dysfunction and ROS generation. Consecutively, it leads to apoptosis and neurodegeneration. SBE treatment ameliorates memory deficits and improves learning and memory function. SBE also exhibited remarkable neuroprotective effects against Aβ 1–42 induced neurotoxicity via the apoptosis pathway (Figure 8). This study offers SBE at a dose of 100 mg/kg which suggests the possibility of development as a health functional food for the improvement of learning and memory impairment.

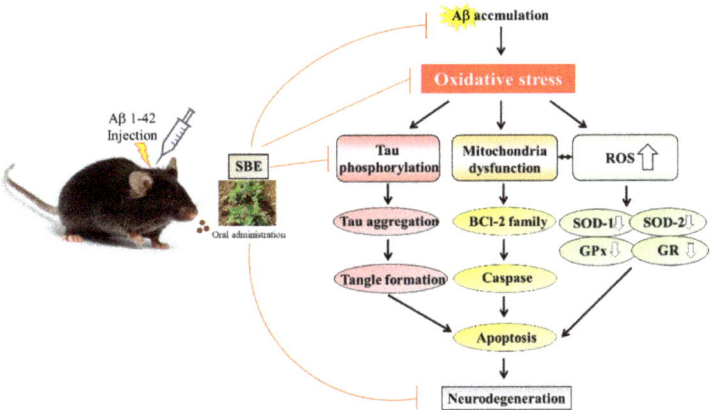

Figure 8. The proposed mechanism by which SBE ameliorates learning and memory in mice following an injection of amyloid-β 1–42 (Aβ 1–42).

Author Contributions: H.J.L. conducted the experiments and participated in the interpretation and writing of the manuscript. D.Y.L. and H.L.K. performed the data analysis and quality control assessment respectively. S.H.Y. planned and led the project, and contributed the data review, editing and manuscript finalization. All authors have read and agreed to the published version of the manuscript.

Funding: This study was carried out with the support of the 'Cooperative Research Program for Agriculture Science and Technology Development (Project no. PJ013215012020)' Rural Development Administration, Republic of Korea.

Conflicts of Interest: The authors declare no conflict of interest in this study.

References

1. Wen, H.; Fu, Z.; Wei, Y.; Zhang, X.; Ma, L.; Gu, L.; Li, J. Antioxidant Activity and Neuroprotective Activity of Stilbenoids in Rat Primary Cortex Neurons via the PI3K/Akt Signaling Pathway. *Molecules* **2018**, *23*, 2328. [CrossRef] [PubMed]
2. Huang, D.S.; Yu, Y.C.; Wu, C.H.; Lin, J.Y. Protective Effects of Wogonin against Alzheimer's Disease by Inhibition of Amyloidogenic Pathway. *Evid. Based Complement Alternat. Med.* **2017**, *3*, 1–13. [CrossRef] [PubMed]
3. Paul Murphy, M.; LeVine, H. Alzheimer's Disease and the β-Amyloid Peptide. *J. Alzheimers Dis.* **2010**, *19*, 311. [CrossRef] [PubMed]
4. Huang, H.C.; Jiang, Z.F. Accumulated amyloid-beta peptide and hyperphosphorylated tua protein: Relationship and links in Alzheimer's disease. *J. Alzhimers Dis.* **2009**, *16*, 15–17. [CrossRef] [PubMed]
5. Klein, A.M.; Kowall, N.W.; Ferrante, R.J. Neurotoxicity and oxidative damage of beta amyloid 1–42 versus beta amyloid 1–40 in the mouse cerebral cortex. *Ann. N. Y. Acad. Sci.* **1999**, *893*, 314–320. [CrossRef]
6. Kim, D.H.; Jung, W.Y.; Park, S.J.; Kim, J.M.; Lee, S.; Kim, Y.C.; Ryu, J.H. Anti-amnesic effect of ESP-102 on Aβ (1–42)-induced memory impairment in mice. *Pharmacol. Biochem. Behav.* **2010**, *92*, 239–248. [CrossRef]
7. Butterfield, D.A.; Reed, T.; Newman, S.F.; Sultana, R. Roles of amyloid β-peptide-associated oxidative stress and brain protein modifications in the pathogenesis of Alzheimer's disease and mild cognitive impairment. *Free Radic. Biol. Med.* **2007**, *43*, 658–677. [CrossRef]
8. Valle, V.; Oliver, J.; Roca, P. Role of uncoupling proteins in cancer. *Cancers* **2010**, *2*, 567–591. [CrossRef]
9. Ighodaro, O.M.; Akinloye, O.A. First line defence anti-oxidants-superoxide dismutase (SOD), catalase (CAT) and glutathione peroxidase (GPX): Their fundamental role in the entire antioxidant defence grid. *Alex. J. Med.* **2018**, *54*, 287–293. [CrossRef]
10. Suganthy, N.; Malar, D.S.; Devi, K.P. Rhizophora mucronata attenuates beta-amyloid induced cognitive dysfunction, oxidative stress and cholinergic deficit in Alzheimer's disease animal model. *Metab. Brain Dis.* **2016**, *4*, 937–949. [CrossRef]

11. Lee, H.J.; Spandidos, D.A.; Tsatsakis, A.; Margina, D.; Izotov, B.N.; Yang, S.H. Neuroprotective effects of Scrophularia buergeriana extract against glutamate-induced toxicity in SH-SH5Y cells. *Int. J. Mol. Med.* **2019**, *43*, 2144–2152. [PubMed]
12. Jeong, E.J.; Ma, C.J.; Lee, K.Y.; Kim, S.H. KD-501, a standardized extract of Scrophulaira buergeriana has both cognitive-enhancing and antioxidant activities in mice given scopolamine. *J. Ethnopharmacol.* **2009**, *121*, 98–105. [CrossRef] [PubMed]
13. Liu, Z.; Li, P.; Wu, J.; Wang, Y.; Li, P.; Hou, X.; Zhang, Q.; Wei, N.; Zhao, Z.; Liang, H.; et al. The Cascade of Oxidative Stress and Tau Protein Autophagic Dysfunction in Alzheimer's Disease. In *Alzheimer's Disease—Challenges for the Future*; IntechOpen: London, UK, 2015; pp. 27–45. [CrossRef]
14. Brion, J.P. Neurofibrillary Tangles and Alzheimer's Disease. *Eur. Neurol.* **1998**, *40*, 130–140. [CrossRef] [PubMed]
15. Gu, Q.; Wang, J.D.; Xia, H.H.; Lin, M.C.; He, H.; Zou, B.; Tu, S.P.; Yang, Y.; Liu, X.G.; Lam, S.K.; et al. Activation of the caspase-8/Bid and Bax pathways in aspirin-induced apoptosis in gastric cancer. *Carcinogenesis* **2015**, *26*, 541–546. [CrossRef]
16. Selznick, L.A.; Zheng, T.S.; Flavell, R.A.; Rakic, P.; Roth, K.A. Amyloid beta-induced neuronal death is bax-dependent but caspase-independent. *J. Neuropathol. Exp. Neurol.* **2000**, *59*, 271–279. [CrossRef]
17. Westphal, D.; Dewson, G.; Czabotar, P.E.; Kluck, R.M. Molecular biology of Bax and Bak activation and action. *Biochim. Biophys. Acta* **2011**, *1813*, 521–531. [CrossRef]
18. Oltavai, Z.N.; Milliman, C.L.; Korsmeyer, S.J. Bcl-2 heterodimerizes in vivo with a conserved homolog, Bax, that accelerates programmed cell death. *Cell* **1993**, *74*, 609–619.
19. Finucane, D.M.; Boosy Wetzel, E.; Waterhouse, N.J.; Cotter, T.G.; Green, D.R. Bax-induced caspase activation and apoptosis via cytochrome c release from mitochondria is inhibitable by Bcl-xL. *J. Biol. Chem.* **1999**, *274*, 2225–2233. [CrossRef]
20. Lee, H.J.; Lee, S.K.; Lee, D.R.; Choi, B.K.; Le, B.; Yang, S.H. Ameliorating effect of Citrus aurantium and nobiletin on β-amyloid (1–42)-induced memory impairment in mice. *Mol. Med. Rep.* **2019**, *20*, 3448–3455. [CrossRef]
21. Zhu, H.; Yan, H.; Tang, N.; Li, X.; Pang, P.; Li, H.; Chen, W.; Guo, Y.; Shu, S.; Cai, Y.; et al. Impairment of spatial memory in an Alzheimer's disease model via degeneration of hippocampal cholinergic synapses. *Nat. Commun.* **2017**, *22*, 1676. [CrossRef]
22. Zhang, S.; Hu, X.; Guan, W.; Luan, L.; Li, B.; Tang, Q.; Fan, H. Isoflurane anesthesia promotes cognitive impairment by inducing expression of β-amyloid protein-related factors in the hippocampus of aged rats. *PLoS ONE* **2017**, *12*, e0175654. [CrossRef] [PubMed]
23. Tucker, L.B.; Velosky, A.G.; McCabe, J.T. Applications of the Morris water maze in translational traumatic brain injury research. *Neurosci. Biobehav. Rev.* **2018**, *88*, 187–800. [CrossRef] [PubMed]
24. Laniski, F.R.; Alves, C.B.; Souza, A.C.; Pinto, S.; Roman, S.S.; Rhoden, C.R.; Alves, M.P.; Luchese, C. Protective effect of meloxicam-loaded nanocapsules against amyloid-β peptide-induced damage in mice. *Behav. Brain Res.* **2012**, *230*, 100–107. [CrossRef] [PubMed]
25. Butterfield, D.A.; Swomely, A.M.; Sultana, R. Amyloid β-peptide (1–42)-induced oxidative stress in Alzheimer disease: Importance in disease pathogenesis and progression. *Antioxid. Redox Signal.* **2013**, *19*, 823–835. [CrossRef] [PubMed]
26. Ganguly, G.; Chakrabarti, S.; Chatterjee, U.; Saso, L. Proteinpathy, oxidative stress and mitochondrial dysfunction: Cross talk in Alzheimer's disease and Parkinson's disease. *Drug Des. Devel. Ther.* **2017**, *11*, 797–810. [CrossRef]
27. Huang, W.J.; Zhang, X.; Chen, W.W. Role of oxidative stress in Alzheimer's disease (Review). *Biomed. Rep.* **2016**, *4*, 519–522. [CrossRef]
28. Resende, R.; Moreira, P.I.; Proenca, T.; Deshpande, A.; Busciglio, J.; Pereira, C.; Oliveria, C.R. Brain oxidative stress in a triple-transgenic mouse model of Alzheimer disease. *Free Radic. Biol. Med.* **2008**, *15*, 2051–2057. [CrossRef]
29. Farajdokht, F.; Amani, M.; Mizaei Bravil, F.; Alihemmati, A.; Mohaddes, G.; Babri, S. Troxerutin protects hippocampal neurons against amyloid beta-induced oxidative stress and apoptosis. *EXCEL J.* **2017**, *16*, 1081–1089.

30. Razaul, H.; Sarder, N.U.; Amir, H. Amyloid beta (Aβ) and Oxidative stress: Progression of Alzheimer's Disease. *Adv. Biotech. Micro.* **2018**, *11*, 7–16. [CrossRef]
31. Iqbal, K.; Liu, F.; Gong, C.X.; Alonso Adel, C.; Grundke-Iqbal, I. Mechanisms of tau-induced neurodegeneration. *Acta Neuropathol.* **2009**, *118*, 53–69. [CrossRef]

Publisher's Note: MDPI stays neutral with regard to jurisdictional claims in published maps and institutional affiliations.

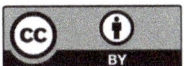 © 2020 by the authors. Licensee MDPI, Basel, Switzerland. This article is an open access article distributed under the terms and conditions of the Creative Commons Attribution (CC BY) license (http://creativecommons.org/licenses/by/4.0/).

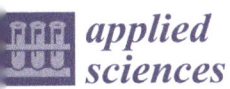

Article

Scrophularia buergeriana Extract (Brainon) Improves Scopolamine-Induced Neuronal Impairment and Cholinergic Dysfunction in Mice through CREB-BDNF Signaling Pathway

Hae-Jin Lee [1,†], Hae-Lim Kim [1,†], Dae-Young Lee [2], Dong-Ryung Lee [3], Bong-Keun Choi [3] and Seung-Hwan Yang [1,*]

1. Department of Biotechnology, Chonnam National University, Yeosu 59626, Korea; haecutejin@naver.com (H.-J.L.); ics1357@naver.com (H.-L.K.)
2. Department of Herbal Crop Research, National Institute of Horticultural and Herbal Science, Rural Development Administration (RDA), Eumseong 27709, Korea; dylee0809@korea.kr
3. Nutrapharm Tech, Jungwon-gu, Seongnam, Gyunggi 13201, Korea; drlee@nutrapharm.co.kr (D.-R.L.); cbcbcbk@nutrapharm.co.kr (B.-K.C.)
* Correspondence: ymichigan@jnu.ac.kr; Tel.: +82-61-659-7306
† These authors contributed equally to this work.

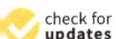

Citation: Lee, H.-J.; Kim, H.-L.; Lee, D.-Y.; Lee, D.-R.; Choi, B.-K.; Yang, S.-H. *Scrophularia buergeriana* Extract (Brainon) Improves Scopolamine-Induced Neuronal Impairment and Cholinergic Dysfunction in Mice through CREB-BDNF Signaling Pathway. *Appl. Sci.* **2021**, *11*, 4286. https://doi.org/10.3390/app11094286

Academic Editor: Hari Prasad Devkota

Received: 11 March 2021
Accepted: 7 May 2021
Published: 10 May 2021

Publisher's Note: MDPI stays neutral with regard to jurisdictional claims in published maps and institutional affiliations.

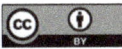

Copyright: © 2021 by the authors. Licensee MDPI, Basel, Switzerland. This article is an open access article distributed under the terms and conditions of the Creative Commons Attribution (CC BY) license (https://creativecommons.org/licenses/by/4.0/).

Abstract: We evaluated the effectiveness of *Scrophularia buergeriana* extract (Brainon) on cognitive dysfunction and determined its underlying mechanisms in a scopolamine (SCO)-treated mouse model of memory impairment. Brainon treatment for 28 days ameliorated the symptoms of memory impairment as indicated by the results of both passive avoidance performance and the Morris water mazes. Brainon lowered acetylcholinesterase activity and raised acetylcholine levels in the hippocampus. The treatment elevated the protein levels of brain-derived neurotrophic factor (BDNF) and phosphorylated cAMP response element-binding (CREB). Additionally, the excessive generation of SCO-induced reactive oxygen species (ROS) and subsequent oxidative stress were suppressed by the enhancement of superoxide dismutase (SOD)-1 and SOD-2 proteins. mRNA levels of upregulated interleukin (IL)-1β, IL-6, and tumor necrosis factor (TNF)-α, as well as the apoptotic protein Bcl-2-associated X protein (Bax), cleaved caspase-9, and cleaved poly adenosine diphosphate-ribose polymerase (PARP) expression after SCO injection were downregulated by Brainon treatment. Collectively, these findings suggested that Brainon possesses anti-amnesic effects through the CREB-BDNF pathway. Moreover, it exerted antioxidant, anti-inflammatory, and anti-apoptotic effects in SCO-induced mice exhibiting cognitive impairment and memory loss.

Keywords: *Scrophularia buergeriana*; anti-amnesic effect; cholinergic neurotransmission; anti-oxidant; anti-inflammation; anti-apoptotic

1. Introduction

The characterization of Alzheimer's diseases (AD) represents amyloid β accumulation, hyperphosphorylation of the tau protein, increased inflammation and oxidative stress leading to neuronal death, which is accompanied by an impairment in memory and cognitive abilities [1,2]. Moreover, a decrease in the neurotransmitter, acetylcholine (Ach), in the AD brain is a crucial factor responsible for dementia [1].

Scopolamine (SCO) is a muscarinic receptor blocker and tropane alkaloid drug that interrupts cholinergic nerve transmission, causing memory disability and cognitive deficits in the central nervous system (CNS) [1,3–6]. Normal cholinergic activity in the CNS influences hippocampal nerve regeneration and memory impairment via the cAMP response element-binding protein (CREB)-brain-derived neurotrophic factor (BDNF) signaling [7]. SCO administration causes cholinergic neuronal pathway dysregulation, including increased acetylcholinesterase (AChE) activity, suppression of ACh release and impairment of the memory circuit, and decreased CREB-BDNF levels. Moreover, the neuronal inflammatory cascade, oxidative stress generation, and neuron cell death, including cholinergic malfunction, are causative factors in patients with neurodegenerative disorders. The hippocampus is susceptible to oxidative stress, and excessive oxidative stress induces memory deficiency by damaging synaptic plasticity and causing inflammation and neuronal cell death [7,8]. SCO-treated mice showed oxidative stress-induced neuronal inflammation and apoptosis in the brain [9]. Therefore, SCO injection of animals is utilized as a useful pharmacological experimental model for cognitive degeneration and memory disorders in AD [2–5].

Scrophularia buergeriana Miquel (SB), belonging to the Scrophulariaceae family, is indigenous to Korea and also found abundantly in China and Japan. In traditional medicine, dried SB roots have long been used to alleviate high fever, swollen skin, obstipation, pharyngitis, neuro-inflammation, and throat infection [10]. SB roots have been found to contains various components such as E-harpagoside, 8-O-E-p-methoxycinnamoyl harpagide (MCA-Hg), E-p-methoxy-cinnamic acid (p-MCA), cinnamic acid, and angoroside C. Moreover, we confirmed that Brainon exhibited significant neuroprotective effects against neurotoxicity caused SH-SY5Y cells by glutamate [11]. We previously demonstrated that Brainon exerts anti-amnesic effects via inhibition of amyloid beta accumulation and hyperphosphorylation of tau protein in memory deficit mice by β-amyloid [12].

Therefore, we administrated 30 or 100 mg/kg Brainon based on the previous study [12] and confirmed the cognitive-improving activities of Brainon using passive avoidance performance and Morris water maze (MWM) task based on this research. To demonstrate the potential mechanism of Brainon, we confirmed the CREB-BDNF signaling pathway, AChE activity, and ACh levels in mice hippocampal tissue. Moreover, the anti-inflammatory and antioxidant effects of Brainon, as well as its effects on neuronal death, were evaluated in SCO-caused memory-impaired mice.

2. Materials and Methods

2.1. Preparation of Sample

Brainon was supplied by Nutrapharm Tech Co., Ltd., (Seongnam, Korea). SB roots were dried and extracted using 70% EtOH. The resulting solution was filtered, concentrated, and dried to yield Brainon extract (SB extract; SBE). The detailed process has been described previously [11,12]. To dissolve the Brainon, we used 0.5% carboxy-methylcellulose (CMC) and then applied for the in vivo study.

2.2. Animals

The experimental protocol and process were admitted by the Animal Care and Use Committee (Permission number: 2019-05-003) of ChemOn Inc. (YoungIn, Korea). Eight-week-old male C57BL/6N mice were offered (Orient Bio, Seongnam, Korea) and housed under regulated conditions (temperature: 23 ± 3 °C, 12 h light/dark cycle, $55 \pm 15\%$ humidity, lighting intensity 150–300 Lux). They freely utilized food and drinking water and had an acclimation period for a week before the experiment started.

2.3. Design of Experiment

The experimental mice were randomized into 5 groups after 1-week adaptation ($n = 8$ per group): Normal group, SCO-treated group, SCO with Brainon (30 or 100 mg/kg/day). Ginkgo Biloba Extract (GBE, 50 mg/kg/day), which was found to have an improving effect on memory deficit [13,14], was used as a positive control agent. 0.5% CMC was used to dissolve Brainon and GBE and administered (10 mL/kg/day) for 28 days via gastric gavage. The passive avoidance test was performed for 3 days (days 15–17), whereas the MWM task was performed for 7 days (days 22–28). Memory deficiency was caused by SCO injection (1 mg/kg, i.p.) within 30 min following the oral administration of Brainon and GBE extract. Behavior test was conducted for 30 min after the SCO injection.

2.4. Step-Through Passive Avoidance Performance

The device (Twin County Med Associates, Hudson, NY, USA) for the passive avoidance test consisted of two identical compartments, separated into light and dark areas with an automated door and electric floor. Experiments were conducted at the same time every day for 3 days. The mice were placed in the dark compartments for 120 s before being moved back to the lit compartments. If the mice moved to a dark area, they were immediately transferred back to the lit compartment (day 15). During the acquisition trial (day 16), mice could move freely without lighting for 60 s for familiarization. After adaptation training, they were permitted to enter the two compartments and move freely for 120 s and, when moved to the dark area, a 0.20 mA scrambled shock was treated. Animals that did not move were removed from the tests. On the retention trial (day 17), the mice were located in the light section and the automated board was opened, and the transfer time to the dark section was analyzed.

2.5. MWM Trial

To confirm the long-term spatial memory ability of the mice, an MWM test was conducted from days 22 to 28. The MWM tasks consisted of a training session for 2 days (days 22 and 23), a behavioral session for the following 5 days (days 24–27), and a probe trial session for 1 day (day 28). Mice were allowed 60 s to find the hidden platform located at one of the water pool's release points. If the mice could not locate the platform, they were manually located on the platform for 30 s. All mice were tested in two trials per day and the platform location in the water pool was randomly altered between trials. Learning and memory capabilities were confirmed by measuring the escape latency. The platform was eliminated from the pool and probe trials were performed to confirm the spatial memory ability by checking the platform crossing number of the mice for 60 s at day 28. Figure 1 is a schematic of the experimental design.

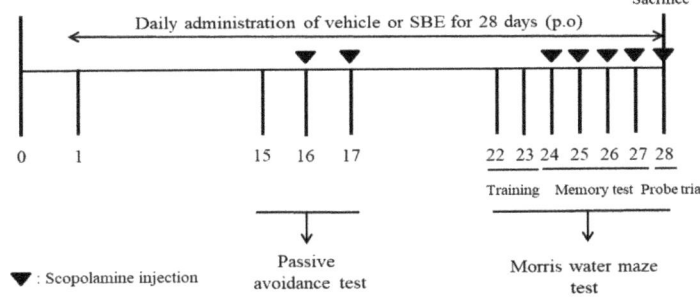

Figure 1. Experiment process of scopolamine-treated memory deficiency in mice.

2.6. AChE Activity and Contents of ACh

The hippocampi were homogenized with cold phosphate-buffered saline and centrifuged (1500× g) for 15 min at 4 °C. Centrifuged supernatant was gathered to confirm AChE activity and ACh levels utilizing commercial kits (Abcam, Cambridge, UK), in accordance with the manufacturer's manuals.

2.7. Preparation of Total RNA and Quantitative RT-PCR

Mice hippocampi were pulverized, and the total RNA was isolated utilizing a RNeasy Mini kit following the manufacturer's manuals (Qiagen GmbH, Hilden, Germany). cDNA synthesis was carried out utilizing a CellScript^{TM} All-in-One cDNA Master Mix (Cell-Safe, Yongin, Korea) at 25 °C (5 min) and 42 °C (15 min). qPCR was conducted using a QuantStudio 3 Real-time PCR device (Thermo Fisher Scientific Inc., Waltham, MA, USA). The synthesized primers for PCR are shown in Table 1. Conditions of cycling were 95 °C (10 min), followed by 50 cycles of 95 °C (15 s) and 72 °C (60 s). The target gene levels were determined by the comparative Ct method utilizing LightCycler 96 Software 1.1 (Roche Diagnostics, Basel, Switzerland).

Table 1. Real-time PCR primer sequences.

Gene		Primer Sequence
IL-1β	Forward	5′-ATG GCA GTT CCT GAA CTC AAC T-3′
	Reverse	5′-CAG GAC AG TAT AGA TTC TTT CCT TT-3′
IL-6	Forward	5′-GAT GCT ACC AAA CTG GAT ATA ATC-3′
	Reverse	5′-GGT CCT TAG CCA CTC CTT CTG TG-3′
TNF-α	Forward	5′-ATG AGC ACA GAA AGC ATG ATC CGC-3′
	Reverse	5′-CCT CCT TAG CCA CTC CTT CTG TG-3′
GAPDH	Forward	5′-CGG TGC TGA GTA TGT CGT GGA GTC T-3′
	Reverse	5′-GTT ATT ATG GGG GTC TGG GAT GGA A-3′

2.8. Extraction of Protein and Western Blot Analysis

The hippocampi were homogenized with RIPA reagent (DYNE Bio, Seongnam, Korea) and the homogenates were centrifuged (10,000× g) for 15 min at 4 °C. Supernatant of hippocampal tissue was harvested, and protein concentrations were quantified utilizing a commercially available BCA protein assay kit (Thermo, Waltham, MA, USA). 30 μg of total protein was electrophoresed on SDS-PAGE and moved onto membranes (Millipore Corp., Bedford, MA, USA). For blocking, the membranes were kept for 1 h at 23 °C then incubated with the first antibodies for SOD-1, SOD-2, GAPDH (Santa Cruz Biotechnology, Santa Cruz, CA, USA), Bax, Bcl-2, cleaved PARP, cleaved caspase-9, phosphor-CREB, CREB (Cell Signaling Technology, Inc., Danvers, MA, USA), and BDNF (Abcam, Cambridge, UK) at a 1:1000 dilution at 23 °C for 1 h. The incubated membranes were washed and further reacted with second antibodies (1:1000; GenDEPOT, Barker, TX, USA) at 23 °C for 1 h. The membranes were processed for detection using ECL solution (Atto, Tokyo, Japan) and the band intensity was measured utilizing Image-Pro Plus (Media Cybernetics, Inc., Rockville, MD, USA).

2.9. Statistical Analysis

Statistical analysis between groups was conducted using Student's t-test and one-way analysis of variance followed by multiple comparisons Dunnett's post-hoc test utilizing Origin 7.0 (OriginLab, Northhampton, MA, USA). Results are expressed as the means ± standard error of the mean. Significant differences between groups were considered statistically significant at $p < 0.05$ and $p < 0.01$.

3. Results

3.1. Composition of Brainon

The marker compound in Brainon was confirmed by high-performance liquid chromatography (HPLC) analysis. Quantitative analysis of Brainon revealed that Angoroside C content was determined at approximately 0.5% (Data not shown), and the optimized Brainon was used for the following experiments.

3.2. Brainon Recovers Scopolamine-Treated Step-through Latency in the Passive Avoidance Test

To assess the effectiveness of Brainon on learning and fear-motivated memory, we conducted the passive avoidance task. The SCO-injected group had a considerably shorter step-through latency compared with Normal group (Figure 2). However, Brainon 30 and 100 mg/kg treatment considerably restored ($p < 0.05$) the scopolamine-caused cognitive deficit and GBE 50 mg/kg administration also improved ($p < 0.05$) memory function when comparison with SCO-injected group only.

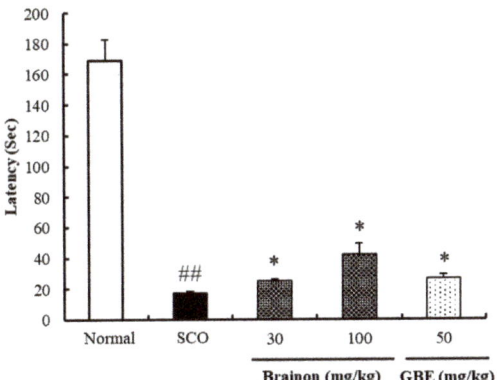

Figure 2. Effects of Brainon scopolamine-treated memory deficit in passive avoidance performance. Values are represented as means ± SEM ($n = 8$). ## $p < 0.01$ vs. Normal group; * $p < 0.05$ vs. SCO-treated group.

3.3. Brainon Improves SCO-Induced Spatial Memory Deficiency in the Morris Water Maze Task

To examine the effects of Brainon on the spatial memory impairment of mice, escape latency, swim distance, and the platform crossing numbers were assessed in all test groups. Figure 3A revealed that the escape latency of the SCO-treated group was significantly prolonged for 4 days (days 24–27) compared to that in the Normal group ($p < 0.01$). In contrast, 100 mg/kg Brainon and 50 mg/kg GBE shortened ($p < 0.05$) the escape latency on days 26 and 27; 100 mg/kg Brainon also decreased ($p < 0.05$) the escape latency compared to that in the SCO-treated group from day 25. Swimming distance to find the platform in the MWM task showed similar results to those of the escape latency (Figure 3B). The mice in the Brainon 30 ($p < 0.05$), 100 ($p < 0.01$), and GBE 50 ($p < 0.05$) mg/kg groups swam shorter distances to locate the platform in comparison with the SCO-treated groups on day 26. We confirmed that the dose of 30 mg/kg ($p < 0.05$) and 100 mg/kg ($p < 0.05$) Brainon on day 27 reduced the swimming distance in mice when finding the platform. In the probe trials (Figure 3C) on day 28, the platform crossing numbers of the mice in the SCO-treated group was considerably lower comparison with that of the mice in the Normal group ($p < 0.01$). On the other hand, administration with 30 and 100 mg/kg of Brainon ($p < 0.01$) and 50 mg/kg GBE ($p < 0.01$) increased the platform crossing numbers comparison with that observed in the SCO-injected group. Our results demonstrate that Brainon administration enhanced spatial, learning, and memory functions in SCO-treated memory-deficient mice.

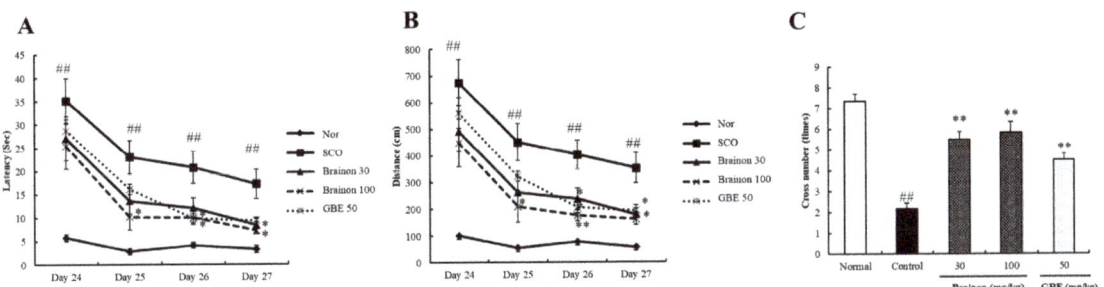

Figure 3. Effects of Brainon scopolamine treated spatial memory deficiency in the MWM trial. (**A**) The escape latency (s) and (**B**) swim distance of mice was investigated for 4 days (**C**) The platform crossing number was carried out on probe trial. Values are represented as means ± SEM ($n = 8$). ## $p < 0.01$ vs. Normal group; * $p < 0.05$ and ** $p < 0.01$ vs. SCO-treated group.

3.4. Brainon Decreases AChE Activity and Increases ACh Levels in SCO-Induced Hippocampal Tissues

To evaluate the effects of Brainon on AChE and ACh levels, we determined AChE activity and ACh levels in SCO-treated hippocampal tissue. Figure 4A shows that AChE activity in the Normal group was lower than that of the SCO-treated group. Exposure to 100 mg/kg Brainon ($p < 0.01$) and 50 mg/kg GBE ($p < 0.01$) considerably lowered AChE activity comparison with that in the SCO-injected group. However, the ACh levels were found to differ (Figure 4B). SCO treatment significantly downregulated ACh levels in the hippocampus. On the contrary, treatment with 30 ($p < 0.05$) and 100 ($p < 0.01$) mg/kg Brainon increased ACh levels in a dose dependent comparison with that in the SCO-injected group.

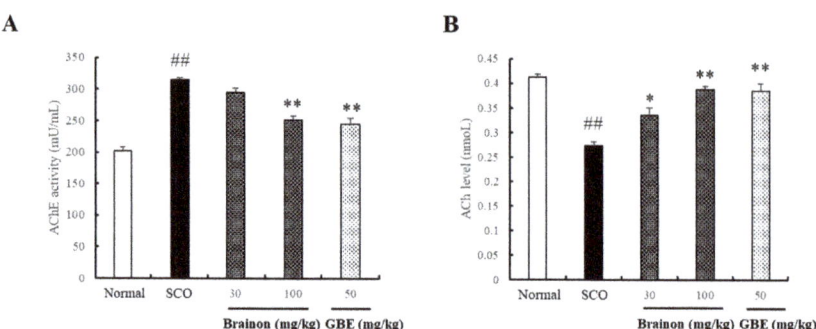

Figure 4. Effects of Brainon on acetylcholinesterase (AChE) activity and acetylcholine (ACh) level in mice hippocampal tissues. The hippocampal tissues were homogenized, and the supernatant was used for calculation of (**A**) AChE activity and (**B**) ACh level. Values were calculated in units per mg protein are represented as means ± SEM ($n = 3$). ## $p < 0.01$ vs. Normal group; * $p < 0.05$ and ** $p < 0.01$ vs. SCO-treated group.

3.5. Brainon Increases BDNF Protein Expression and CREB Phosphorylation Levels in SCO-Induced Hippocampal Tissue

To demonstrate the effectiveness of Brainon on the memory-associated proteins in SCO-treated cognitive impairment, we measured the BDNF expression and phosphorylated CREB levels using western blotting. Figure 5 shows that SCO treatment significantly decreased the expression of BDNF and phosphorylated CREB in the hippocampus comparison with that in the Normal group ($p < 0.01$). However, in the hippocampus, 100 mg/kg Brainon ($p < 0.01$) and 50 mg/kg GBE ($p < 0.01$) prevented a decrease in BDNF protein compared to that in the SCO-treated group. In addition, treatment with 30 ($p < 0.01$) and 100 ($p < 0.01$) mg/kg of Brainon increased the levels of phosphorylated CREB in a dose dependent comparison to the hippocampal tissue in the SCO-injected group.

3.6. Brainon Upregulates the Expression of SOD-1 and SOD-2 in SCO-Induced Hippocampal Tissue

To examine the effects of Brainon on antioxidant enzymes, we determined SOD-1 and SOD-2 levels in SCO-treated hippocampal tissue of mice. SCO treatment significantly decreased SOD-1 and SOD-2 levels in comparison with that in the Normal group. However, administration with 30 ($p < 0.01$) and 100 ($p < 0.01$) mg/kg Brainon increased SOD-1 levels by 1.6- and 3.6-fold, respectively, whereas administration with 50 mg/kg ($p < 0.01$) of GBE recovered the decreased SOD-1 levels 3.9-fold with SCO treatment. Furthermore, treatment with 100 mg/kg ($p < 0.01$) Brainon and 50 mg/kg ($p < 0.01$) GBE also enhanced SOD-2 levels by 1.9- and 2.1-fold, respectively, in comparison with the mice in the SCO-injected group (Figure 6).

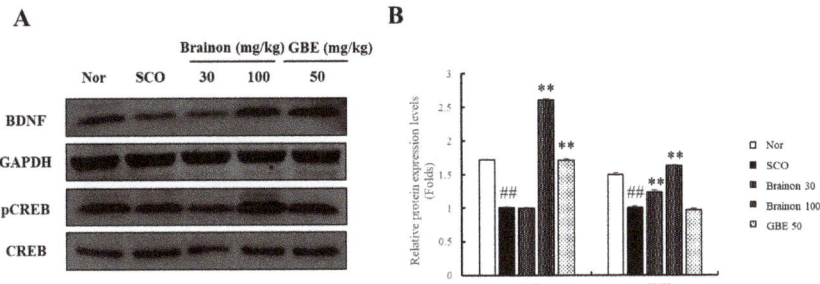

Figure 5. Effects of Brainon on CREB-BDNF pathway in the memory deficit mice hippocampal tissues. (**A**) Brain-derived neurotrophic factor (BDNF) and phosphorylation of cAMP-response element-binding protein (CREB) was measured via western blotting. (**B**) The protein band density was determined using the software. Phosphorylation levels of the CREB protein were normalized using the CREB, and BDNF protein was normalized using the GAPDH. Values are expressed as means ± SEM (n = 3). ## p < 0.01 vs. Normal group; ** p < 0.01 vs. SCO-treated group.

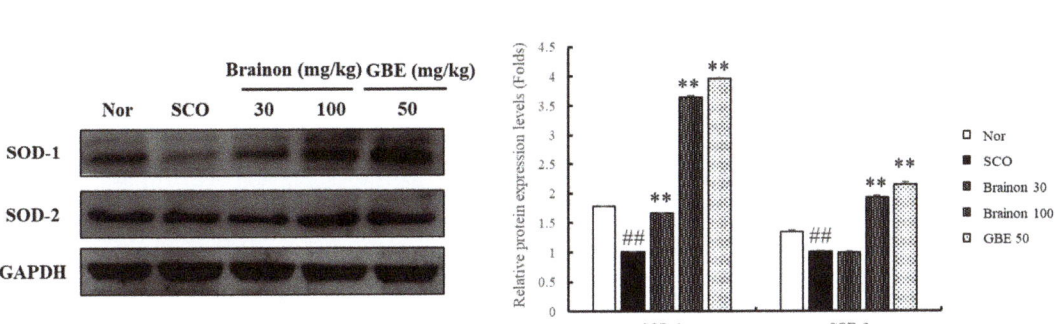

Figure 6. Effects of Brainon on anti-oxidant related protein levels in the hippocampal tissues of memory deficit mice. (**A**) Superoxide dismutase (SOD)-1, and SOD-2 protein expression were evaluated via western blotting. (**B**) The protein band density was measured utilizing by the software. Protein was normalized using the GAPDH. Values are represented as means ± SEM (n = 3). ## p < 0.01 vs. Normal group; ** p < 0.01 vs. SCO-treated group.

3.7. Brainon Decreases Interleukin (IL)-1β, IL-6, and Tumor Necrosis Factor (TNF)-α mRNA Expression in SCO-Induced Hippocampal Tissue

The effects of Brainon on the expression of IL-1β, IL-6, and TNF-α mRNA in the hippocampi of SCO-treated mice were confirmed using real-time qPCR (Figure 7). SCO treatment significantly increased expression of IL-1β, IL-6, and TNF-α mRNA compared to that in the Normal group (p < 0.01). Figure 7 shows that the expression of IL-1β mRNA significantly decreased after treatment with 100 mg/kg Brainon (p < 0.01) and 50 mg/kg GBE (p < 0.01) by 30% and 18%, respectively, compared to the SCO-injected group. In comparison with the SCO-injected group, expression of IL-6 mRNA was reduced dose dependently after treatment with 30 (p < 0.05) and 100 (p < 0.01) mg/kg Brainon by 25% and 29%, respectively, and even further reduced by 35% after treatment with 50 (p < 0.01) mg/kg GBE. Treatment with 100 mg/kg Brainon (p < 0.01) and 50 mg/kg GBE (p < 0.01) considerably alleviated TNF-α mRNA expression by 22% and 28%, respectively, compared to that in the SCO-injected group.

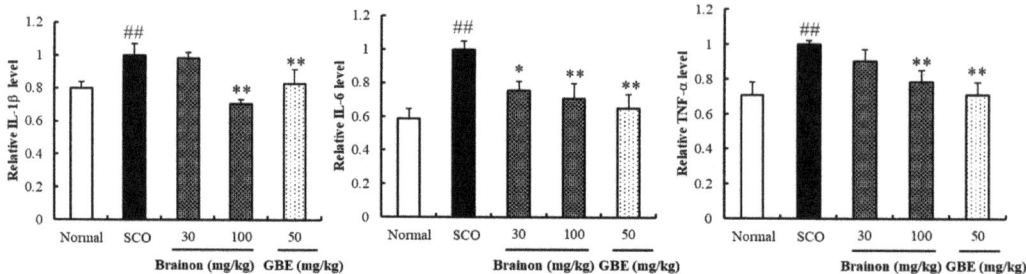

Figure 7. Effects of Brainon on anti-inflammation related mRNA expression in the memory deficit mice hippocampal tissues. Interleukin (IL)-1β, IL-6, and tumor factor necrosis (TNF)-α was evaluated by real-time qPCR. The levels of IL-1β, IL-6, and TNF-α mRNA were normalized utilizing the glyceraldehyde 3-phosphate dehydrogenase (GAPDH) as control. Values are represented as means ± SEM ($n = 3$). ## $p < 0.01$ vs. Normal group; * $p < 0.05$ and ** $p < 0.01$ vs. SCO-treated group.

3.8. Brainon Suppresses Apoptosis-Related Protein Levels in SCO-Induced Hippocampal Tissue

To demonstrate the effects of Brainon on SCO-induced apoptosis, we examined Bax, Bcl-2, cleaved caspase-9, and cleaved-PARP protein expression in the mouse hippocampus. As shown in Figure 8, SCO injection markedly upregulated protein levels of Bax, cleaved caspase-9, and cleaved-PARP comparison with that in the Normal control group. On the contrary, Bcl-2 protein levels downregulated in the SCO-treated group. Meanwhile, treatment with 30 ($p < 0.01$) and 100 mg/kg Brainon ($p < 0.01$), and 50 mg/kg GBE ($p < 0.01$) significantly prevented the SCO-caused increase in the expression of Bax and cleaved-PARP proteins. Treatment with 100 mg/kg ($p < 0.01$) Brainon also decreased the expression of cleaved-caspase 9 proteins but 50 mg/kg GBE did not reduce cleaved-caspase 9. Furthermore, treatment with 100 mg/kg Brainon ($p < 0.01$) restored the SCO-caused reduction in Bcl-2 protein expression in the hippocampi.

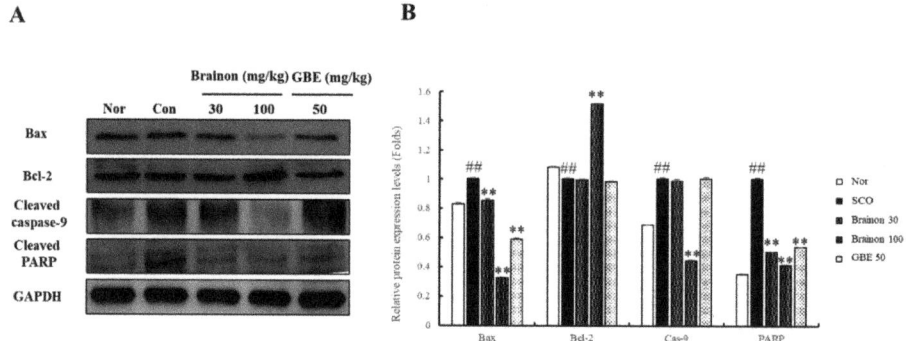

Figure 8. Effects of Brainon on cell death-related protein expression in the memory deficit mice hippocampal tissues. (**A**) Bcl-2-associated X protein (Bax), B-cell lymphoma 2 (Bcl-2), cleaved caspase-9 and cleaved poly (adenosine diphosphate (ADP)-ribose) polymerase (PARP) protein was analyzed using western blotting. (**B**) The density of the protein bands was determined utilizing the software. Protein was normalized using the GAPDH. Values are represented as means ± SEM ($n = 3$). ## $p < 0.01$ vs. Normal group; ** $p < 0.01$ vs. SCO-treated group.

4. Discussion

Dementia is a complex condition involving the disruption of cortical function along with adverse effects on memory, reasoning, orientation, learning capacity, and emotional stability. Progressive dementia is associated with AD, a prevalent neurodegenerative disorder, characterized by excessive accumulation of neuritic plaques and neuronal loss, including abnormal tau proteins and β-amyloid. A depletion of the neurotransmitter, ACh, occurs in patients with AD. Degeneration of the cholinergic neurons is also an crucial factor that contributes toward the development of dementia [15].

In this study, mice were tested to a passive avoidance test and an MWM task in a spatial memory trial to assess their learning abilities and memory deficits [6]. SCO treatment significantly decreased cognitive function as reported in a previous study [16]. However, Brainon treatment recovered the decreased step-through latency and reduced escape latency and swim distance in passive avoidance performance and MWM trials, respectively.

ACh establishes synaptic connections between neurons; it plays an important role in the CNS and is related to cognition and memory [17]. ACh is hydrolyzed by AChE. Increased ACh levels resulting from AChE inhibition enhance learning and memory by improving cholinergic deficiency [15,18]. Acting as a non-selective muscarinic cholinergic receptor antagonist, SCO causes cholinergic dysfunction that leads to impaired learning and memory. It is known that AChE inhibitors antagonize the effects of scopolamine on spatial memory in the radial arm maze [19] in the Morris Water maze and in passive avoidance tests [20,21]. This suggests a strong correlation between anti-AChE activity and the ability to oppose these amnestic effects of scopolamine [22]. We administered SCO to mice to induce cholinergic neurodegeneration alongside cognitive deficiency and confirmed the decline in ACh levels and increase in AChE activity [23]. We discovered that Brainon treatment significantly enhanced ACh levels and decreased AChE activity in the hippocampi of SCO-injected mice.

SCO-induced neurodegeneration results in a decrease in cholinergic activity and BDNF as well as the inhibition of phosphorylated CREB expression in the hippocampal tissue [4]. High BDNF expression in the CNS, particularly in the hippocampus, is a neurotrophic factor that modulates the growth and survival of neurons. BDNF enhances synaptic plasticity and regulates memory formation by increasing the activity of enzymes related to ACh synthesis [24]. CREB also leads to neuronal synaptic plasticity through the expression of downstream targets of Bcl-2 and neuroprotective effectiveness against reactive oxygen species (ROS)-caused cell toxicity [25,26]. Disturbance of phosphorylated CREB indicates neurodegenerative disorders, such as AD as well as Huntington's and Parkinson's disease [25,27]. In this study, we assessed the relevance of the CREB–BDNF signaling mechanism in AD. Brainon upregulated BDNF protein levels as well as phosphorylated CREB protein levels in the hippocampi comparison with those in the SCO-treated group.

ROS induces oxidative stress and is significant in the pathology of AD [9,28]. Excessive oxidative damage induces neuroinflammation and results in neurotoxicity, contributing to clinical symptoms of AD, including cognitive deficits [29,30] Antioxidant enzymes, such as SOD-1 and SOD-2, play a protective role against oxidative stress by catalyzing the conversion of superoxide anions to oxygen and hydrogen peroxide. Results from previous studies show that ACh exerts a neuroprotective effect against oxidative stress by increasing the expression of SOD, and that ACh levels are positively related with those of SOD [31,32]. In the present study, treatment with Brainon recovered the antioxidant defense system by increasing SOD and ACh levels in the hippocampal tissues of SCO-induced mice.

ROS-caused oxidative stress is considerably correlated with neuroinflammation, which exacerbates neurodegenerative disorders and contributes to the progression of AD. SCO administration upregulated IL-1β, IL-6, and TNF-α levels in mouse hippocampi, and these findings were consistent with the results from previous studies [33,34]. However, Brainon suppressed the SCO-induced neuroinflammatory cytokines in the SCO-treated mouse hippocampi. ROS, the primary cause of oxidative stress, is also responsible for the initiation of apoptosis. It promotes the overexpression of the proapoptotic protein, Bax, leading to cell death. The antiapoptotic protein, Bcl-2, which has effects opposite to those of Bax, is regulated by CREB. Bax upregulation and Bcl-2 downregulation promote neuronal cell death by increasing caspase activator release in the hippocampal tissue [12,35,36]. Our results suggested that SCO activated Bax, cleaved caspase-9, and cleaved-PARP, while downregulating protein expression of Bcl-2. Moreover, we found that Brainon alleviated the overexpression of Bax and the activation of cleaved caspase-9, cleaved-PARP, and on the other hand increased protein expression of Bcl-2 in SCO-treated mice.

To summarize, Brainon was found to have an anti-amnesic effect, which could be regulated by cholinergic activity and the CREB-BDNF signaling pathway, and by virtue of its antioxidant, anti-inflammation, and anti-apoptotic properties.

5. Conclusions

In this study, we proved that Brainon effectively restored memory in the SCO-induced mouse model by improving the function of the cholinergic system and CREB-BDNF pathway. Brainon exerted antioxidant effects by inhibiting ROS generation and upregulating the SOD proteins. Decreased ROS levels by Brainon treatment resulted in anti-inflammatory effects by the downregulation of IL-1β, IL-6, and TNF-α, as well as anti-apoptotic effects with decreased protein levels of Bax, cleaved caspase-9, and cleaved-PARP. This study indicated that Brainon is a potential treatment option for patients with neurodegenerative diseases. Moreover, it could potentially be developed as a safe healthcare supplement to improve cognitive disorder and reverse memory loss.

Author Contributions: H.-J.L. performed the experiments and participated in the writing and interpretation of the manuscript. H.-L.K. and D.-Y.L. conducted the data analysis and quality control assessment respectively. D.-R.L. and B.-K.C. conceptualization and discussed the conclusion and edited the manuscript. S.-H.Y. planned and led the project, and contributed the data review, editing and manuscript finalization. All authors have read and agreed to the published version of the manuscript.

Funding: This study was carried out with the support of the 'Cooperative Research Program for Agriculture Science and Technology Development (Project No. PJ013215012020)' Rural Development Administration, Republic of Korea.

Institutional Review Board Statement: The study was conducted according to the guidelines and approved by the Institutional Animal Care and Use committee of ChemOn Inc. (YoungIn, Korea) (Permission number: 2019-05-003).

Informed Consent Statement: Not applicable.

Data Availability Statement: Not applicable.

Acknowledgments: Not applicable.

Conflicts of Interest: Author D.-R.L. is director of research institute of Nutrapharm Tech Co., Ltd. Author B.-K.C. is chief executive officer of Nutrapharm Tech Co., Ltd. The authors declare no conflict of interest.

References

1. Demirci, K.; Nazıroğlu, M.; Övey, İ.S.; Balaban, H. Selenium attenuates apoptosis, inflammation and oxidative stress in the blood and brain of aged rats with scopolamine-induced dementia. *Metab. Brain Dis.* **2017**, *32*, 321–329. [CrossRef] [PubMed]
2. El-Amarasy, S.A.; Abd-Elsalam, R.M.; Ahmed-Farid, O.A. Ameliorative Effect of Silymarin on Scopolamine-induced Dementia in Rats. *Open Access Maced. J. Med. Sci.* **2018**, *17*, 1215–1224. [CrossRef]
3. Lee, B.; Sur, B.; Shim, I.; Lee, H.; Hahm, D.H. Phellodendron amurense and Its Major Alkaloid Compound, Berberine Ameliorates Scopolamine-Induced Neuronal Impairment and Memory Dysfunction in Rats. *Korean J. Physiol. Pharmacol.* **2012**, *16*, 79–89. [CrossRef]
4. Lee, B.; Sur, B.; Shim, J.; Hahm, D.H.; Lee, H. Acupuncture stimulation improves scopolamine-induced cognitive impairment via activation of cholinergic system and regulation of BDNF and CREB expression in rats. *BMC Complement. Altern. Med.* **2014**, *14*, 338. [CrossRef] [PubMed]
5. Lee, B.; Sur, B.; Park, J.; Shin, H.; Kwon, S.; Yeom, M.; Kim, S.J.; Shim, I.; Yin, C.S.; Lee, H.; et al. Fucoidan Ameliorates Scopolamine-induced Neuronal Impairment and Memory Dysfunction in Rats via Activation of Cholinergic System and Regulation of cAMP-response Element-binding Protein and Brain-derived Neurotrophic Factor Expressions. *J. Korean Soc. Appl. Biol. Chem.* **2012**, *55*, 711–720. [CrossRef]
6. Shabani, S.; Mirshekar, M.A. Diosmin is neuroprotective in a rat model of scopolamine-induced cognitive impairment. *Biomed. Pharmacother.* **2018**, *108*, 1376–1383. [CrossRef]

8. Lee, J.S.; Kim, H.G.; Lee, H.W.; Han, J.M.; Lee, S.K.; Kim, D.W.; Saravanakumar, A.; Son, C.G. Hippocampal memory enhancing activity of pine needle extract against scopolamine-induced amnesia in a mouse model. *Sci. Rep.* **2015**, *5*, 9651. [CrossRef]
9. Karthivashan, G.; Park, S.Y.; Kweon, M.H.; Kim, J.; Haque, M.E.; Cho, D.Y.; Kim, I.S.; Cho, E.A.; Ganesan, P.; Choi, D.K. Ameliorative potential of desalted *Salicornia europaea* L. extract in multifaceted Alzheimer's-like scopolamine-induced amnesic mice model. *Sci. Rep.* **2018**, *8*, 7174. [CrossRef]
10. Budzynska, B.; Czubara, A.B.; Slomka, M.K.; Wozniak, K.S.; Michalak, A.; Musik, I.; Biala, G. Effects of imperatorin on scopolamine-induced cognitive impairment and oxidative stress in mice. *Psychopharmacology* **2015**, *232*, 931–942. [CrossRef]
11. Kim, J.K.; Kim, Y.H.; Lee, H.H.; Lim, S.S.; Park, K.W. Effect of *Scrophularia buergeriana* Extract on the Degranulation of Mast Cells and Ear Swelling Induced by Dinitrofluorobenzene in Mice. *Inflammation* **2011**, *35*, 183–191. [CrossRef]
12. Lee, H.J.; Spandidos, D.A.; Tsatsakis, A.; Margina, D.; Izotov, B.N.; Yang, S.H. Neuroprotective effects of *Scrophularia buergeriana* extract against glutamate-induced toxicity in SH-SY5Y cells. *Int. J. Mol. Med.* **2019**, *43*, 2144–2152. [CrossRef] [PubMed]
13. Lee, H.J.; Lee, D.Y.; Kim, H.L.; Yang, S.H. *Scrophularia buergeriana* Extract Improves Memory Impairment via Inhibition of the Apoptosis Pathway in the Mouse Hippocampus. *Appl. Sci.* **2020**, *10*, 7987. [CrossRef]
14. DeFeudis, F.V.; Drieu, K. "Stress-alleviating" and "vigilance-enhancing" actions of *Ginkgo biloba* extract (EGb 761). *Drug Dev. Res.* **2004**, *62*, 1–25. [CrossRef]
15. Tang, F.; Nag, S.; Shiu, S.Y.W.; Pang, S.F. The effects of melatonin and *Ginkgo biloba* extract on memory loss and choline acetyltransferase activities in the brain of rats infused intracerebroventricularly with β-amyloid 1–40. *Life Sci.* **2002**, *71*, 2625–2631. [CrossRef]
16. Puri, A.; Srivastava, P.; Pandey, P.; Yadav, R.S.; Bhatt, P.C. Scopolamine induced behavioral and biochemical modifications and protective effect of *Celastrus paniculatous* and *Angelica glauca* in rats. *Int. J. Nutr. Pharmacol. Neurol. Dis.* **2014**, *4*, 158–163. [CrossRef]
17. Ko, Y.H.; Kwon, S.H.; Lee, S.Y.; Jang, C.G. Isoorientin improves scopolamine-induced cognitive impairments by restoring the cholinergic system, antioxidant defense, and p-CREB/BDNF signaling in the hippocampus and frontal cortex. *Arch. Pharm. Res.* **2019**, *42*, 722–731. [CrossRef]
18. Lian, W.; Fang, J.; Xu, L.; Zhou, W.; Kang, D.; Xiong, W.; Jia, H.; Liu, A.L.; Du, G.H. DL0410 Ameliorates Memory and Cognitive Impairments Induced by Scopolamine via Increasing Cholinergic Neurotransmission in Mice. *Molecules* **2017**, *22*, 410. [CrossRef]
19. Kim, D.E.; Han, D.Y.; Kim, S.H.; Chung, D.K. Anti-amnesic and Antioxidant Effect of Yeongkyekamjotanggayonggolmoryo Aqueous Extracts on Scopolamine-induced Memory Impairment in Mice. *J. Orient. Neuropsychiatry* **2018**, *29*, 121–134. [CrossRef]
20. Braida, D.; Paladini, E.; Griffini, P.; Lamperti, M.; Maggi, A.; Sala, M. An inverted U-shaped curve for heptylphysostigmine on radial maze performance in rats: Comparison with other cholinesterase inhibitors. *Eur. J. Pharmacol.* **1996**, *302*, 13–20. [CrossRef]
21. Bejar, C.; Wang, R.H.; Weinstock, M. Effect of rivastigmine on scopolamine-induced memory impairment in rats. *Eur. J. Pharmacol.* **1999**, *383*, 231–240. [CrossRef]
22. Dawson, G.R.; Bentley, G.; Draper, F.; Rycroft, W.; Iversen, S.D.; Pagella, P.G. The behavioral effects of heptyl physostigmine, a new cholinesterase inhibitor, in tests of long-term and working memory in rodents. *Pharmacol. Biochem. Behav.* **1991**, *39*, 865–871. [CrossRef]
23. Kang, S.Y.; Lee, K.Y.; Park, M.J.; Kim, Y.C.; Markelonis, G.J.; Oh, T.H.; Kim, Y.C. Decursin from Angelica gigas mitigates amnesia induced by scopolamine in mice. *Neurobiol. Learn. Mem.* **2003**, *79*, 11–18. [CrossRef]
24. Bhuvanendran, S.; Kumari, Y.; Othman, I.; Shaikh, M.F. Amelioration of Cognitive Deficit by Embelin in a Scopolamine-Induced Alzheimer's Disease-Like Condition in a Rat Model. *Front. Pharmacol.* **2018**, *25*, 665. [CrossRef] [PubMed]
25. Jegal, K.H.; Park, S.J.; Kim, C.Y.; Park, J.H.; Jang, J.H. Effect of Poria Cocos on the Scopolamine-induced Memory Impairment and Its Underlying Molecular Mechanism. *Korean J. Orient. Physiol. Pathol.* **2010**, *24*, 228–235.
26. Mantamadiotis, T.; Lemberger, T.; Bleckmann, S.C.; Kern, B.; Kretz, O.; Villabla, A.M.; Tronche, F.; Kellendonk, C.; Gau, D.; Kapfhammer, J.; et al. Disruption of CREB function in brain leads to neurodegeneration. *Nat. Genet.* **2002**, *31*, 47–54. [CrossRef] [PubMed]
27. Li, Q.; Zhao, H.F.; Zhang, Z.F.; Liu, Z.G.; Pei, X.R.; Wang, J.B.; Cai, M.Y.; Li, Y. Long-term administration of green tea catechins prevents age-related spatial learning and memory decline in C57BL/6J mice by regulating hippocampal cyclic amp-response element binding protein signaling cascade. *Neuroscience* **2009**, *159*, 1208–1215. [CrossRef] [PubMed]
28. Ravichandran, V.A.; Kim, M.; Han, S.K.; Cha, Y.S. *Stachys sieboldii* Extract Supplementation Attenuates Memory Deficits by Modulating BDNF-CREB and Its Downstream Molecules, in Animal Models of Memory Impairment. *Nutrients* **2018**, *10*, 917. [CrossRef]
29. Akesenov, M.Y.; Markesbery, W.R. Changes in thiol content and expression of glutathione redox system genes in the hippocampus and cerebellum in Alzheimer's disease. *Neurosci. Lett.* **2001**, *302*, 141–145. [CrossRef]
30. Bartus, R.T. On neurodegenerative diseases, models, and treatment strategies: Lessons learned and lessons forgotten a generation following the cholinergic hypothesis. *Exp. Neurol.* **2000**, *163*, 495–529. [CrossRef]
31. Bonda, D.J.; Wang, X.; Perry, G.; Nunomura, A.; Tabaton, M.; Zhu, X.; Smith, M.A. Oxidative stress in Alzheimer's disease: A possibility for prevention. *Neuropharmacology* **2010**, *59*, 290–294. [CrossRef]
32. Zhang, W.; Bai, M.; Hao, J.H.; Mao, N.; Su, C.; Miao, J.; Li, Z. Early memory deficits precede plaque deposition in APPswe/Ps1dE9 mice: Involvement of oxidative stress and cholinergic dysfunction. *Free Radic. Biol. Med.* **2012**, *52*, 1443–1452. [CrossRef] [PubMed]

32. Frinchi, M.; Nuzzo, D.; Scaduto, P.; Carlo, M.D.; Massenti, M.F.; Belluardo, N.; Mudò, G. Anti-inflammatory and antioxidant effects of muscarinic acetylcholine receptor (mAChR) activation in the rat hippocampus. *Sci. Rep.* **2019**, *9*, 14233. [CrossRef]
33. Guo, C.; Shen, J.; Meng, Z.; Yang, X.; Li, E. Neuroprotective effects of polygalacic acid on scopolamine-induced memory deficits in mice. *Phytomedicine* **2016**, *23*, 149–155. [CrossRef] [PubMed]
34. Iqbal, S.; Shah, F.A.; Naeem, K.; Nadeem, H.; Sarwar, S.; Ashraf, Z.; Imran, M.; Khan, T.; Anwar, Y.; Li, S. Succinamide Derivatives Ameliorate Neuroinflammation and Oxidative Stress in Scopolamine-Induced Neurodegeneration. *Biomolecules* **2020**, *10*, 443. [CrossRef] [PubMed]
35. Muhammad, T.; Ali, T.; Ikram, M.; Khan, A.; Alam, S.I.; Kim, M.O. Melatonin Rescue Oxidative Stress-Mediated Neuroinflammation/Neurodegeneration and Memory Impairment in Scopolamine-Induced Amnesia Mice Model. *J. Neuroimmune Pharmacol* **2019**, *14*, 278–294. [CrossRef]
36. Puangmalai, N.; Thangnipon, W.; Ampornkul, R.S.; Suwanna, N.; Tuchinda, P.; Nobathian, S. Neuroprotection of N-benzylcinnamide on scopolamine-induced cholinergic dysfunction in human SH-SY5Y neuroblastoma cells. *Neural Regen. Res* **2017**, *12*, 1492–1498. [CrossRef]

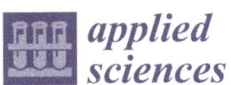

Article

Anti-Osteoarthritic Effects of *Terminalia Chebula* Fruit Extract (AyuFlex®) in Interleukin-1β-Induced Human Chondrocytes and in Rat Models of Monosodium Iodoacetate (MIA)-Induced Osteoarthritis

Hae Lim Kim [1], Hae Jin Lee [1], Dong-Ryung Lee [2], Bong-Keun Choi [2] and Seung Hwan Yang [1,*]

[1] Department of Biotechnology, Chonnam National University, Yeosu 59626, Korea; ics1357@naver.com (H.L.K.); haecutejin@naver.com (H.J.L.)
[2] NUON Co., Ltd., Jungwon-gu, Seongnam, Gyunggi 13201, Korea; drlee@nuon.kr (D.-R.L.); cbcbcbk@nuon.kr (B.-K.C.)
* Correspondence: ymichigan@jnu.ac.kr; Tel.: +82-61-659-7306

Received: 21 November 2020; Accepted: 2 December 2020; Published: 4 December 2020

Abstract: Osteoarthritis (OA) is a general joint illness caused by the destruction of joint cartilage, and is common in the population of old people. Its occurrence is related to inflammatory reactions and cartilage degradation. AyuFlex® is an aqueous extract of *Terminalia chebula* fruit, and *T. chebula* has been utilized extensively in several traditional oriental medications for the management of diverse diseases. Pre-clinical and clinical research has shown its antioxidant and anti-inflammatory effectiveness. Nevertheless, the mechanism underlying the anti-arthritic effects of AyuFlex® remains unclear. In the current research, we proposed the ameliorating effects of AyuFlex® with respect to the incidence of OA and described the latent signalization in interleukin (IL)-1β-treated chondrocytes and MIA-incurred OA in a rat model. *In vitro*, AyuFlex® decreased oxidative stress and induction of pro-inflammatory cytokines and mediators as well as matrix metalloproteinases (MMPs), while also increasing the levels of collagen synthesis-related proteins. Mechanistically, we identified that AyuFlex® disrupted nuclear factor kappa B (NF-κB) and mitogen-activated protein kinase (MAPK) activation via the inhibition of NF-κB p65 and extracellular regulated protein kinase (ERK) phosphorylation. The ameliorating effects of AyuFlex® were also observed in vivo. AyuFlex® significantly inhibited the MIA-incurred increase in OA symptoms such as oxidative stress, cartilage damage, and changes in cytokines and MMPs revelation in arthrodial cartilage. Therefore, our results suggest that AyuFlex® attenuates OA progression in vivo, indicating that AyuFlex® can be suggested as an excellent therapeutic remedy for the care of OA.

Keywords: *Terminalia chebula* fruit; osteoarthritis; AyuFlex®; cartilage collapse; MMPs; inflammation response

1. Introduction

Osteoarthritis (OA) is a lingering joint illness accompanied by inflammation of the synovium and cartilage degeneration, causing physical disability in the elderly. Functional foods and medicines have been commonly utilized to care for OA, but pharmacological treatment of OA has limited effects [1,2]. Non-steroidal anti-inflammatory drugs (NSAIDs) are usually utilized for reducing inflammation and pain in OA. However, a long-time consumption of NSAIDs adversely affects the gastrointestinal and cardiovascular systems [3,4]. To this day, the etiology of OA is not obvious, and no effectual therapeutic treatment has been developed for OA. Therefore, safer and more effective novel agents are needed for the treatment of OA [1].

The extracellular matrix (ECM) is mostly an organization of type I and II collagen, and aggrecan, which are the main constituents of ordinary cartilage that support the arthrodial cartilage to adapt to biomechanical forces during joint activity [5]. ECM is created and retained by the chondrocytes and is controlled by SOX9, which encodes the main transcription factor for ECM homeostasis [6,7]. Many studies have shown that inflammatory reactions generally play an enormous role in the OA and contributes to chondrocyte movement and phenotype and ECM degradation [7–9]. Overexpression of pro-inflammatory cytokines like IL-1β and IL-6 are implicated in the etiology of OA by upregulating the matrix metalloproteinases (MMPs) and triggering ECM collapse. In particular, IL-1β exerts inflammatory reactions by considerably upregulating the production of pro-inflammatory factors, and catabolic factors, for example, leukotriene B_4 (LTB_4), nitric oxide (NO), and MMPs to degrade the ECM [10–12].

MAPK mechanisms have been revealed to play an apparent part in terms of OA biology such as matrix composition and homeostasis of cartilage [13,14]. Additionally, NF-κB mechanisms are a core controller of pro-inflammatory and catabolic factor production. When the NF-κB mechanisms are activated, NF-κB p65 is phosphorylated in the cytoplasm and ultimately translocated to the nucleus [15,16]. Practically, transitions in these mechanisms have been identified to play a crucial role in articular chondrocyte function as well as form part of OA etiology and illness progression [17].

The fruit of *Terminalia chebula* Retz. (Fam. Combretaceae) has been widely utilized in Ayurvedic, Iranian medicine, and Unani as a treatment for diverse diseases such as asthma, bleeding piles, sore throat, vomiting, and gout [18–20]. Moreover, *T. chebula* has been widely known to exhibit antioxidant effects by inhibiting ROS and NO production [21–24]. Clinical research has also proven that oxidative stress and inflammation contribute to OA, low back pain (LBP), and motor-related joint discomfort. The *T. chebula* fruit exhibits antioxidant efficacy and downregulates inflammatory cytokines; however, its therapeutic effects warrant further investigation [25–29].

Meanwhile, recent preclinical and clinical studies have revealed that the standardized aqueous extract of *T. chebula* fruit (AyuFlex®) could markedly suppress OA progression [25,30–35]. However, the underlying mechanism, the anti-arthritic effect of AyuFlex®, remains obscure. Therefore, in our study, we devised experiments to clarify the effectiveness and applications of AyuFlex®, and to evaluate the protective effectiveness of arthrodial cartilage in IL-1β-treated chondrocytes and MIA-incurred OA in a rat model.

2. Materials and Methods

2.1. AyuFlex® Preparation and Component Analyze

AyuFlex®, a water-soluble product derived from the edible fruits of *T. chebula* (Natreon Inc., New Brunswick, NJ, USA) [35], presents a phytochemical profile that includes ellagic acid as standardized using high-performance liquid chromatography (HPLC). Dimethyl sulfoxide (DMSO) was utilized to dissolve the AyuFlex® and was then diluted in chondrocyte culture medium for in vitro studies.

2.2. Culture and Sample Processing of Primary Human Chondrocytes (HCHs)

Primary human chondrocytes (HCHs) were provided by PromoCell Bioscience Alive GmbH (Heidelberg, Germany) and also retained in HCH culture medium complemented with fetal calf (FC) serum in CO_2 incubator. When 80–90% confluence was reached, HCHs were subcultured, and cells of passage 1 were utilized for the experiment thereafter. HCHs was cultured in a 6-well plate at 1×10^5 cells per well. After 24 h, the HCH cells were exposed at each concentration of AyuFlex® (5, 10, and 20 μg/mL) and in combination with IL-1β (10 ng/mL) in a humidified incubator for 24 h. HCHs exposed with growth media including only DMSO served as the vehicle control (final concentration of DMSO 0.1%).

2.3. Cell Viability Analysis

Cell viability was conducted utilizing the 3-(4, 5-dimethylthiazol-2-yl)-2, 5-diphenyl tetrazolium bromide (MTT) assay. HCHs were exposed with each concentration of AyuFlex® (5, 10, and 20 µg/mL) during 24 h. The MTT reagent (5 mg/mL) was dispensed into each well, and the cells were maintained in a humidified incubator for 3 h. The culture supernatants were suctioned from each well, and DMSO was utilized to melt the formazan crystals. The optical density (OD) was analyzed at a wavelength of 570 nm utilizing microplate reader equipment (Tecan, Mannedorf, Switzerland).

2.4. Western Blotting

After lysing HCHs with CelLytic reagent (Sigma-Aldrich, St. Louis, MO, USA), the lysates were kept at 4 °C and centrifuged at 10,000× g for 15 min. The content of the proteins was calculated by utilizing a Bradford reagent (Bio-Rad Laboratories, Hercules, CA, USA). To separate, the proteins were applied by sodium dodecyl sulfate-polyacrylamide gel electrophoresis (SDS-PAGE) on 10% gels and then blotted to Immobilon-P membranes (Millipore, Bedford, MA, USA). The membranes were blocked with 5% skim milk in tris-buffered saline comprising 0.1% Tween-20 (TBS-T) for 1 h at 23 °C, and next with primary antibodies for β-actin, COL1A1, NF-κB p65, phospho-NF-κB p65, ERK, phospho-ERK (1:1000; Cell Signaling Technology, Inc., Danvers, MA, USA), 5-LOX, IL-6, MMP-2, -3, and -13, aggrecan (1:1000; Abcam, Cambridge, MA, USA), SOX9, COL2A1 (1:500; Santa Cruz Biotechnology, Santa Cruz, CA, USA), iNOS (1:1000; Invitrogen Life Technologies, Carlsbad, CA, USA), and leukotriene B_4 (LTB_4; 1:500; Enzo Life Sciences, Farmingdale, NY, USA) overnight at 4 °C. Following incubation with primary antibodies, the membranes were reacted with the goat anti-rabbit or -mouse IgG(H+L)-horseradish peroxidase (HRP) secondary antibodies for 1 h at room temperature (RT). Protein bands were detected with the chemiluminescent (ECL) reagent (GenDEPOT, Barker, TX, USA), and the intensity of bands was sensed utilizing a LuminoGraph chemiluminescent imaging instrument (Atto, Tokyo, Japan). As control for normalization, β-actin was utilized. Bands on the membranes were quantified utilizing the ImageJ program (developed at the NIH).

2.5. Animals

Sixty male Sprague-Dawley (SD) rats (6-week-old; 130-190 g) were offered from Samtako Bio, Inc. (Osan, Korea). Whole animals were acclimated for seven days and normal animals were sorted out for experiments. The experiment was progressed under optimal conditions (22 ± 2 °C and 12 h light/dark cycles). Animals were free to consume sterile water and food. The study was conducted in compliance following the national guidelines for the management and utilization of experimental animals permitted by the Animal Ethics Committee (permission number: IV-RB-02-1910-21 of INVIVO Co. Ltd. (Chungnam, Korea)). Once a week, alterations in body weight and alterations in water and food consumption were observed.

2.6. Monosodium iodoacetate (MIA)-Incurred Osteoarthritis (OA) and Drug Administration

The left knee was shaved and then 50 µL of 0.9% sodium chloride including 3 mg monosodium iodoacetate (MIA) was injected once into the synovial cavity utilizing an insulin syringe to induce OA. After three days, the rats were randomly arranged to six groups, comprising eight rats each. A non-MIA-stimulated control group was also used: (1) Non-MIA-stimulated control + Vehicle; (2) MIA-stimulated control + Vehicle; (3) MIA + AyuFlex® 25 mg/kg; (4) MIA + AyuFlex® 50 mg/kg; (5) MIA + AyuFlex® 100 mg/kg; and (6) MIA + Ibuprofen 20 mg/kg. The test substances were homogenized in a carboxymethyl cellulose sodium salt (CMC-Na) of 0.5%. Then, the test substances were administrated orally once a day for three weeks.

2.7. Progression of OA and Hind Paw Weight-Bearing Distribution

After 0, 7, 14, and 21 days after treatment of the test substances, the whole rats were left free to roam the cage, and the walking and knee joint swelling aspect, for instance, gait disorder was precisely assessed in rats. Limping and swelling were categorized as: No change (0), Mild swelling (1), Moderate swelling (2), and Severe swelling (3). All evaluations were performed by an identical proficient evaluator, who blinded the type of test substance administered to the rats during the study period.

The normal balance of weight bearing capacity in the hind paws was impaired after OA occurrence. Rats were cautiously located in the measurement chamber of the incapacitance meter tester (IITC Life Science, Woodland Hills, CA, USA) to assess alterations in weight-bearing tolerance and the force applied by each hind limb was averaged for 10 s. The following formula: % weight distribution of left hind paw = weight on left hind limb/(weight on right hind limb + weight on left hind limb) × 100 was used to analyze the percentage distribution of the left hind paw.

2.8. Histological Examination of Joints

To determine the effectiveness of AyuFlex® on knee joint cartilage atrophy, we evaluated the histological alteration in a rat model with MIA-incurred OA. After euthanizing the animals at the end of the experiments, the knee joint was incised, fixed with 10% formalin for 24 h at 4 °C, and decalcified using 5% hydrochloric acid (Sigma-Aldrich, St. Louis, MO, USA) for four days. After removal of calcification, acetone was utilized to dehydrate the specimens, which were then embedded in paraffin. Paraffin-embedded knee joints were sliced 5 μm thick along the sagittal axis. Hematoxylin and Eosin (H&E) and Safranin-O fast green staining (Sigma-Aldrich, St. Louis, MO, USA) were utilized to stain the sliced sections. Whole stained sections were scanned utilizing the Motic EasyScan (Meyer Instrument, Houston, TX, USA) and were assessed and graded on a 0-13 scale depending on the Mankin scoring system by a double-blinded observer.

2.9. Cartilage Protein Expression

Cartilage tissue was excised and cleaned three times in cold PBS. Cartilage was frozen by liquid nitrogen briefly and then pulverized. Protein was extracted with RIPA reagent (Tris-HCl of 50 mM, pH 7.5; sodium chloride (NaCl) of 150 mM; ethylenediaminetetraacetic acid (EDTA) of 2 mM; Triton X-100 of 1%; sodium deoxycholate of 0.5%; SDS of 0.1%; protease inhibitor of 0.1% (Roche, Mannheim, Germany)) and then centrifuged at 10,000× g during 15 min at 4 °C. Protein concentration was calculated by the same method as described above. The protein expression profiles of β-actin, 5-LOX, LTB$_4$, IL-6, MMP-2, -3, and -13, iNOS, SOX9, aggrecan, COL1A1, and COL2A1 were confirmed by western blotting as described above.

2.10. Statistical Analysis

The results are presented as the means ± standard error of the mean (SEM) and were assessed with the SPSS program (version 22.0, SPSS Inc., Chicago, IL, USA). Student's t-test and one-way analysis of variance (ANOVA) were utilized to compare different treatment groups, followed by multiple comparisons correction through Dunnett's post-hoc test utilizing Origin 7.0 software (OriginLab, Northampton, MA, USA). The differences between mean values were regarded significant or intensely significant if $p < 0.05$ and $p < 0.01$, respectively.

3. Results

3.1. Effects of AyuFlex® on Cell Viability in Primary Human Chondrocytes (HCHs)

The influence of AyuFlex® on the cell viability of HCHs was confirmed by using the MTT analysis. AyuFlex® did not show cytotoxicity at any of the concentrations (5, 10, and 20 μg/mL) investigated in this study (Figure 1).

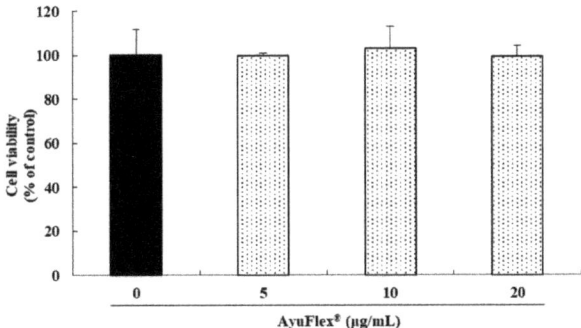

Figure 1. Effects of AyuFlex® on cell viability in primary human chondrocytes (HCHs). HCHs were treated with each concentration of AyuFlex® (5, 10, and 20 µg/mL) for 24 h. Cell viability was evaluated utilizing the 3-(4, 5-dimethylthiazol-2-yl)-2, 5-diphenyl tetrazolium bromide (MTT) assay.

3.2. AyuFlex® Repressed the Expression of iNOS, 5-LOX, LTB$_4$, and IL-6 in IL-1β-Treated HCHs

To confirm the anti-inflammatory effects of AyuFlex®, HCHs were simultaneously treated with each concentration of AyuFlex® (5, 10, and 20 µg/mL) and IL-1β (10 ng/mL) for 24 h. The protein presenting of iNOS, 5-LOX, LTB$_4$, and IL-6 was investigated by western blotting. IL-1β was revealed to significantly induce the protein expression of iNOS, 5-LOX, LTB$_4$, and IL-6 against the vehicle control. In contrast, the expression of iNOS, 5-LOX, LTB$_4$, and IL-6 in HCHs treated with a combination of AyuFlex® and IL-1β decreased in the range of 14–46% ($p < 0.01$), 20–26% ($p < 0.01$), 44–58% ($p < 0.01$), and 58–74% ($p < 0.01$), respectively (Figure 2).

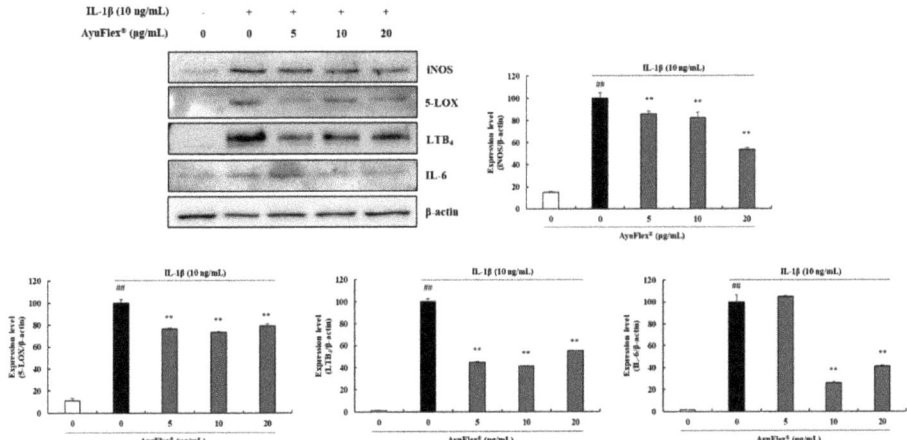

Figure 2. AyuFlex® repressed the expression of iNOS, 5-LOX, LTB$_4$, and IL-6 in IL-1β-treated HCHs. HCHs were treated with IL-1β (10 ng/mL) single or in combination with AyuFlex® (5, 10, and 20 µg/mL) for 24 h. Effects of AyuFlex® on the expression of iNOS (135 kDa), 5-LOX (78 kDa), LTB$_4$ (36 kDa), and IL-6 (25 kDa) in IL-1β-treated HCHs were analyzed. Protein bands were quantified utilizing ImageJ. As a control for normalization, β-actin was utilized. ## $p < 0.01$, in comparison with the vehicle control group. ** $p < 0.01$, in comparison with the IL-1β-treated control group.

3.3. AyuFlex® Diminished the Production of MMP-2, -3, and -13 in IL-1β-Treated HCHs

As MMPs play major roles in cartilage destruction, we appraised the effects of AyuFlex® on MMP-2, -3, and -13 expression in IL-1β-treated HCHs by western blot analysis. Our results revealed that IL-1β considerably upregulated the expression of MMP-2, -3, and -13 contrasted with that in the untreated- and vehicle control treated-HCHs. Treatment of HCHs with a combination of AyuFlex® and IL-1β considerably reduced the protein expression of MMP-2, -3, and -13 in the range of 20–43% ($p < 0.01$), 39–72% ($p < 0.01$), and 38–77% ($p < 0.01$), respectively (Figure 3).

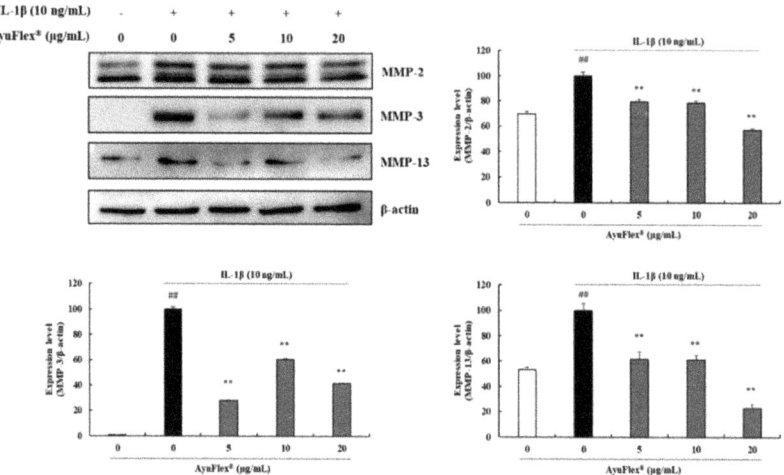

Figure 3. AyuFlex® diminished the production of MMP-2, -3, and -13 in IL-1β-treated HCHs. HCHs were treated with IL-1β (10 ng/mL) single or in combination with AyuFlex® (5, 10, and 20 μg/mL) for 24 h. The expression of MMP-2 (62, 72 kDa), MMP-3 (54 kDa), and MMP-13 (54 kDa) was detected by western blot analysis. Protein bands were quantified utilizing ImageJ. As the control for normalization, β-actin was utilized. ## $p < 0.01$, in comparison with the vehicle control group. ** $p < 0.01$, in comparison with the IL-1β-treated control group.

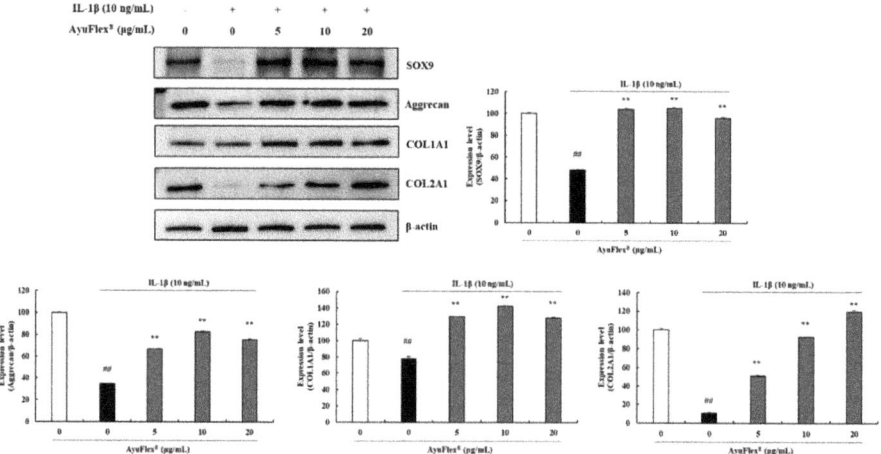

Figure 4. AyuFlex® treatment attenuated the degradation of collagen synthesis-involved proteins in IL-1β-treated HCHs. HCHs were exposed with IL-1β (10 ng/mL) single or in combination with AyuFlex® (5, 10, and 20 μg/mL) for 24 h. The expression of SOX9 (65 kDa), aggrecan (110 kDa), COL1A1 (220 kDa), and COL2A1 (190 kDa) was determined by western blotting. Protein bands were quantified utilizing ImageJ. As the control for normalization, β-actin was utilized. ## $p < 0.01$, in comparison with the vehicle control group. ** $p < 0.01$, in comparison with the IL-1β-treated control group.

3.4. AyuFlex® Treatment Attenuated the Degradation of Collagen Synthesis-Involved Proteins in IL-1β-Treated HCHs

The effects of AyuFlex® on the expression of collagen synthesis-involved proteins in IL-1β-treated HCHs was investigated using western blotting. The protein levels of SOX9, aggrecan, COL1A1, and COL2A1 were assessed. As shown in Figure 4, IL-1β significantly reduced SOX9, aggrecan, COL1A1, and COL2A1 expression in contrast with that in the vehicle control. As shown in Figure 4, AyuFlex® treatment considerably upregulated the expression of SOX9, aggrecan, COL1A1, and COL2A1 compared to that in IL-1β-stimulated HCHs. Treatment with AyuFlex® (5, 10, and 20 μg/mL) increased SOX9, aggrecan, COL1A1, and COL2A1 expression compared with that in the IL-1β-stimulated HCHs (1.9–2.1-fold, $p < 0.01$; 1.9–2.3-fold, $p < 0.01$; 1.6–1.8-fold, $p < 0.01$; 4.7–11.1-fold, $p < 0.01$, respectively).

3.5. Effects of AyuFlex® on the NF-κB and MAPK Mechanisms in IL-1β-Treated HCHs

The impacts of AyuFlex® on IL-1β-triggered NF-κB and MAPK activation was confirmed with western blotting. In Figure 5A,B, it was confirmed that IL-1β conspicuously triggered phosphorylation of NF-κB p65 and ERK. In contrast, treatment with AyuFlex® alleviated this IL-1β-induced phosphorylation of NF-κB p65 and ERK in HCHs (42–49% and 53–63%, respectively), without affecting the total form of NF-κB p65 and ERK expression.

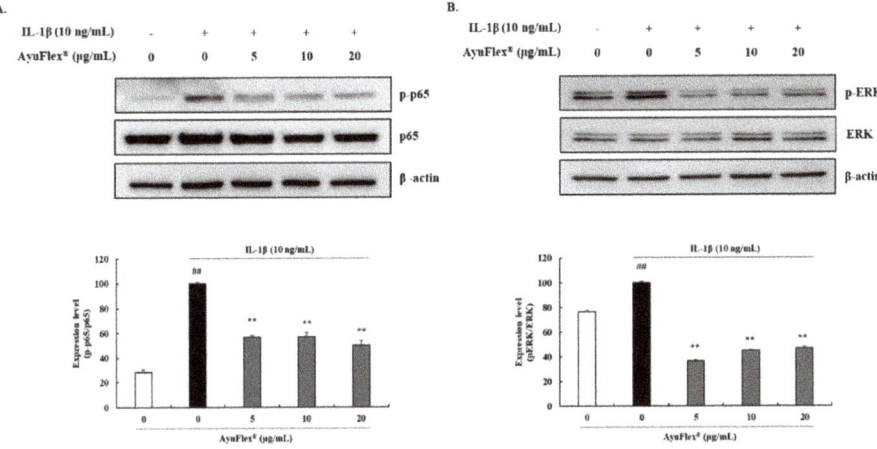

Figure 5. Effects of AyuFlex® on the NF-κB and MAPK mechanisms in IL-1β-treated HCHs. HCHs were pretreated with AyuFlex® (5, 10, and 20 μg/mL) for 24 h and then incubated with IL-1β (10 ng/mL) for 30 min. (**A**) The expression of NF-κB p65 (65 kDa) and phospho-NF-κB p65 (65 kDa) was examined with western blotting. (**B**) The expression of ERK (42, 44 kDa) and phospho-ERK (42, 44 kDa) was determined by western blotting. Western blot bands were quantified utilizing ImageJ. As the control for normalization, β-actin was utilized. ## $p < 0.01$, in comparison with the vehicle control group. ** $p < 0.01$, in comparison with the IL-1β-treated control group.

3.6. Effects of AyuFlex® on Changes in the Body Weight of Rats with Monosodium Iodoacetate (MIA)-Incurred Osteoarthritis (OA)

The effects of AyuFlex® on body weight in rats with MIA-incurred OA was investigated. The body weight of all animals was measured once a week and the changes were recorded for three weeks. No significant differences were observed between the six groups (Figure 6) for three weeks, and these results demonstrated that the body weight was not influenced by AyuFlex®.

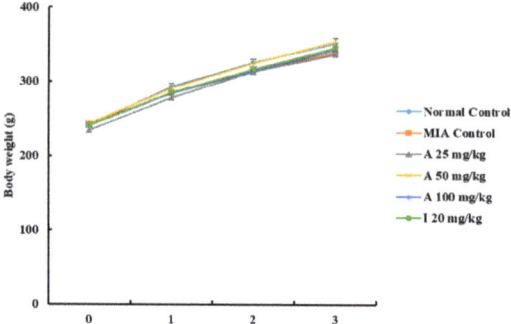

Figure 6. Effects of AyuFlex® on changes in body weight of rats with monosodium iodoacetate (MIA)-incurred osteoarthritis (OA). Body weight was evaluated once a week for three weeks and the data are presented as the mean ± SEM (n = 8/group). A, AyuFlex®; I, Ibuprofen. No significant difference was discovered between any of the groups.

3.7. Effects of AyuFlex® on Weight-Bearing Distribution in the Hind Paw for 21 Days in MIA-Incurred OA in Rats

To confirm progression of OA, hind paw weight-bearing capabilities and the ratio of weight distribution between the right (healthy) and left (MIA-incurred osteoarthritis) limbs was confirmed utilizing an incapacitance meter tester at days 0, 7, 14, and 21. The ratio in the MIA control group on day 7 was obviously lower than that in the normal control group, and this difference was endured until day 21. However, the ratio of the weight distribution between the left and right limbs increased in the AyuFlex® (26%, 36%, 40%) and ibuprofen (32%) groups in comparison with the MIA control group on day 7. In particular, the weight distribution of the animals treated with AyuFlex® at 25 mg/kg (42.60 ± 0.72), 50 mg/kg (45.50 ± 0.29), and 100 mg/kg (46.21 ± 0.77) returned to the normal level and showed similar results to the ibuprofen (45.34 ± 0.74) group at day 21 (Table 1). Our results revealed that AyuFlex® might alleviate OA-associated pain symptoms.

Table 1. Effects of AyuFlex® on weight-bearing distribution in the hind paw for 21 days in MIA-incurred OA in rats. The results are expressed as the mean ± SEM (n = 8/group). A, AyuFlex®; I, Ibuprofen. * $p < 0.05$, ** $p < 0.01$, in comparison with MIA-induced control group; ## $p < 0.01$, in comparison with the non-MIA induced control group.

Treatment	Weight Bearing Distribution (%)			
	Day 0	Day 7	Day 14	Day 21
Normal Control	51.33 ± 0.95	49.91 ± 0.58	51.05 ± 0.75	48.80 ± 0.49
MIA Control	30.08 ± 2.86 ##	27.54 ± 3.47 ##	33.45 ± 1.18 ##	39.01 ± 1.31 ##
A 25 mg/kg	32.07 ± 2.40	34.84 ± 2.87	36.95 ± 3.17	42.60 ± 0.72 *
A 50 mg/kg	31.75 ± 2.70	37.63 ± 2.46 *	39.18 ± 1.41 **	45.50 ± 0.29 **
A 100 mg/kg	30.56 ± 2.80	38.57 ± 2.31 *	40.57 ± 1.17 **	46.21 ± 0.77 **
I 20 mg/kg	31.41 ± 3.45	36.45 ± 3.30	41.53 ± 1.20 **	45.34 ± 0.74 **

3.8. Effects of AyuFlex® on Arthritis Index (AI) for 21 Days in MIA-Incurred OA in Rats

To assess OA-associated symptoms such as limping and swelling, we observed every animal on a weekly basis. The MIA control group showed a high AI index including swelling and limping score than all other groups, which gradually decreased over time (Table 2). Rats treated with AyuFlex® at 50 mg/kg and 100 mg/kg had noticeably downregulated the AI index after day 14 compared with those treated with MIA (control group) (respectively, $p < 0.01$). Furthermore, AyuFlex® administered at 50 mg/kg and 100 mg/kg downregulated the AI index to a similar level as ibuprofen—the positive control—after day 14. We confirmed that the increased AI index due to OA was significantly reduced by AyuFlex®.

Table 2. Effects of AyuFlex® on arthritis index (AI) for 21 days in MIA-incurred OA in rats. The results are expressed as the mean ± SEM (n = 8/group). A, AyuFlex®; I, Ibuprofen. ** p < 0.01, in comparison with the MIA-induced control group; ## p < 0.01, in comparison with the non-MIA induced control group.

Treatment	Arthritis Index			
	Day 0	Day 7	Day 14	Day 21
Normal Control	0.00	0.00	0.00	0.00
MIA Control	2.06 ± 0.34 ##	2.07 ± 0.30 ##	1.56 ± 0.06 ##	1.51 ± 0.12 ##
A 25 mg/kg	2.10 ± 0.19	2.05 ± 0.25	1.28 ± 0.14	1.08 ± 0.08 **
A 50 mg/kg	1.95 ± 0.20	1.50 ± 0.21	1.14 ± 0.07 **	0.90 ± 0.04 **
A 100 mg/kg	2.00 ± 0.20	1.48 ± 0.26	0.99 ± 0.01 **	0.91 ± 0.05 **
I 20 mg/kg	1.94 ± 0.21	1.61 ± 0.31	1.04 ± 0.08 **	0.74 ± 0.12 **

3.9. Effects of AyuFlex® on the Expression of iNOS, 5-LOX, LTB$_4$, and IL-6 in Arthrodial Cartilage

To indicate the impacts of AyuFlex® on OA-upregulated inflammation, the protein expression of iNOS, 5-LOX, LTB$_4$, and IL-6 was detected in the cartilage tissue. MIA-incurred OA enormously increased the protein levels of iNOS, 5-LOX, LTB$_4$, and IL-6 in comparison with that in the normal control. The expression of iNOS, 5-LOX, LTB$_4$, and IL-6 was significantly reduced in response to AyuFlex® and ibuprofen than in response to the MIA-injected group. The 25 mg/kg AyuFlex®-treated group mitigated the expression levels of iNOS, 5-LOX, LTB$_4$, and IL-6 increased by MIA injection (19%, 7%, 3%, and 35%, respectively). Treatment with 50 mg/kg AyuFlex® obviously decreased (p < 0.01, for all conditions) the expression of iNOS, 5-LOX, LTB$_4$, and IL-6 by 55%, 38%, 43%, and 39%, respectively, with respect to the expression levels in the MIA-treated group. The 100 mg/kg AyuFlex® significantly alleviated (p < 0.01, for all conditions) the iNOS, 5-LOX, LTB$_4$, and IL-6 expression levels to 67%, 32%, 34%, and 44%, respectively, of those observed in the MIA-treated group (Figure 7).

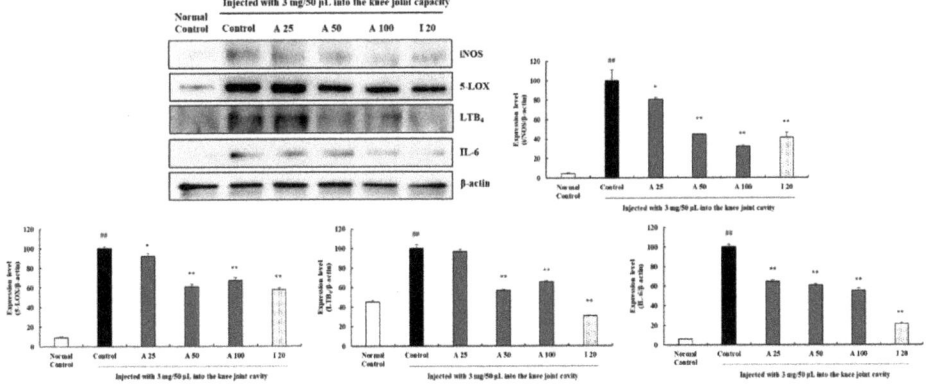

Figure 7. Effects of AyuFlex® on the expression of iNOS, 5-LOX, LTB$_4$, and IL-6 in arthrodial cartilage. The expression of iNOS (135 kDa), 5-LOX (78 kDa), LTB$_4$ (36 kDa), and IL-6 (25 kDa) was measured by western blotting. Protein bands were quantified utilizing ImageJ. As the control for normalization, β-actin was utilized. The results are expressed as the mean ± SEM of independent experiments (n = 3/group). A, AyuFlex®; I, Ibuprofen. * p < 0.05 and ** p < 0.01, in comparison with the MIA-induced control group; ## p < 0.01, in comparison with the non-MIA induced control group.

3.10. Effects of AyuFlex® on Joint Pathology in MIA-Incurred OA in Rats

To observe the morphological alterations and seriousness of the articular destruction in the joint tissue, H&E and Safranin-O staining were conducted in rats with MIA-incurred OA. H&E staining revealed that the MIA control group revealed serious alterations in the cartilage, synovial membrane, and fibrous tissue. However, it was confirmed that administration with AyuFlex® and ibuprofen effectually relieved the structural morphological alterations in arthrodial cartilage when it was compared with the MIA (control group; Figure 8A). Additionally, we stained the proteoglycan layer with safranin-O to confirm the cartilage breakdown (Figure 8B). In the MIA control group, normal cartilage (red) was destructed and the proteoglycan layer was reduced. Conversely, the proteoglycan layer was clearly visible in animals treated with AyuFlex® at 50 mg/kg, 100 mg/kg, and ibuprofen. In addition, using the Mankin scoring system, the seriousness of OA lesions was scored as shown in Figure 8C. The Mankin score was reduced in the AyuFlex® 100 mg/kg treated group by 60% and was noticeably reduced in the AyuFlex® 50 mg/kg and ibuprofen 20 mg/kg treated groups by 64% and 71%, respectively, compared with that in response to MIA (control group).

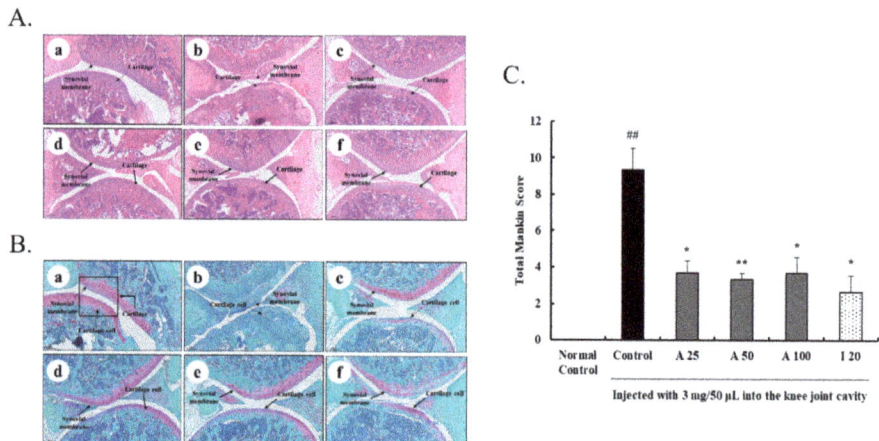

Figure 8. Effects of AyuFlex® on joint pathology in MIA-incurred OA in rats. (**A**) Knee joints were stained with H&E and (**B**) Safranin-O, (**C**) and graded on a scale 0-13 scale using the Mankin scoring system. (a) Normal Control group, (b) MIA Control group, (c) MIA + AyuFlex® 25 mg/kg, (d) MIA + AyuFlex® 50 mg/kg, (e) MIA + AyuFlex® 100 mg/kg, and (f) MIA + Ibuprofen 20 mg/kg. The results are expressed as the mean ± SEM (n = 5/group). A, AyuFlex®; I, Ibuprofen. Scale bar = 300 µm. * $p < 0.05$ and ** $p < 0.01$ in comparison with the MIA-stimulated control group; ## $p < 0.01$, in comparison with the non-MIA induced control group.

3.11. AyuFlex® Decreased the Production of MMP-2, -3, and -13 in Arthrodial Cartilage

To identify the effects of AyuFlex® on MMPs in the cartilage tissues of OA incurred rats, the protein levels of MMP-2, -3, and -13 were evaluated. As shown in Figure 9, the injection of MIA considerably upregulated MMP-2, -3, and -13 expression than the normal control group. The protein expression of MMP-2, -3, and -13 was significantly reduced with AyuFlex® and ibuprofen treatment compared with the MIA treatment (control group). When compared with the MIA-injected group, the 25 mg/kg AyuFlex®-treated group reduced the expression levels of MMP-2, -3, and -13, by 0.1%, 14%, and 36%, respectively. Treatment with 50 mg/kg AyuFlex® substantially decreased ($p < 0.01$, for all conditions) the expression of MMP-2, -3, and -13, by 32%, 32%, and 48%, respectively, with respect to the expression levels in the MIA-treated group. The 100 mg/kg AyuFlex® evidently downregulated ($p < 0.01$, for all conditions) the MMP-2, -3, and -13 expression levels to 24%, 33%, and 52%, respectively, of those observed in the MIA-treated group (Figure 9).

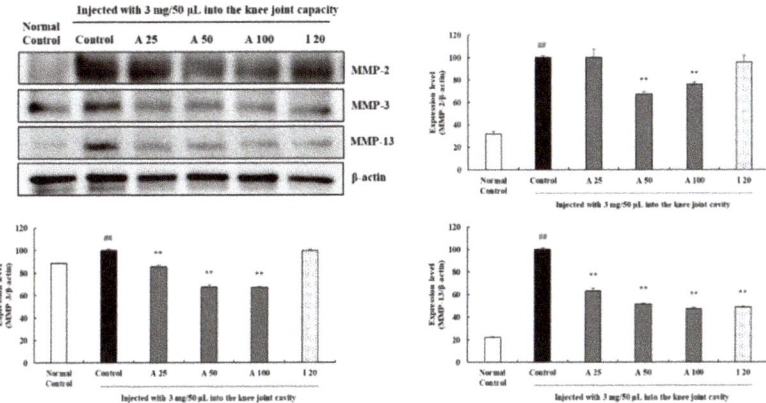

Figure 9. AyuFlex® decreased the production of MMP-2, -3, and -13 in arthrodial cartilage. The expression of MMP-2 (62, 72 kDa), MMP-3 (54 kDa), and MMP-13 (54 kDa) was determined by western blotting. Protein bands were quantified using ImageJ. As the control for normalization, β-actin was utilized. The results are expressed as the mean ± SEM of independent experiments ($n = 3$/group). A, AyuFlex®; I, Ibuprofen. ** $p < 0.01$, in comparison with the MIA-induced control group; ## $p < 0.01$, in comparison with the non-MIA induced control group.

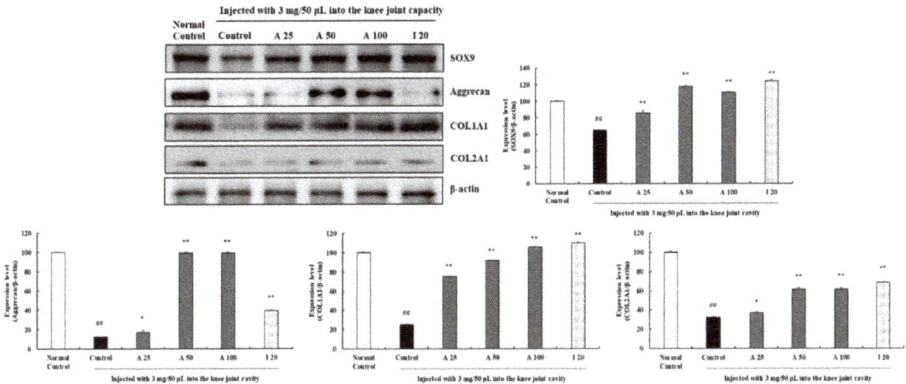

Figure 10. AyuFlex® treatment attenuated the degradation of collagen synthesis-involved proteins in arthrodial cartilage. The expression of SOX9 (65 kDa), aggrecan (110 kDa), COL1A1 (220 kDa), and COL2A1 (190 kDa) was determined by western blotting. Protein bands were quantified utilizing ImageJ. As the control for normalization, β-actin was utilized. The results are expressed as the mean ± SEM of independent experiments ($n = 3$/group). A, AyuFlex®; I, Ibuprofen. * $p < 0.05$ and ** $p < 0.01$, in comparison with the MIA-induced control group; ## $p < 0.01$, in comparison with the non-MIA induced control group.

3.12. AyuFlex® Treatment Attenuated the Degradation of Collagen Synthesis-Involved Proteins in Arthrodial Cartilage

To investigate the impacts of AyuFlex® on the expression of collagen synthesis-involved proteins in cartilage tissues of OA induced rats, the protein levels of SOX9, aggrecan, COL1A1, and COL2A1 were evaluated. As shown in Figure 10, injection of MIA considerably diminished SOX9, aggrecan, COL1A1, and COL2A1 expression compared with that in the normal control group. When it was compared with the MIA-injected group, the 25 mg/kg AyuFlex®-treated group upregulated the expression levels of SOX9, aggrecan, COL1A1, and COL2A1 by 1.3-fold, 1.3-fold, 3.0-fold, and 1.1-fold, respectively. Treatment with 50 mg/kg AyuFlex® considerably upregulated ($p < 0.01$, for all conditions) the expression of SOX9, aggrecan, COL1A1, and COL2A1 by 1.8-fold, 8.0-fold, 3.6-fold, and 1.9-fold, respectively, with respect to the expression levels in the MIA-treated group. The 100 mg/kg AyuFlex® significantly increased ($p < 0.01$, for all conditions) the SOX9, aggrecan, COL1A1, and COL2A1 expression levels to 1.7-fold, 8.0-fold, 4.2-fold, and 1.9-fold, respectively, of those observed in the MIA-treated group (Figure 10).

4. Discussion

OA is one of the most general chronic degenerative joint illnesses in the population of old people, which is featured by the destruction of the arthrodial cartilage. Over time, the subchondral bone thickness and various inflammatory mediators are produced in the synovial membrane [36,37]. For this reason, steroids and non-steroidal anti-inflammatory medications are mainly utilized to alleviate the progression of arthritis. However, these anti-inflammatory drugs alleviate only joint pain and swelling and have side effects when administered for a long time. Therefore, there is a need for efficacious and safe medication that not only alleviates the symptoms of OA, but also delays the progression of the disease [38].

The fruit of T. chebula has been utilized widely in a variety of traditional oriental medicine for the therapy of different diseases. It exhibits significant bioactive effects such as antioxidant and anti-inflammatory activities [18–29]. In many studies, T. chebula has been revealed to exhibit antioxidant effects by inhibiting ROS and NO production [21–24]. Therefore, we investigated the anti-osteoarthritic effects of a standardized aqueous extract of the T. chebula fruit (AyuFlex®) in IL-1β-treated chondrocytes and in a rat model of MIA-incurred OA.

IL-1β, one of the most crucial inflammatory cytokines, is mainly utilized for OA research. Chondrocytes stimulated by IL-1β provoke 5-LOX and iNOS, producing large amounts of LTB_4 and NO [39]. iNOS is a major nitric oxide synthase (NOS) enzyme and is responsible for synthesizing NO [40]. In addition, 5-LOX induces LTB_4, which upregulates the induction and secretion of pro-inflammatory cytokines such as IL-6 from the synovial membranes. The accumulated NO and LTB_4 can stimulate cells to synthesize and release MMPs that inhibit the production of type I and II collagen, eventually leading to cartilage degradation [41–45]. Therefore, this inflammatory factor affects both bone absorption and joint pain. In this study, we showed that AyuFlex® downregulated iNOS and 5-LOX expression in chondrocytes stimulated by IL-1β. Furthermore, it was confirmed that AyuFlex® also inhibited LTB_4 and IL-6 expression. These findings demonstrate that AyuFlex® inhibited LTB_4 and IL-6 production, and these results may be connected with the regulation of iNOS and 5-LOX expression, thereby reducing the progression of OA.

Moreover, recent studies have explained that IL-1β remarkably upregulated the synthesis of cartilage matrix-degrading enzymes, for example, MMPs. MMPs have been considered one of the major enzymes that breakdown aggrecan and collagen in cartilage. Several studies have demonstrated that the appearance of MMPs is upregulated in cartilage tissues of OA patients. MMPs are enzymes that mediate the diverse role in tissue remodeling such as conversion, degradation, and destruction of the ECM [46–49]. Therefore, drugs that can suppress MMP expression can be used for the treatment of arthritis. Interestingly, our study showed that AyuFlex® prevents IL-1β-induced MMP-2, -3, and -13 expression at the protein level in chondrocytes. Collagens and proteoglycans are the essential constituent of the ECM. Most of the collagen in arthrodial cartilage is type I and II collagen, which offers the tensile strength in tissue [50,51]. The main proteoglycan in arthrodial cartilage is aggrecan, which offers structural support by keep moisture in the matrix. SOX9 is an indispensable transcription factor for controlling the appearance of many cartilage ECM genes such as COL1A1 and COL2A1 [52]. Aggrecan and collagens I and II are synthesized and secreted by chondrocytes to prevent mechanical destruction under normal circumstances. When cartilage destruction occurs, aggrecan and collagens I and II undergo significant breakdown due to increased production of proteases. These conditions promote the progression of OA [53]. Meanwhile, proteins related to matrix synthesis including aggrecan, SOX9, and collagens I and II were markedly inhibited by IL-1β. The results of the current study show that AyuFlex® can inhibit the reduction of aggrecan, SOX9, and the collagen I and II levels in IL-1β-stimulated chondrocytes. These results indicate that AyuFlex® suppresses MMPs due to downregulation of oxidative stress and inflammation development by IL-1β.

MAPK and NF-κB are two major mechanisms in the onset of OA. Activated MAPK elevated MMPs, and this mechanism is associated with cartilage destruction. The transcription factor NF-κB triggers a variety inflammatory reaction in OA. Previous studies have also shown that NF-κB is an crucial regulatory factor in the production of iNOS expression in chondrocytes [13–16]. As this signaling pathway is closely related to OA, it is recognized as a promising target in OA. Many recent studies have revealed that substances such as resveratrol and curcumin are activated as intracellular signaling molecules during anti-inflammatory action through these various signaling pathways [54–57]. Therefore, the mechanisms of NF-κB and MAPK are very important in inhibiting OA progress and we evaluated the efficacy of AyuFlex® in NF-κB and MAPK mechanisms based on these studies. In our study, IL-1β conspicuously demoted the phosphorylation of ERK and NF-κB p65. In contrast, this process could be reversed by AyuFlex® without affecting the total protein expression.

Taken together, AyuFlex® showed antioxidant, anti-inflammatory, and anti-degenerative effects in OA in an in vitro model. However, in vitro studies are not sufficient to prove the therapeutic effect of AyuFlex® on OA. Therefore, we confirmed the effects of AyuFlex® in protection against cartilage destruction in a rat model with MIA-incurred OA.

MIA is known to inhibit glycolytic signaling in cells by obstructing with glyceraldehyde-3-phosphatase activity and causes inflammation along with cartilage degeneration. Inflammatory stimulation triggers the release of cytokine and its complex biochemical interaction with other mediators, leading to OA and promoting illness symptoms, for example, pain, swelling, and stiffness [58–61]. MIA-incurred OA is an established model to affirm the anti-osteoarthritic effectiveness of candidate therapeutic agents on OA pathology. Therefore, a rat model with MIA-induced OA has been used in many studies associated with OA.

Weight bearing distribution is utilized for pain measurement and as an index of joint discomfort. MIA injections reduce it in the affected limb, indicating joint pain [62,63]. In this study, it was found that treatment with AyuFlex® and ibuprofen considerably upregulated the weight bearing distribution, indicating symptoms of pain relief. In addition, after inducing MIA, general OA symptoms such as swelling and limping in the knee joint were confirmed. In our present study, we discovered that AyuFlex® and ibuprofen treatment protected against OA symptoms in rats with MIA-incurred OA. These results indicate that the administration of AyuFlex® and ibuprofen showed a marked improvement in OA symptoms and pain-related behavior.

Exacerbation of OA symptoms is accompanied by pain and joint destruction, which is related to the expression of inflammatory cytokines [64]. Therefore, we confirmed the expression of iNOS, 5-LOX, LTB$_4$, and IL-6 proteins in cartilage tissues in rats with MIA-incurred OA to affirm the antioxidant and anti-inflammatory effects of AyuFlex®. In our study, we confirmed that AyuFlex® treatment reduced the MIA-triggered increase in cytokine levels, and these results indicate that AyuFlex® may reduce the inflammatory response, and then the mediators can decrease cartilage damage. Therefore, based on the in vitro and in vivo studies, the use of AyuFlex® can provide anti-inflammatory effects in OA treatment.

Additionally, cartilage and proteoglycan damage were confirmed in rats with MIA-incurred OA through H&E and Safranin-O staining of the arthrodial cartilage. AyuFlex® treatment markedly inhibited MIA-induced synovial membrane damage and cartilage destruction. Moreover, it was confirmed that the expression of MMP proteins such as MMP-2, -3, and -13 was increased by MIA in cartilage tissue, whereas AyuFlex® treatment reduced MMP expression. These results indicate that AyuFlex® suppresses MMPs due to downregulation of oxidative stress and inflammation development by MIA. Therefore, based on in vitro and in vivo studies, it is suggested that the use of AyuFlex® could inhibit the decomposition of cartilage by inhibiting MMPs in OA treatment. Arthrodial cartilage damage occurs because the main component of the extracellular matrix, proteoglycan, is degraded by the MMPs. In the present study, we observed collagen synthesis-related proteins in the arthrodial cartilage. We also confirmed that AyuFlex® reduced cartilage destruction through an increase in SOX9, aggrecan, and collagen I and II levels in arthrodial cartilage. Furthermore, based on in vitro and in vivo studies, AyuFlex® revealed collagen preserving properties shown by the significantly suppressed MMPs and upregulated collagen synthesis-related proteins.

Therefore, in our research, AyuFlex® showed anti-osteoarthritic effects through the suppression of NF-κB and MAPK mechanisms, which contribute to a further understanding of the effectiveness of AyuFlex® on OA treatment. In addition, if there are additional studies such as in vivo studies of MIA-induced rat models for ellagic acid, an indicator component of AyuFlex®, we believe that the efficacy of AyuFlex® in the treatment of OA could be further demonstrated.

5. Conclusions

We report here for the first time that AyuFlex® inhibits oxidative stress, inflammation, and cartilage degradation and improves cartilage regeneration through suppressing the phosphorylation of the ERK and NF-κB p65 signaling pathways triggered by IL-1β in human chondrocytes. Moreover, we discovered the anti-osteoarthritic effects of AyuFlex® in rats with MIA-incurred OA by reducing the levels of oxidative stress, pro-inflammatory mediators, and pro-inflammatory cytokines. Additionally, AyuFlex® decreased the expression of MMPs and suppressed the destruction of synovial membrane and arthrodial cartilage, thereby suppressing the progression of OA. Furthermore, AyuFlex® revealed collagen preserving properties as shown by the significantly upregulated collagen synthesis-related proteins. These results from the in vitro and in vivo studies demonstrated that the biochemical actions of AyuFlex® relieve pain by reducing oxidative stress, inflammation, and cartilage breakdown in arthritis. These results from our study suggest that AyuFlex® could be used as a safe and effective herbal formulation in the treatment of OA among the natural products.

Author Contributions: H.L.K. and H.J.L. performed the experiments and wrote the original draft preparation. D.-R.L. and B.-K.C. conceptualized and discussed the conclusions and edited the manuscript. S.H.Y. undertook the manuscript editing and supervision. All authors have read and agreed to the published version of the manuscript.

Funding: This research received no external funding.

Acknowledgments: The authors thank Natreon Inc., New Brunswick, NJ, USA and Maypro Industries LLC, Purchase, NY, USA for providing samples, encouragement, and generous support.

Conflicts of Interest: The authors declare no conflict of interest.

References

1. Lane, N.E.; Shidara, K.; Wise, B.L. Osteoarthritis year in review 2016: Clinical. *Osteoarthr. Cartil.* **2017**, *25*, 209–215. [CrossRef] [PubMed]
2. Glyn-Jones, S.; Palmer, A.J.R.; Agricola, R.; Price, A.J.; Vincent, T.L.; Weinans, H.; Carr, A.J. Osteoarthritis. *Lancet* **2015**, *386*, 376–387. [CrossRef]
3. Yang, H.J.; Kim, M.J.; Qiu, J.Y.; Zhang, T.; Wu, T.Z.; Wu, X.; Jang, D.-J.; Park, S.M. Rice Porridge Containing Welsh Onion Root Water Extract Alleviates Osteoarthritis-Related Pain Behaviors, Glucose Levels, and Bone Metabolism in Osteoarthritis-Induced Ovariectomized Rats. *Nutrients* **2019**, *11*, 1503. [CrossRef] [PubMed]
4. Cho, S.H. Effect of Green Lipped Mussel Extract Oil Complex (Gwanjeolpalpal) on Monosodium Iodoacetate-Induced Osteoarthritis in Animal Model. *J. Korean Soc. Food Sci. Nutr.* **2019**, *48*, 206–214. [CrossRef]
5. Olivotto, E.; Otero, M.; Marcu, K.B.; Goldring, M.B. Pathophysiology of osteoarthritis: Canonical NF-κB/IKKβ-dependent and kinase-independent effects of IKKα in cartilage degradation and chondrocyte differentiation. *RMD Open* **2015**, *1* (Suppl. S1), e000061. [CrossRef]
6. DeLise, A.Á.; Fischer, L.; Tuan, R.S. Cellular interactions and signaling in cartilage development. *Osteoarthr. Cartil.* **2000**, *8*, 309–334. [CrossRef]

7. Van der Kraan, P.M.; Van den Berg, W.B. Chondrocyte hypertrophy and osteoarthritis: Role in initiation and progression of cartilage degeneration? *Osteoarthr. Cartil.* **2012**, *20*, 223–232. [CrossRef]
8. Dreier, R. Hypertrophic differentiation of chondrocytes in osteoarthritis: The developmental aspect of degenerative joint disorders. *Arthritis Res. Ther.* **2010**, *12*, 216. [CrossRef]
9. Goldring, S.R.; Goldring, M.B. The role of cytokines in cartilage matrix degeneration in osteoarthritis. *Clin. Orthop. Relat. Res.* **2004**, *427*, S27–S36. [CrossRef]
10. Kelwick, R.; Desanlis, I.; Wheeler, G.N.; Edwards, D.R. The ADAMTS (A Disintegrin and Metalloproteinase with Thrombospondin motifs) family. *Genome Biol.* **2015**, *16*, 113. [CrossRef]
11. Goldring, M.B.; Otero, M. Inflammation in osteoarthritis. *Curr. Opin. Rheumatol.* **2011**, *23*, 471. [CrossRef] [PubMed]
12. Santangelo, K.; Nuovo, G.J.; Bertone, A.L. In vivo reduction or blockade of interleukin-1β in primary osteoarthritis influences expression of mediators implicated in pathogenesis. *Osteoarthr. Cartil.* **2012**, *20*, 1610–1618. [CrossRef] [PubMed]
13. Zhen, X.; Wei, L.; Wu, Q.; Zhang, Y.; Chen, Q. Mitogen-activated protein kinase p38 mediates regulation of chondrocyte differentiation by parathyroid hormone. *J. Biol. Chem.* **2001**, *276*, 4879–4885. [CrossRef] [PubMed]
14. Watanabe, H.; de Caestecker, M.P.; Yamada, Y. Transcriptional cross-talk between Smad, ERK1/2, and p38 mitogen-activated protein kinase pathways regulates transforming growth factor-β-induced aggrecan gene expression in chondrogenic ATDC5 cells. *J. Biol. Chem.* **2001**, *276*, 14466–14473. [CrossRef] [PubMed]
15. Kumar, A.; Takada, Y.; Boriek, A.M.; Aggarwal, B.B. Nuclear factor-κB: Its role in health and disease. *J. Mol. Med.* **2004**, *82*, 434–448. [CrossRef]
16. Csaki, C.; Mobasheri, A.; Shakibaei, M. Synergistic chondroprotective effects of curcumin and resveratrol in human articular chondrocytes: Inhibition of IL-1β-induced NF-κB-mediated inflammation and apoptosis. *Arthritis Res. Ther.* **2009**, *11*, R165. [CrossRef]
17. Loeser, R.F.; Erickson, E.A.; Long, D.L. Mitogen-activated protein kinases as therapeutic targets in osteoarthritis. *Curr. Opin. Rheumatol.* **2008**, *20*, 581. [CrossRef]
18. Bag, A.; Bhattacharyya, S.K.; Chattopadhyay, R.R. The development of *Terminalia chebula* Retz. (Combretaceae) in clinical research. *Asian Pac. J. Trop. Biomed.* **2013**, *3*, 244–252. [CrossRef]
19. Jokar, A.; Masoomi, F.; Sadeghpour, O.; Nassiri-Toosi, M.; Hamedi, S. Potential therapeutic applications for *Terminalia chebula* in Iranian traditional medicine. *J. Tradit. Chin. Med.* **2016**, *36*, 250–254. [CrossRef]
20. Sato, Y.; Oketani, H.; Singyouchi, K.; OHTSUBO, T.; KIHARA, M.; SHIBATA, H.; HIGUTI, T. Extraction and purification of effective antimicrobial constituents of *Terminalia chebula* RETS. against methicillin-resistant Staphylococcus aureus. *Biol. Pharm. Bull.* **1997**, *20*, 401–404. [CrossRef]
21. Hazra, B.; Sarkar, R.; Biswas, S.; Mandal, N. Comparative study of the antioxidant and reactive oxygen species scavenging properties in the extracts of the fruits of *Terminalia chebula*, *Terminalia belerica* and Emblica officinalis. *BMC Complement Altern. Med.* **2010**, *10*, 20. [CrossRef] [PubMed]
22. Bag, A.; Kumar Bhattacharyya, S.; Kumar Pal, N.; Ranjan Chattopadhyay, R. Anti-inflammatory, anti-lipid peroxidative, antioxidant and membrane stabilizing activities of hydroalcoholic extract of *Terminalia chebula* fruits. *Pharm. Biol.* **2013**, *51*, 1515–1520. [CrossRef] [PubMed]
23. Kalaiselvan, S.; Rasool, M. Triphala exhibits anti-arthritic effect by ameliorating bone and cartilage degradation in adjuvant-induced arthritic rats. *Immunol. Investig.* **2015**, *44*, 411–426. [CrossRef] [PubMed]
24. Saha, S.; Verma, R.J. Antioxidant activity of polyphenolic extract of *Terminalia chebula* Retzius fruits. *J. Taibah Univ. Sci.* **2016**, *10*, 805–812. [CrossRef]
25. Kishore, K.K.; Kishan, P.V.; Ramakanth, G.S.H.; Chandrasekhar, N.; Usharani, P. A study of *Terminalia chebula* extract on endothelial dysfunction and biomarkers of oxidative stress in patients with metabolic syndrome. *Eur. J. Biomed. Pharm. Sci.* **2016**, *3*, 181–188.
26. Vnukov, V.V.; Panina, S.B.; Krolevets, I.V.; Milutina, N.P.; Ananyan, A.A.; Zabrodin, M.A.; Plotnikov, A.A. Features of oxidative stress in the blood and the synovial fluid associated with knee osteoarthritis. *Adv. Gerontol.* **2015**, *28*, 284–289.
27. Siems, W.; Bresgen, N.; Brenke, R.; Siems, R.; Kitzing, M.; Harting, H.; Eckl, P.M. Pain and mobility improvement and MDA plasma levels in degenerative osteoarthritis, low back pain, and rheumatoid arthritis after infrared A-irradiation. *Acta Biochim. Pol.* **2010**, *57*, 313–319. [CrossRef]

28. Heidari, B.; Hajian-Tilaki, K.; Babaei, M. Determinants of pain in patients with symptomatic knee osteoarthritis. *Casp. J. Intern. Med.* **2016**, *7*, 153.
29. Klyne, D.M.; Barbe, M.F.; Hodges, P.W. Systemic inflammatory profiles and their relationships with demographic, behavioural and clinical features in acute low back pain. *Brain Behav. Immun.* **2017**, *60*, 84–92. [CrossRef]
30. Murdock, N.; Gupta, C.R.; Vega, N.; Kotora, K.; Miller, J.; Goad, T.J.; Lasher, A.M.; Canerdy, D.T.; Kalidindi, S.R. Evaluation of *Terminalia chebula* extract for anti-arthritic efficacy and safety in osteoarthritic dogs. *J. Vet. Sci. Technol.* **2016**, *7*. [CrossRef]
31. Kumar, C.U.; Pokuri, V.K.; Pingali, U. Evaluation of the analgesic activity of standardized aqueous extract of *Terminalia Chebula* in healthy human participants using hot air pain model. *J. Clin. Diagn. Res.* **2015**, *9*, FC01. [CrossRef] [PubMed]
32. Murdock, N. Therapeutic Efficacy and Safety Evaualtion of Terminalia Chebula Extract in Moderately Arthritic Canines. Master's Thesis, Murray State University, Murray, KY, USA, 2015.
33. Nutalapati, C.H.; Chiranjeevi, U.K.; Kishan, P.V.; Kiran, K.K.; Pingali, U. A randomized, double-blind, placebo-controlled, parallel group clinical study to evaluate the analgesic effect of aqueous extract of *Terminalia chebula*, a proprietary chromium complex, and their combination in subjects with joint discomfort. *Asian J. Pharm. Clin. Res.* **2016**, *9*, 264–269.
34. Pokuri, V.K.; Kumar, C.U.; Pingali, U. A randomized, double-blind, placebo-controlled, cross-over study to evaluate analgesic activity of *Terminalia chebula* in healthy human volunteers using a mechanical pain model. *J. Anaesthesiol. Clin. Pharmacol.* **2016**, *32*, 329.
35. Lopez, H.L.; Habowski, S.M.; Sandrock, J.E.; Raub, B.; Kedia, A.; Bruno, E.J.; Ziegenfuss, T.N. Effects of dietary supplementation with a standardized aqueous extract of *Terminalia chebula* fruit (AyuFlex®) on joint mobility, comfort, and functional capacity in healthy overweight subjects: A randomized placebo-controlled clinical trial. *BMC Complement Altern. Med.* **2017**, *17*, 475. [CrossRef]
36. Zhang, Y.; Li, R.; Zhong, Y.; Zhang, S.; Zhou, L.; Shang, S. Fuyuan decoction enhances SOX9 and COL2A1 expression and Smad2/3 phosphorylation in IL-1β-activated chondrocytes. *Evid. Based Complement Alternat. Med.* **2015**, *2015*, 821947. [CrossRef] [PubMed]
37. Loeser, R.F. Aging and osteoarthritis: The role of chondrocyte senescence and aging changes in the cartilage matrix. *Osteoarthr. Cartil.* **2009**, *17*, 971–979. [CrossRef]
38. Altman, R.D. Practical considerations for the pharmacologic management of osteoarthritis. *Am. J. Manag. Care* **2009**, *15* (Suppl. S8), S236–S243.
39. Koch, B.; Baum, W.; Burmester, G.R.; Rohwer, P.; Reinke, M.; Zacher, J.; Kalden, J.R. Prostaglandin E2, interleukin 1 and gamma interferon production of mononuclear cells of patients with inflammatory and degenerative joint diseases. *Z. Rheumatol.* **1989**, *48*, 194–199.
40. Sasaki, K.; Hattori, T.; Fujisawa, T.; Takahashi, K.; Inoue, H.; Takigawa, M. Nitric oxide mediates interleukin-1-induced gene expression of matrix metalloproteinases and basic fibroblast growth factor in cultured rabbit articular chondrocytes. *J. Biochem.* **1998**, *123*, 431–439. [CrossRef]
41. Boileau, C.; Pelletier, J.P.; Tardif, G.; Fahmi, H.; Laufer, S.; Lavigne, M.; Martel-Pelletier, J. The regulation of human MMP-13 by licofelone, an inhibitor of cyclo-oxygenases and 5-lipoxygenase, in human osteoarthritic chondrocytes is mediated by the inhibition of the p38 MAP kinase signalling pathway. *Ann. Rheum. Dis.* **2005**, *64*, 891–898. [CrossRef]
42. Hardy, M.M.; Seibert, K.; Manning, P.T.; Currie, M.G.; Woerner, B.M.; Edwards, D.; Koki, A.; Tripp, C.S. Cyclooxygenase 2-dependent prostaglandin E2 modulates cartilage proteoglycan degradation in human osteoarthritis explants. *Arthritis Rheum.* **2002**, *46*, 1789–1803. [CrossRef]
43. Brinckerhoff, C.E.; Matrisian, L.M. Matrix metalloproteinases: A tail of a frog that became a prince. *Nat. Rev. Mol. Cell Biol.* **2002**, *3*, 207–214. [CrossRef] [PubMed]
44. Klein, T.; Bischoff, R. Physiology and pathophysiology of matrix metalloproteases. *Amino Acids* **2011**, *41*, 271–290. [CrossRef]
45. Cheleschi, S.; Pascarelli, N.A.; Valacchi, G.; Di Capua, A.; Biava, M.; Belmonte, G.; Giordani, A.; Sticozzi, C.; Anzini, M.; Fioravanti, A. Chondroprotective effect of three different classes of anti-inflammatory agents on human osteoarthritic chondrocytes exposed to IL-1β. *Int. Immunopharmacol.* **2015**, *28*, 794–801. [CrossRef]

46. Madhavan, S.; Anghelina, M.; Rath-Deschner, B.; Wypasek, E.; John, A.; Deschner, J.; Piesco, N.; Agarwal, S. Biomechanical signals exert sustained attenuation of proinflammatory gene induction in articular chondrocytes. *Osteoarthr. Cartil.* **2006**, *14*, 1023–1032. [CrossRef] [PubMed]
47. Nummenmaa, E.; Hämäläinen, M.; Moilanen, T.; Vuolteenaho, K.; Moilanen, E. Effects of FGF-2 and FGF receptor antagonists on MMP enzymes, aggrecan, and type II collagen in primary human OA chondrocytes. *Scand. J. Rheumatol.* **2015**, *44*, 321–330. [CrossRef] [PubMed]
48. Tetlow, L.C.; Adlam, D.J.; Woolley, D.E. Matrix metalloproteinase and proinflammatory cytokine production by chondrocytes of human osteoarthritic cartilage: Associations with degenerative changes. *Arthritis Rheum.* **2001**, *44*, 585–594. [CrossRef]
49. Dean, D.D.; Martel-Pelletier, J.; Pelletier, J.P.; Howell, D.S.; Woessner, J.F. Evidence for metalloproteinase and metalloproteinase inhibitor imbalance in human osteoarthritic cartilage. *J. Clin. Investig.* **1989**, *84*, 678–685. [CrossRef]
50. Wieland, H.A.; Michaelis, M.; Kirschbaum, B.J.; Rudolphi, K.A. Osteoarthritis—An untreatable disease? *Nat. Rev. Drug Discov.* **2005**, *4*, 331–344. [CrossRef]
51. Heinegård, D. Fell-Muir Lecture: Proteoglycans and more–from molecules to biology. *Int. J. Exp. Pathol.* **2009**, *90*, 575–586. [CrossRef]
52. Bell, D.M.; Leung, K.K.; Wheatley, S.C.; Ng, L.J.; Zhou, S.; Ling, K.W.; Sham, M.H.; Koopman, P.; Tam, P.P.L.; Cheah, K.S. SOX9 directly regulates the type-II collagen gene. *Nat. Genet.* **1997**, *16*, 174–178. [CrossRef] [PubMed]
53. Wilusz, R.E.; Sanchez-Adams, J.; Guilak, F. The structure and function of the pericellular matrix of articular cartilage. *Matrix Biol.* **2014**, *39*, 25–32. [CrossRef]
54. Shakibaei, M.; Csaki, C.; Nebrich, S.; Mobasheri, A. Resveratrol suppresses interleukin-1β-induced inflammatory signaling and apoptosis in human articular chondrocytes: Potential for use as a novel nutraceutical for the treatment of osteoarthritis. *Biochem. Pharmacol.* **2008**, *76*, 1426–1439. [CrossRef] [PubMed]
55. Buhrmann, C.; Mobasheri, A.; Matis, U.; Shakibaei, M. Curcumin mediated suppression of nuclear factor-κB promotes chondrogenic differentiation of mesenchymal stem cells in a high-density co-culture microenvironment. *Arthritis Res. Ther.* **2010**, *12*, R127. [CrossRef] [PubMed]
56. Shakibaei, M.; Mobasheri, A.; Buhrmann, C. Curcumin synergizes with resveratrol to stimulate the MAPK signaling pathway in human articular chondrocytes in vitro. *Genes Nutr.* **2011**, *6*, 171–179. [CrossRef]
57. Buhrmann, C.; Popper, B.; Aggarwal, B.B.; Shakibaei, M. Resveratrol downregulates inflammatory pathway activated by lymphotoxin α (TNF-β) in articular chondrocytes: Comparison with TNF-α. *PLoS ONE* **2017**, *12*, e0186993. [CrossRef]
58. Jeong, J.-W.; Lee, H.H.; Kim, J.S.; Choi, E.-O.; Hyun, H.-B.; Kim, H.J.; Kim, M.Y.; Ahn, K.I.; Kim, G.-Y.; Lee, K.W.; et al. Mori Folium water extract alleviates articular cartilage damages and inflammatory responses in monosodium iodoacetate-induced osteoarthritis rats. *Mol. Med. Rep.* **2017**, *16*, 3541–3848. [CrossRef]
59. Sabri, M.I.; Ochs, S. Inhibition of glyceraldehyde-3-phosphate dehydrogenase in mammalian nerve by iodoacetic acid. *J. Neurochem.* **1971**, *18*, 1509–1514. [CrossRef]
60. Van der Kraan, P.M.; Vitters, E.L.; van de Putte, L.B.; van den Berg, W.B. Development of osteoarthritic lesions in mice by "metabolic" and "mechanical" alterations in the knee joints. *Am. J. Pathol.* **1989**, *135*, 1001–1014.
61. Lee, A.S.; Ellman, M.B.; Yan, D.; Kroin, J.S.; Cole, B.J.; van Wijnen, A.J.; Im, H.J. A current review of molecular mechanisms regarding osteoarthritis and pain. *Gene* **2013**, *527*, 440–447. [CrossRef]
62. Bove, S.E.; Calcaterra, S.L.; Brooker, R.M.; Huber, C.M.; Guzman, R.E.; Juneau, P.L.; Schrier, D.J.; Kilgore, K.S. Weight bearing as a measure of disease progression and efficacy of anti-inflammatory compounds in a model of monosodium iodoacetate-induced osteoarthritis. *Osteoarthr. Cartil.* **2013**, *11*, 821–830. [CrossRef]
63. Woo, Y.J.; Joo, Y.B.; Jung, Y.O.; Ju, J.H.; Cho, M.L.; Oh, H.J.; Jhun, J.Y.; Park, M.K.; Park, J.S.; Kang, C.M.; et al. Grape seed proanthocyanidin extract ameliorates monosodium iodoacetate-induced osteoarthritis. *Exp. Mol. Med.* **2011**, *43*, 561–570. [CrossRef] [PubMed]

64. Kwon, J.Y.; Lee, S.H.; Na, H.-S.; Jung, K.A.; Choi, J.W.; Cho, K.-H.; Lee, C.-Y.; Kim, S.J.; Park, S.-H.; Shin, D.-Y.; et al. Kartogenin inhibits pain behavior, chondrocyte inflammation, and attenuates osteoarthritis progression in mice through induction of IL-10. *Sci. Rep.* **2018**, *8*, 1–11. [CrossRef] [PubMed]

Publisher's Note: MDPI stays neutral with regard to jurisdictional claims in published maps and institutional affiliations.

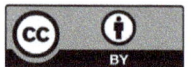 © 2020 by the authors. Licensee MDPI, Basel, Switzerland. This article is an open access article distributed under the terms and conditions of the Creative Commons Attribution (CC BY) license (http://creativecommons.org/licenses/by/4.0/).

Liensinine Prevents Vascular Inflammation by Attenuating Inflammatory Mediators and Modulating VSMC Function

Moon Young Jun [1], Rajendra Karki [1], Keshav Raj Paudel [1], Nisha Panth [2], Hari Prasad Devkota [3] and Dong-Wook Kim [1,*]

1. Department of Oriental Medicine Resources, Mokpo National University, Muan-gun, Jeonnam 534-729, Korea; herb1999@mokpo.ac.kr (M.Y.J.); Rajendra.Karki@stjude.org (R.K.); keshavraj.paudel@uts.edu.au (K.R.P.)
2. College of Pharmacy and Natural Medicine Research Institute, Mokpo National University, Muan-gun, Jeonnam 58554, Korea; n.panth@centenary.org.au
3. Graduate School of Pharmaceutical Sciences, Kumamoto University, 5-1 Oe-honmachi, Chou-ku, Kumamoto City, Kumamoto 862-0973, Japan; devkotah@kumamoto-u.ac.jp
* Correspondence: dbkim@mokpo.ac.kr

Abstract: Liensinine is a bisbenzylisoquinoline alkaloid found in various parts of the lotus (*Nelumbo nucifera* Gaertn.) including seeds. In this study, we explored the preventive activity of liensinine on vascular inflammation via attenuation of inflammatory mediators in macrophage and targeting the proliferation and migration of human vascular smooth muscle cells (VSMC). Anti-oxidative activity was evaluated by using the 1,1-diphenyl-2-picrylhydrazyl (DPPH) free radical scavenging assay method and measuring the peroxidation of serum lipid. Inflammatory markers were studied by evaluating the release of nitric oxide (NO) and the protein levels of inducible nitric oxide synthase (iNOS) and cyclooxygenase (COX-2) in macrophage cells (RAW264.7) and interleukin (IL)-6 production in VSMC. Similarly, anti-proliferative activity in VSMC was evaluated by 3-(4,5-dimethylthiazol-2-yl)-2,5-diphenyltetrazolium bromide (MTT) assay. The enzymatic activity of matrix metalloproteinase (MMP)-9 in VSMC was evaluated by gelatin zymography. Liensinine possesses significant anti-oxidative activity as revealed by the DPPH assay and inhibition of serum lipid peroxidation. Likewise, liensinine decreased NO generation in RAW 264.7 cells. In VSMC, liensinine suppressed platelet-derived growth factor stimulated proliferation and tumor necrosis factor-α (TNF-α) induced MMP-9 enzymatic activity as well as IL-6 expression. Our results revealed the potential preventive effect of liensinine on vascular inflammation, suggesting it as a promising compound for the prevention of vascular inflammation.

Keywords: vascular inflammation; liensinine; VSMC; macrophage; proliferation; migration

1. Introduction

Atherosclerosis is defined as a chronic vascular inflammatory disorder that progresses with the lipid oxidation due to hypercholesteremia, diabetes mellitus, hypertension and various other disorders [1]. Oxidized lipids induce the secretion of various cytokines and recruit macrophages and T-lymphocytes at the site of a lesion [2]. Further, accelerated vascular smooth muscle cell (VSMC) migration and proliferation contribute to atherosclerotic plaque development [3,4]. It is also stimulated by oxidative stress, which produces different inflammatory cytokines; tumor necrosis factor-α(TNF-α), interleukin-6 (IL-6) and growth factor such as platelet-derived growth factor-BB (PDGF-BB). According to the previous study, treatment of IL-6 to C57Bl/6 mice increased fatty streak cores by approximately five times as revealed by oil red o staining of aortic sinus serial section, and increased the release of inflammatory cytokine, IL-1β and TNF-αin the plasma [5]. Moreover, TNF-αand PDGF-BB are already reported to stimulate the migration of human aortic VSMC from media to the intima of blood vessels [6]. These migrated cells are extensively proliferated under the influence of inducing agents like PDGF, TNF-αand lipopolysaccharide (LPS) in the intimal layer of arteries forming atheroma [7–9]. Mitogen-activated protein kinases (MAPKs), a family of serine-threonine kinases, regulate cell adhesion, migration and proliferation on human aortic VSMC in response to external stimuli including TNF-α [10] and PDGF-BB [11,12]. The role of matrix metalloproteinase (MMP) is well known due to their function for disrupting matrices composed of gelatin or elastin, which could permit human aortic VSMC migration by destroying the elastic lamina present between the intima and media [13,14]. Vascular inflammation is a result of toxic insult by the mediators released by the macrophage. Initially, monocytes normally circulating in the blood vessel are migrated to tunica media due to endothelial dysfunction. At this site, they engulf the oxidized low-density lipoprotein (ox-LDL) and become activated after changing the morphology from macrophage to foam cell, as recognized by the accumulation of fatty streaks on lipid laden molecules [15,16]. Activated macrophages release inflammatory mediators like nitric oxide (NO) via the inducible nitric oxidase pathway, and prostaglandins via cyclooxygenase pathway. Collectively, these endogenous inflammatory agents trigger the formation of a necrotic core at the site of an atherosclerosis lesion [17,18].

Liensinine is a bisbenzylisoquinoline alkaloid found in various part of the lotus (*Nelumbo nucifera* Gaertn.) including seeds (Figure 1). Liensinine and other bisbenzylisoquinoline alkaloids present in lotuses are reported as potent anticancer, anti-inflammatory, antioxidant, cardiovascular protective and neuroprotective agents [19–21]. Traditionally, the seed embryo of the lotus has been used as medicine in China for cardiovascular diseases, nervous disorders and sleeplessness [22]. Previously, we reported the anti-atherosclerotic activity of *Nelumbo nucifera* leaf extract and its alkaloid rich fraction through inhibition of neointimal hyperplasia in rats and inhibiting VCMC proliferation and migration [12,23]. In the current study, we aim to determine the similarly beneficial activity of the liensinine against vascular inflammation through anti-inflammatory, anti-proliferative, anti-migratory and anti-oxidative activities.

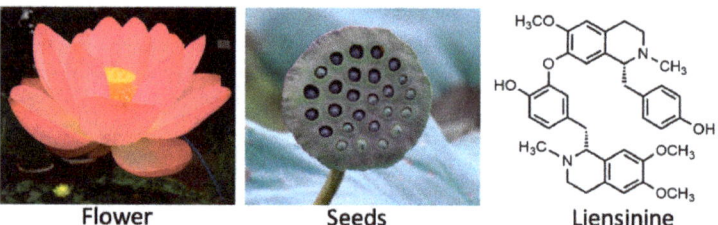

Figure 1. The flower and seeds of *Nelumbo nucifera* and the chemical structure of liensinine.

2. Materials and Methods

2.1. Reagents

Liensinine (Cas number: 2586-96-1) was purchased from Sigma Aldrich. 3-(4,5-Dimethylthiazol-2-yl)-2,5-diphenyltetrazolium bromide (MTT) and lipopolysaccharide (LPS) were obtained from Sigma Aldrich (St Louis, MO, USA). PDGF-BB and TNF-α were purchased from R & D systems (Minneapolis, MN, USA). All remaining common laboratory chemical reagents or solvents were purchased from Sigma-Aldrich, South Korea.

2.2. Cell Culture

VSMC from human aorta obtained from ATCC, USA and RAW264.7 cells purchased from Korean cell line bank (Seoul, Korea) were cultured in complete cell culture media with Dulbecco's modified Eagle's medium (DMEM), 10% fetal bovine serum (FBS), and 1% antibiotics (penicillin + streptomycin) in a standard cell incubator with 5% CO_2. The cells were incubated in media with 0.1% FBS for 24 h to allow them to synchronize at G0 phase for each assay. Liensinine was solubilized in dimethyl sulfoxide (DMSO) and diluted in a serum-free medium for treatment of cells. The final % of DMSO while treating cells were below 0.1%.

2.3. DPPH Assay and Thiobarbituric Acid Reactive Substance (TBARS) Assay for Lipid Peroxidation Assay

The anti-oxidant activity of liensinine was evaluated using a DPPH free radical scavenging assay and measurement of serum lipid peroxidation was carried out using TBARS assay following the methods as described previously [11].

2.4. Proliferation Assay

PDGF-BB was used as a proliferation inducer in VSMC and % proliferation was measured by MTT colorimetric assay as described previously [24]. VSMC were treated with liensinine 1 h before PDGF-BB and incubated for 24 h to allow proliferation. Freshly prepared MTT in phosphate buffer saline was added and incubated for an additional 4 h. The purple color formazan developed due to the reduction of MTT by viable VSMC were dissolved with DMSO. Then, a colorimetric reading was taken by measuring absorbance at 540 nm with a microplate reader. The anti-proliferative effect of liensinine was evaluated by comparison with the control group (treated with PDGF-BB) as 100%.

2.5. Gelatin Zymography

Gelatin zymography was carried out to examine the enzymatic activity of MMP-9 as described previously [14]. Briefly, VSMC were seeded in 60 mm petri plates at the density of 1×10^6 cells. Liensinine was added at a predetermined concentration for 1 h and cells were treated with TNF-α (100 ng/mL) for the next 24 h. The supernatant cell culture media was collected and 30 μg of protein equivalent was used for electrophoresis in 10% SDS-PAGE with 0.25% gelatin. Next, the gels were incubated in renaturating buffer (2.5% Triton X-100) for half-an-hour and incubated again in developing buffer at 37 °C for 16–24 h. In order to visualize the bands of MMP2 and MMP-9, gels were stained with 0.05% Coomassie Brilliant Blue followed by incubation in destaining buffer. Photographs of the gel were taken to observe the proteolysis of gelatin by MMP-2 and MMP-9.

2.6. Determination of IL-6 Release in TNF-α Stimulated VSMC

VSMC was pretreated with 1–30 μM of liensinine for 1 h and further treated with TNF-α for the next 24 h. The level of IL-6 released by cells was measured in culture supernatant using an ELISA kit of IL-6, according to manufacturer's protocol.

2.7. Cell Viability/Cytotoxicity Assay, NO Release and Immunoblot of iNOS, and COX-2 Protein Expression in RAW264.7 Cells

RAW264.7 cell viability or cytotoxicity assay was carried out using the MTT colorimetric assay as described in Section 2.4 (without any stimulant). The NO levels in RAW264.7 cells were evaluated as mentioned previously [25]. Briefly, the cells were treated with 1–20 μM of liensinine for 1 h, then induced with LPS at 1 μg/mL for the next 24 h. The level of NO in culture supernatant was measured by mixing a 1:1 ratio (100 μL) of supernatant: Griess reagent. The colored product was measured calorimetrically by reading absorbance at 540 nm. For protein expression of iNOS and COX-2 in RAW 264.7 cells, immunoblotting was carried out [26].

2.8. Statistical Analysis

Data analysis and graphs were prepared using SigmaPlot or Microsoft Excel. The data are represented as mean ± standard error mean. Multiple groups were compared using one-way analysis of variance (ANOVA) and Duncan's post-hoc test. p-values of < 0.05 were considered as statistically significant.

3. Results

3.1. Liensinine Scavenges DPPH Free Radicals and Inhibits Serum Lipid Peroxidation

Liensinine showed concentration-dependent DPPH free radical scavenging activity as displayed in Figure 2a. The inhibitory concentration 50 (IC_{50}) of liensinine was found to be 1.8 µg/mL. Figure 2b shows the measurement of serum lipid peroxidation. Liensinine at concentrations of 30 and 40 µg/mL showed remarkable reduction of serum lipid peroxidation in terms of TBARS value.

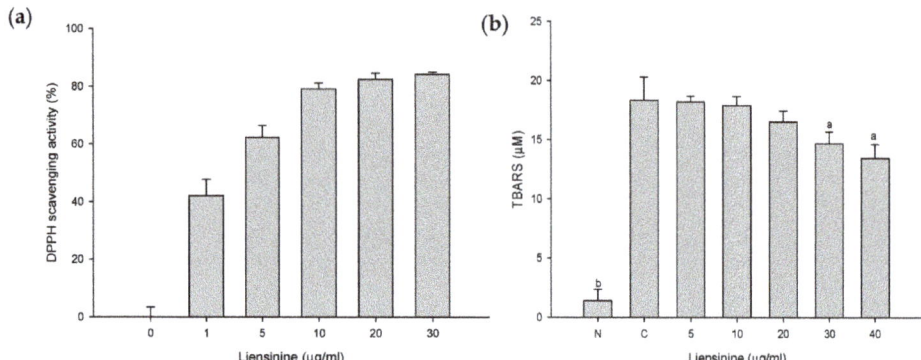

Figure 2. The antioxidant potency of liensinine. (**a**) 1,1-diphenyl-2-picrylhydrazyl (DPPH) free radical scavenging activity (IC$_{50}$ = 1.8 µg/mL and r^2 = 0.94) (**b**) Serum lipid peroxidation inhibitory activity. N represents the normal group (without copper sulphate). ^{a} p < 0.05 and ^{b} p < 0.01 vs. C (the control group; presence of copper sulfate only). n = 3 replicates.

3.2. Liensinine Inhibits VSMC Proliferation

PDGF-BB is a potent growth factor over-expressed in human coronary arteries during atherosclerosis and restenosis [27]. Figure 3 shows the potent anti-proliferative activity of liensinine against PDGF-BB stimulated VSMC proliferation. Liensinine, at a concentrations of 20 and 30 µg/mL notably decreased the % cell proliferation to 67.16% and 47.02%, respectively, vs. 100% of control (PDGF-BB only).

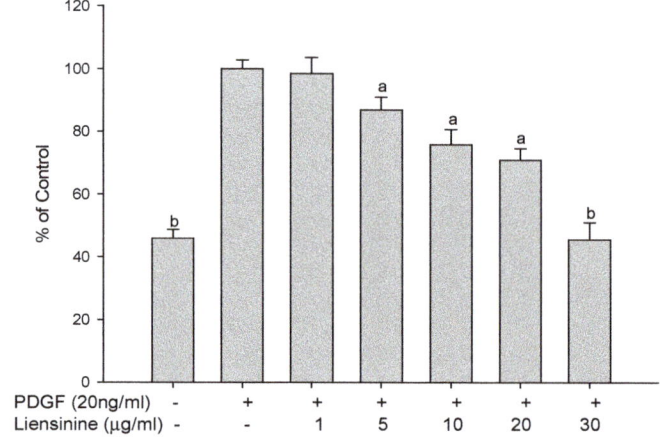

Figure 3. The effect of liensinine on platelet-derived growth factor-BB (PDGF-BB) induced proliferation of human vascular smooth muscle cells (VSMC). VSMC were pretreated with different concentration of liensinine for 1 h followed by stimulation with 20 ng/mL of PDGF-BB for 24 h. The effect on proliferation of VSMC was evaluated by MTT assay. ^{a} p < 0.05 and ^{b} p < 0.01 vs. Control (only PDGF). n = 3 replicates.

3.3. Liensinine Inhibits MMP-9 Enzymatic Action

The degradation of the extracellular matrix by enzymatic action of MMPs (stimulated by various mitogens) is responsible for VSMC migration. TNF-α is one such mitogen/activator that stimulates MMP-9 enzyme activity in VSMCs [28]. The effect of liensinine on the MMP-9 proteolytic degradation of gelatin in VSMCs is displayed in Figure 4. The MMP-9 band was drastically increased by TNF-α (compared to without TNF-α) and decreased concentration dependently by liensinine (compared to TNF-α).

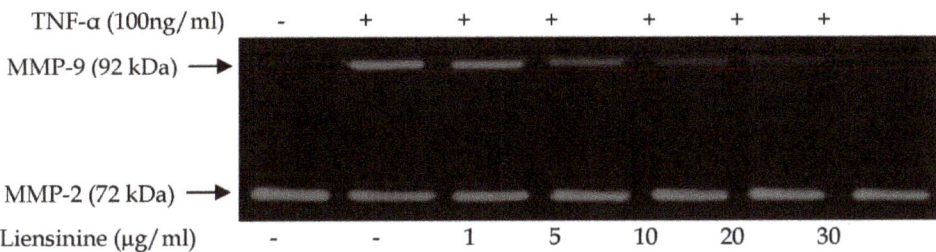

Figure 4. The effect of liensinine on matrix metalloproteinase (MMPs) secretion in TNF-α stimulated VSMC. VSMC were pretreated with different concentrations of liensinine and stimulated with TNF-α. The effect of liensinine on MMPs proteolytic/enzymatic activity was observed by gelatin zymography. The photographs of the gel were taken after Coomassie Brilliant Blue staining. n = 3 replicates.

3.4. Liensinine Inhibits IL-6 in VSMC

As shown in Figure 5, TNF-α significantly increased the IL-6 production in VSMC by 3-fold compared to the control (without TNF-α) while liensinine at a concentration of 10, 20, 30 µg/mL significantly inhibited the IL-6 release.

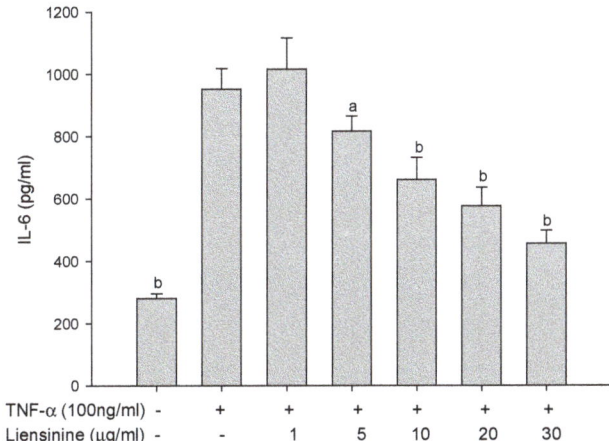

Figure 5. The effect of liensinine in IL-6 release in TNF-α stimulated VSMC. VSMC were pretreated with different concentrations of liensinine and stimulated with TNF-α. The effect of liensinine on IL-6 release was measured by IL-6 ELISA Kit. Liensinine concentration-dependently inhibited the IL-6 release in VSMC. [a] $p < 0.05$ and [b] $p < 0.01$ vs. Control (only TNF-α). n = 3 replicates.

3.5. Liensinine Suppresses NO Production and Inhibit Protein Expression of iNOS and COX-2 in RAW264.7

First, we checked the cytotoxicity of various concentrations of liensinine in RAW264.7 cells. Liensinine up to 20 µM did not exert any significant decrease in RAW264.7 cell viability (Figure 6a). The 24 h treatment of cells with LPS increased the production of NO (95.2 ± 9.8 µM) by approximately 3-fold compared to those without LPS treatment. Liensinine showed inhibition of NO release in a concentration-dependent manner (Figure 6b).

Consistent with NO production, there was an overexpression of iNOS (Figure 6c,d) and COX-2 (Figure 6c,e) proteins after LPS treatment, while liensinine (5–20 μM) treatment resulted in a notable reduction in protein expression.

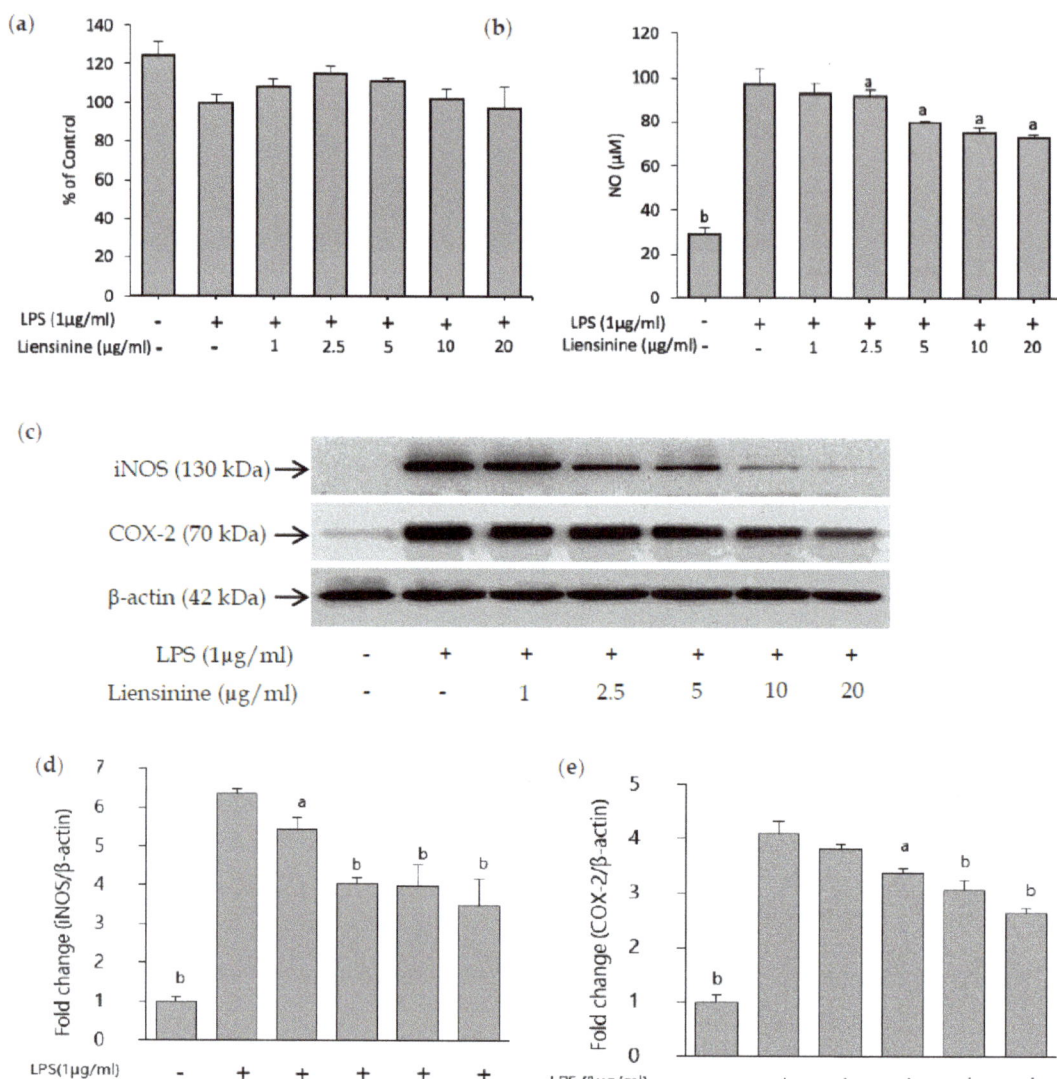

Figure 6. The effects of liensinine on cell viability, nitric oxide (NO) release, and protein expression of iNOS and COX-2. (**a**) Cytotoxicity/cell viability was done by MTT colorimetric assay. (**b**) The effect of liensinine on NO release was determined by Griess reagent assay. (**c**) The expression of the inflammatory proteins iNOS and COX-2 was done by immunoblot. β-actin was used as housekeeping/reference control to calculate relative fold change. (**d**) The fold change of iNOS. (**e**) The fold change of COX-2. [a] $p < 0.05$ and [b] $p < 0.01$ vs. Control (only LPS). n = 3 replicates.

4. Discussion

In our study, we have shown that liensinine inhibits the key features of vascular inflammation mediated by altered VSMC function due to PDGF and TNF-α, and macrophage function by LPS (Figure 7). During vascular inflammation, toxic insults to the blood vessel wall are mediated by oxidative stress, lipid peroxidation, and inflammation mediators released by VSMC and activated macrophage facilitates atherosclerosis progression [29,30]. Under stressful conditions, our bodies generate free radicals such as superoxide anion, which in turn convert NO to peroxynitrite. Peroxynitrite facilitates the oxidative modification of cholesterol to produce enormous quantities of lipid peroxidation byproducts [18]. Blood/serum lipids such as low-density lipoprotein (LDL) are involved in the progression/pathogenesis of numerous diseases including atherosclerosis. Oxidized-LDL upregulates the scavenger receptors on macrophages followed by the increased engulfment of ox-LDL and conversion of macrophages to foam cells characterized by accumulation of fatty streaks [31,32]. Therefore, pharmacological intervention inhibiting serum lipid peroxidation can slow down the process of vascular inflammation. We have previously shown that alkaloid rich fractions of *Nelumbo nucifera* possess strong antioxidant activity and suppress restenosis in a rat model [12]. As liensinine is one of the major alkaloids presents in *Nelumbo nucifera*, we sought to investigate if an antioxidant effect is exerted by liensinine. In our antioxidant activity assay, liensinine showed potent activity as revealed by scavenging the DPPH free radical with IC_{50} of 1.8 µg/mL (Figure 2a) and significantly inhibiting serum lipid peroxidation with 30 and 40 µg/mL concentrations of liensinine (Figure 2b). The DPPH antioxidant activity of liensinine was even better than another major alkaloid, neferine, with IC_{50} of 10.665 µg/mL (17.01 µM) [33].

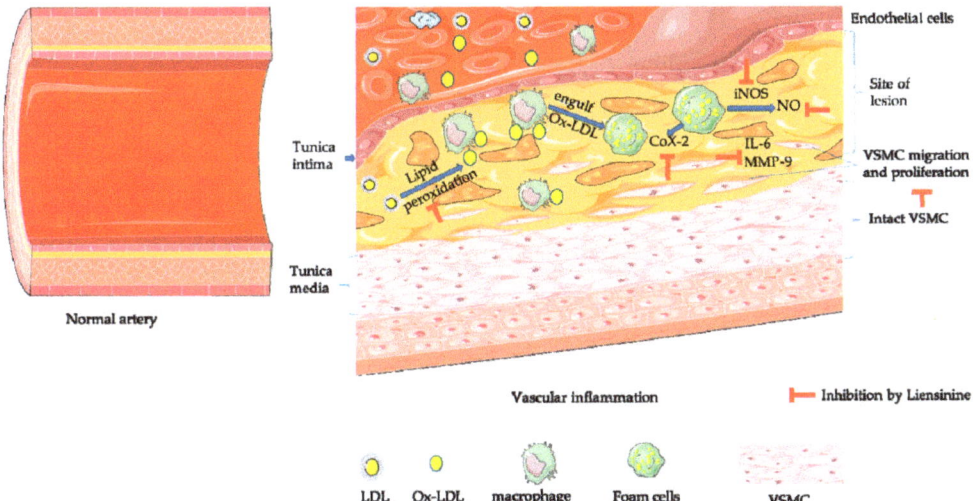

Figure 7. The mechanism of action of liensinine to inhibit vascular inflammation: During the progression of vascular inflammation, low density lipoprotein (LDL) is oxidized to ox-LDL by free radicals and these ox-LDL are engulfed/phagocytized by macrophages. The macrophage converts its phenotype to activated foam cells distinguished by the accumulation of fatty streaks of ox-LDL. These activated macrophages release numbers of inflammation mediators such as nitric oxide (NO), TNF-α, inducible nitric oxide synthase (iNOS) and cyclooxygenase (COX-2). Similarly, the intact vascular smooth cells (VSMC) in the tunica media are activated by cytokines such as TNF-α and growth factor such as PDGF. VSMCs release cytokines such as IL-6 and initiate proliferation mediated by PDGF and migration mediated by matrix metalloproteinase-9 (MMP-9) enzymatic activity at the site of a lesion. Collectively, this process leads to vascular inflammation flowed by atherosclerosis.

In physiological systems, atherogenesis is initiated in major arteries after endothelial dysfunction triggered by oxidative stress, leading to significant changes in the permeability of the vascular intimal layer and resulting in transportation of ox-LDL to the vascular inner layer [34]. After endothelial cells are activated by atherogenic risk factors such as ox-LDL, they overexpress cell adhesion molecules such as intercellular adhesion molecules and vascular cell adhesion molecules to attract circulating cells including monocytes and leukocytes. The transported ox-LDL are engulfed by scavenger receptors of macrophages/monocytes [35]. Macrophages are activated after phagocytosis of ox-LDL and in turn overexpress iNOS and COX-2 [17,36]. It is well established that high iNOS level corresponds with a massive release of NO from macrophages and subsequent inflammatory response [37]. Similarly, LDL also stimulates the production of various prostaglandins through the COX-2 pathway, and these prostaglandins are known to be mitogenic, simulating cell proliferation [38]. Our results showed promising activity of liensinine to suppress NO release from LPS-induced RAW264.7. The 25% reduction of NO by liensinine at a concentration of 20 µg/mL (Figure 6b) was comparable to 20 µM of neferine [33]. Furthermore, liensinine also notably decreased the protein expression of COX-2 and iNOS. The trend of iNOS and COX-2 inhibition shown by liensinine was similar to that shown by glucosamine (a commercially available anti-inflammatory drug) at a concentration of 2.5 to 10 mM in LPS-induced RAW264.7 cells [39].

IL-6 is a well characterized inflammatory mediator and it is released by VSMC after the induction of potent stimulants such as TNF-α [40] and angiotensin II [41]. IL-6 is crucial in vascular remodelling and it, along with ox-LDL, is a potential prognostic marker in predicting cerebral vascular and cardiovascular disorders [42]. In our ELISA result (Figure 5), liensinine suppressed the TNF-α induced IL-6 level in VSMC by approximately 50% at 30 µg/mL concentration. During atherosclerosis, the vascular lumen is narrowed by a fibrous cap composed of (among many other things) VSMC and extracellular matrix. Various growth factors and cytokines produced by endothelial cells and inflammatory cells contribute to the proliferation and migration of VSMC leading to fibrous cap formation [29,43,44]. Cytokines like PDGF can induce proliferation of VSMC to a significantly high level, whereas TNF-α is known to stimulate the migration of VSMC from tunica media to the site of a lesion by increasing MMP-9 expression. MMP-9 is a key gelatinolytic enzyme responsible for the degradation of the elastic lamina barrier of the extra cellular matrix [45,46]. In our previous publications, we have shown that PDGF and TNF-α promote the proliferation and MMP-9-dependent migration of VSMC [11,12,14]. In our result, liensinine inhibited the PDGF-BB induced proliferation/growth of VSMC, revealing its potent anti-proliferating activity. At a 30 µg/mL concentration of liensinine, the proliferation of VSMC was almost completely inhibited to the level of the control (without PDGF) (Figure 3). The potent anti-proliferative activity of liensinine at a concentration of 30 µg/mL is comparable to 50 µM of epigallocatechin-3-O-gallate [47] and 20mM of carnosine [48]. Likewise, liensinine at a concentration of 10, 20 and 30 µg/mL significantly attenuated the expression of MMP-9 induced by TNF-α (Figure 4). We speculate that the notable inhibition of MMP-9 enzymatic activity by *Nelumbo nucifera* leaf extract in our previous study, at a concentration of 250 µg/mL, was in part exerted by liensinine [23]. Taken together, our results provide the mechanistic pathway to attenuate the progression of atherogenesis via controlling vascular inflammation by liensinine possibly by targeting VSMC proliferation, MMP-9 expression and inflammatory mediators released by macrophages (Figure 7).

5. Conclusions

Our results showed that liensinine can effectively prevent the progression of atherosclerosis by modulating the mediators of vascular inflammation via inhibiting the migration and proliferation of VSMC as well as attenuating the release of inflammatory mediators from RAW264.7. Our research is limited to an in vitro experiment, therefore further research is necessary to explore the protective role of liensinine in the pathophysiology of atherosclerosis. It would be worth conducting an in vivo study in a pre-clinical animal model of atherosclerosis and exploring the promising activity of liensinine.

Author Contributions: Conceptualization, D.-W.K. and M.Y.J.; methodology, R.K. and K.R.P.; software, M.Y.J. and R.K.; investigation, M.Y.J. and R.K.; writing—original draft preparation, R.K., K.R.P.; writing—R.K. and K.R.P.; review and editing, N.P. and H.P.D.; supervision, D.-W.K. All authors have read and agreed to the published version of the manuscript.

Funding: This research received no external funding.

Institutional Review Board Statement: Not applicable.

Informed Consent Statement: Not applicable.

Data Availability Statement: The data presented in this study are available on request from the corresponding author.

Acknowledgments: The authors would like to acknowledge the research support provided by Mokpo National University, Muan-gun, Jeonnam, Korea.

Conflicts of Interest: The authors declare no conflict of interest.

References

1. Stemme, S.; Faber, B.; Holm, J.; Wiklund, O.; Witztum, J.L.; Hansson, G.K. T lymphocytes from human atherosclerotic plaques recognize oxidized low density lipoprotein. *Proc. Natl. Acad. Sci. USA* **1995**, *92*, 3893–3897. [CrossRef] [PubMed]
2. Libby, P.; Ridker, P.M.; Maseri, A. Inflammation and atherosclerosis. *Circulation* **2002**, *105*, 1135–1143. [CrossRef] [PubMed]
3. Choi, K.H.; Kim, J.E.; Song, N.R.; Son, J.E.; Hwang, M.K.; Byun, S.; Kim, J.H.; Lee, K.W.; Lee, H.J. Phosphoinositide 3-kinase is a novel target of piceatannol for inhibiting PDGF-BB-induced proliferation and migration in human aortic smooth muscle cells. *Cardiovasc. Res.* **2010**, *85*, 836–844. [CrossRef] [PubMed]
4. Paudel, K.R.; Kim, D.W. Microparticles-Mediated Vascular Inflammation and its Amelioration by Antioxidant Activity of Baicalin. *Antioxidants* **2020**, *9*, 890. [CrossRef] [PubMed]
5. Huber, S.A.; Sakkinen, P.; Conze, D.; Hardin, N.; Tracy, R. Interleukin-6 exacerbates early atherosclerosis in mice. *Arterioscler. Thromb. Vasc. Biol.* **1999**, *19*, 2364–2367. [CrossRef]
6. Moon, S.K.; Cha, B.Y.; Kim, C.H. ERK1/2 mediates TNF-alpha-induced matrix metalloproteinase-9 expression in human vascular smooth muscle cells via the regulation of NF-kappaB and AP-1: Involvement of the ras dependent pathway. *J. Cell Physiol.* **2004**, *198*, 417–427. [CrossRef]
7. Zhang, X.; Hu, W.; Wu, F.; Yuan, X.; Hu, J. Shikonin inhibits TNF-alpha-induced growth and invasion of rat aortic vascular smooth muscle cells. *Can. J. Physiol. Pharmacol.* **2015**, *93*, 615–624. [CrossRef]
8. Yang, G.; Zhou, X.; Chen, T.; Deng, Y.; Yu, D.; Pan, S.; Song, Y. Hydroxysafflor yellow A inhibits lipopolysaccharide-induced proliferation and migration of vascular smooth muscle cells via Toll-like receptor-4 pathway. *Int. J. Clin. Exp. Med.* **2015**, *8*, 5295–5302.
9. Osman, I.; Segar, L. Pioglitazone, a PPARgamma agonist, attenuates PDGF-induced vascular smooth muscle cell proliferation through AMPK-dependent and AMPK-independent inhibition of mTOR/p70S6K and ERK signaling. *Biochem. Pharmacol.* **2016**, *101*, 54–70. [CrossRef]
10. Paudel, K.R.; Oak, M.H.; Kim, D.W. Smooth Muscle Cell Derived Microparticles Acts as Autocrine Activation of Smooth Muscle Cell Proliferation by Mitogen Associated Protein Kinase Upregulation. *J. Nanosci. Nanotechnol.* **2020**, *20*, 5746–5750. [CrossRef]
11. Lee, H.H.; Paudel, K.R.; Kim, D.W. Terminalia chebula Fructus Inhibits Migration and Proliferation of Vascular Smooth Muscle Cells and Production of Inflammatory Mediators in RAW 264.7. *Evid. Based Complement. Altern. Med.* **2015**, *2015*, 502182. [CrossRef] [PubMed]
12. Jun, M.Y.; Karki, R.; Paudel, K.R.; Sharma, B.R.; Adhikari, D.; Kim, D.W. Alkaloid rich fraction from Nelumbo nucifera targets VSMC proliferation and migration to suppress restenosis in balloon-injured rat carotid artery. *Atherosclerosis* **2016**, *248*, 179–189. [CrossRef] [PubMed]
13. Whatling, C.; McPheat, W.; Hurt-Camejo, E. Matrix management: Assigning different roles for MMP-2 and MMP-9 in vascular remodeling. *Arterioscler. Thromb. Vasc. Biol.* **2004**, *24*, 10–11. [CrossRef] [PubMed]
14. Paudel, K.R.; Karki, R.; Kim, D.W. Cepharanthine inhibits in vitro VSMC proliferation and migration and vascular inflammatory responses mediated by RAW264.7. *Toxicol. In Vitro* **2016**, *34*, 16–25. [CrossRef]
15. Maiolino, G.; Rossitto, G.; Caielli, P.; Bisogni, V.; Rossi, G.P.; Calo, L.A. The role of oxidized low-density lipoproteins in atherosclerosis: The myths and the facts. *Mediat. Inflamm.* **2013**, *2013*, 714653. [CrossRef]
16. Lee, H.H.; Paudel, K.R.; Jeong, J.; Wi, A.J.; Park, W.S.; Kim, D.W.; Oak, M.H. Antiatherogenic Effect of Camellia japonica Fruit Extract in High Fat Diet-Fed Rats. *Evid. Based Complement. Altern. Med.* **2016**, *2016*, 9679867. [CrossRef]

17. Baker, C.S.; Hall, R.J.; Evans, T.J.; Pomerance, A.; Maclouf, J.; Creminon, C.; Yacoub, M.H.; Polak, J.M. Cyclooxygenase-2 is widely expressed in atherosclerotic lesions affecting native and transplanted human coronary arteries and colocalizes with inducible nitric oxide synthase and nitrotyrosine particularly in macrophages. *Arterioscler. Thromb. Vasc. Biol.* **1999**, *19*, 646–655. [CrossRef]
18. Panth, N.; Paudel, K.R.; Parajuli, K. Reactive Oxygen Species: A Key Hallmark of Cardiovascular Disease. *Adv. Med.* **2016**, *2016*, 9152732. [CrossRef]
19. Meng, X.-L.; Chen, M.-L.; Chen, C.-L.; Gao, C.-C.; Li, C.; Wang, D.; Liu, H.-S.; Xu, C.-B. Bisbenzylisoquinoline alkaloids of lotus (Nelumbo nucifera Gaertn.) seed embryo inhibit lipopolysaccharide-induced macrophage activation via suppression of Ca^{2+}-CaM/CaMKII pathway. *Food Agric. Immunol.* **2019**, *30*, 878–896. [CrossRef]
20. Meng, X.-L.; Zheng, L.-C.; Liu, J.; Gao, C.-C.; Qiu, M.-C.; Liu, Y.-Y.; Lu, J.; Wang, D.; Chen, C.-L. Inhibitory effects of three bisbenzylisoquinoline alkaloids on lipopolysaccharide-induced microglial activation. *RSC Adv.* **2017**, *7*, 18347–18357. [CrossRef]
21. Sharma, B.R.; Gautam, L.N.; Adhikari, D.; Karki, R. A Comprehensive Review on Chemical Profiling of Nelumbo Nucifera: Potential for Drug Development. *Phytother. Res.* **2017**, *31*, 3–26. [CrossRef] [PubMed]
22. Paudel, K.R.; Panth, N. Phytochemical Profile and Biological Activity of Nelumbo nucifera. *Evid. Based Complement. Altern. Med.* **2015**, *2015*, 789124. [CrossRef] [PubMed]
23. Karki, R.; Jeon, E.R.; Kim, D.W. Nelumbo nucifera leaf extract inhibits neointimal hyperplasia through modulation of smooth muscle cell proliferation and migration. *Nutrition* **2013**, *29*, 268–275. [CrossRef] [PubMed]
24. Panth, N.; Paudel, K.R.; Gong, D.S.; Oak, M.H. Vascular Protection by Ethanol Extract of Morus alba Root Bark: Endothelium-Dependent Relaxation of Rat Aorta and Decrease of Smooth Muscle Cell Migration and Proliferation. *Evid. Based Complement. Altern. Med.* **2018**, *2018*, 7905763. [CrossRef] [PubMed]
25. Paudel, K.R.; Wadhwa, R.; Mehta, M.; Chellappan, D.K.; Hansbro, P.M.; Dua, K. Rutin loaded liquid crystalline nanoparticles inhibit lipopolysaccharide induced oxidative stress and apoptosis in bronchial epithelial cells in vitro. *Toxicol. In Vitro* **2020**, *68*, 104961. [CrossRef] [PubMed]
26. Kim, T.M.; Paudel, K.R.; Kim, D.W. Eriobotrya japonica leaf extract attenuates airway inflammation in ovalbumin-induced mice model of asthma. *J. Ethnopharmacol.* **2020**, *253*, 112082. [CrossRef]
27. Tanizawa, S.; Ueda, M.; van der Loos, C.M.; van der Wal, A.C.; Becker, A.E. Expression of platelet derived growth factor B chain and beta receptor in human coronary arteries after percutaneous transluminal coronary angioplasty: An immunohistochemical study. *Heart* **1996**, *75*, 549–556. [CrossRef]
28. Karki, R.; Jeon, E.R.; Kim, D.W. Magnoliae Cortex inhibits intimal thickening of carotid artery through modulation of proliferation and migration of vascular smooth muscle cells. *Food Chem. Toxicol.* **2012**, *50*, 634–640. [CrossRef]
29. Ross, R. Atherosclerosis—An inflammatory disease. *N. Engl. J. Med.* **1999**, *340*, 115–126. [CrossRef]
30. Paudel, K.R.; Panth, N.; Kim, D.W. Circulating Endothelial Microparticles: A Key Hallmark of Atherosclerosis Progression. *Scientifica* **2016**, *2016*, 8514056. [CrossRef]
31. Paudel, K.R.; Lee, U.W.; Kim, D.W. Chungtaejeon, a Korean fermented tea, prevents the risk of atherosclerosis in rats fed a high-fat atherogenic diet. *J. Integr. Med.* **2016**, *14*, 134–142. [CrossRef]
32. Steinberg, D. Role of oxidized LDL and antioxidants in atherosclerosis. *Adv. Exp. Med. Biol.* **1995**, *369*, 39–48. [CrossRef] [PubMed]
33. Jung, H.A.; Jin, S.E.; Choi, R.J.; Kim, D.H.; Kim, Y.S.; Ryu, J.H.; Kim, D.W.; Son, Y.K.; Park, J.J.; Choi, J.S. Anti-amnesic activity of neferine with antioxidant and anti-inflammatory capacities, as well as inhibition of ChEs and BACE1. *Life Sci.* **2010**, *87*, 420–430. [CrossRef] [PubMed]
34. Tabas, I.; Williams, K.J.; Boren, J. Subendothelial lipoprotein retention as the initiating process in atherosclerosis: Update and therapeutic implications. *Circulation* **2007**, *116*, 1832–1844. [CrossRef]
35. Stephen, S.L.; Freestone, K.; Dunn, S.; Twigg, M.W.; Homer-Vanniasinkam, S.; Walker, J.H.; Wheatcroft, S.B.; Ponnambalam, S. Scavenger receptors and their potential as therapeutic targets in the treatment of cardiovascular disease. *Int. J. Hypertens.* **2010**, *2010*, 646929. [CrossRef]
36. Karki, R.; Park, C.H.; Kim, D.W. Extract of buckwheat sprouts scavenges oxidation and inhibits pro-inflammatory mediators in lipopolysaccharide-stimulated macrophages (RAW264.7). *J. Integr. Med.* **2013**, *11*, 246–252. [CrossRef]
37. Crow, J.P.; Beckman, J.S. Reactions between nitric oxide, superoxide, and peroxynitrite: Footprints of peroxynitrite in vivo. *Adv. Pharmacol.* **1995**, *34*, 17–43. [CrossRef]
38. Kreuzer, J.; Denger, S.; Jahn, L.; Bader, J.; Ritter, K.; von Hodenberg, E.; Kubler, W. LDL stimulates chemotaxis of human monocytes through a cyclooxygenase-dependent pathway. *Arterioscler. Thromb. Vasc. Biol.* **1996**, *16*, 1481–1487. [CrossRef]
39. Rafi, M.M.; Yadav, P.N.; Rossi, A.O. Glucosamine inhibits LPS-induced COX-2 and iNOS expression in mouse macrophage cells (RAW 264.7) by inhibition of p38-MAP kinase and transcription factor NF-kappaB. *Mol. Nutr. Food Res.* **2007**, *51*, 587–593. [CrossRef]
40. Wang, Z.; Castresana, M.R.; Newman, W.H. NF-kappaB is required for TNF-alpha-directed smooth muscle cell migration. *FEBS Lett.* **2001**, *508*, 360–364. [CrossRef]
41. Funakoshi, Y.; Ichiki, T.; Ito, K.; Takeshita, A. Induction of interleukin-6 expression by angiotensin II in rat vascular smooth muscle cells. *Hypertension* **1999**, *34*, 118–125. [CrossRef] [PubMed]
42. Lobbes, M.B.; Lutgens, E.; Heeneman, S.; Cleutjens, K.B.; Kooi, M.E.; van Engelshoven, J.M.; Daemen, M.J.; Nelemans, P.J. Is there more than C-reactive protein and fibrinogen? The prognostic value of soluble CD40 ligand, interleukin-6 and oxidized low-density lipoprotein with respect to coronary and cerebral vascular disease. *Atherosclerosis* **2006**, *187*, 18–25. [CrossRef]

43. Lusis, A.J. Atherosclerosis. *Nature* **2000**, *407*, 233–241. [CrossRef] [PubMed]
44. Libby, P.; Okamoto, Y.; Rocha, V.Z.; Folco, E. Inflammation in atherosclerosis: Transition from theory to practice. *Circ. J.* **2010**, *74*, 213–220. [CrossRef]
45. Karki, R.; Ho, O.M.; Kim, D.W. Magnolol attenuates neointima formation by inducing cell cycle arrest via inhibition of ERK1/2 and NF-kappaB activation in vascular smooth muscle cells. *Biochim. Biophys. Acta* **2013**, *1830*, 2619–2628. [CrossRef] [PubMed]
46. Karki, R.; Kim, S.B.; Kim, D.W. Magnolol inhibits migration of vascular smooth muscle cells via cytoskeletal remodeling pathway to attenuate neointima formation. *Exp. Cell Res.* **2013**, *319*, 3238–3250. [CrossRef]
47. Lee, M.H.; Kwon, B.J.; Koo, M.A.; You, K.E.; Park, J.C. Mitogenesis of vascular smooth muscle cell stimulated by platelet-derived growth factor-bb is inhibited by blocking of intracellular signaling by epigallocatechin-3-O-gallate. *Oxid. Med. Cell. Longev.* **2013**, *2013*, 827905. [CrossRef]
48. Hwang, B.; Song, J.H.; Park, S.L.; Kim, J.T.; Kim, W.J.; Moon, S.K. Carnosine Impedes PDGF-Stimulated Proliferation and Migration of Vascular Smooth Muscle Cells In Vitro and Sprout Outgrowth Ex Vivo. *Nutrients* **2020**, *12*, 2697. [CrossRef]

Article

A Molecular Insight into the Synergistic Mechanism of *Nigella sativa* (Black Cumin) with β-Lactam Antibiotics against Clinical Isolates of Methicillin-Resistant *Staphylococcus aureus*

Lorina I. Badger-Emeka [1,*], Promise Madu Emeka [2] and Hairul Islam M. Ibrahim [3]

1. Department of Biomedical Sciences, Microbiology Division, College of Medicine, King Faisal University, Hofuf 31982, Saudi Arabia
2. Department of Pharmaceutical Science, College of Clinical Pharmacy, King Faisal University, Hofuf 31982, Saudi Arabia; pemeka@kfu.edu.sa
3. Department of Biological Sciences, College of Science, King Faisal University, Hofuf 31982, Saudi Arabia; himo-hamed@kfu.edu.sa
* Correspondence: lbadgeremeka@kfu.edu.sa; Tel.: +966-(0)-536542793

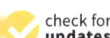

Citation: Badger-Emeka, L.I.; Emeka, P.M.; Ibrahim, H.I.M. A Molecular Insight into the Synergistic Mechanism of *Nigella sativa* (Black Cumin) with β-Lactam Antibiotics against Clinical Isolates of Methicillin-Resistant *Staphylococcus aureus*. *Appl. Sci.* **2021**, *11*, 3206. https://doi.org/10.3390/app11073206

Academic Editor: Hari Prasad Devkota

Received: 15 March 2021
Accepted: 31 March 2021
Published: 2 April 2021

Publisher's Note: MDPI stays neutral with regard to jurisdictional claims in published maps and institutional affiliations.

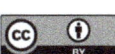

Copyright: © 2021 by the authors. Licensee MDPI, Basel, Switzerland. This article is an open access article distributed under the terms and conditions of the Creative Commons Attribution (CC BY) license (https://creativecommons.org/licenses/by/4.0/).

Abstract: Methicillin-resistant *Staphylococcus aureus* (MRSA) infection is detrimental to hospitalized patients. With diminishing choices of antibiotics and the worry about resistance to colistin in synergistic combined therapy, there are suggestions for the use of herbal derivatives. This investigation evaluated the synergistic effects of *Nigella sativa* (NS) in combination with beta-lactam (β-lactam) antibiotics on extreme drug-resistant (XDR) MRSA isolates. NS concentrations of 10, 7.5, 5.0, 2.5, 1.0, and 0.1 µg/mL, alone and in combination with β-lactam antibiotics, were used to determine the antimicrobial susceptibility of MRSA isolates by the well diffusion method. Time–kill assays were performed using a spectrophotometer, with time–kill curves plotted and synergism ascertained by the fractional inhibitory concentration (FIC). Scanning and transmission electron microscopy were used to gain insight into the mechanism of action of treated groups. Isolates were inhibited by the NS concentrations, with differences in the zones of inhibition being statistically insignificant at $p < 0.05$. There were statistically significant differences in the time–kill assay for the MRSA isolates. In addition, NS combined with augmentin showed better killing than oxacillin and cefuroxime. The mechanism of action shown by the SEM and TEM results revealed cell wall disruption, which probably created interference that led to bacterial lysis.

Keywords: *Nigella sativa*; methicillin-resistant; *Staphylococcus aureus*; synergism; beta-lactam; antibiotics

1. Introduction

The ongoing healthcare problems attributed to multidrug-resistant (MDR) bacterial infections that are difficult to treat continue to plague healthcare systems globally. Methicillin-resistant *Staphylococcus aureus* (MRSA), one bacterium causing such an infection, remains a pathogen in various regions of the world [1]. Like all MDR bacterial infections, MRSA-linked infections can be associated with extended patient hospitalization, high morbidity, and mortality, especially in immunocompromised patients [1–3]. β-lactam antibiotics were the preferred drugs for the treatment of infections resulting from methicillin-resistant *S. aureus*. Vancomycin, a glycopeptide, still serves as the drug of choice in the treatment of MDR *S. aureus* infections. However, the bacterium has developed resistance to the β-lactams as well as vancomycin [4,5]. Thus, there is a decrease in the number of exogenous antibiotics for treating drug-resistant infections [3]. With a diminishing number of antimicrobials of choice, researchers have called for rationalization on the use of available antibiotics. This is intended to help reduce the rate at which MDR and pan-resistant bacterial superbugs are evolving to prevent the world from being taken back to the pre-antibiotic era [6,7]. Other suggestions are to look into alternatives to antimicrobial treatment due to bacterial resistance to systemic monotherapy that has overtaken the rate of production of new antibiotics [8]. One such alternative is the use of a combination of antibiotics [9]. It is postulated that such combined therapeutic measures could lead to successful management of patients with extreme drug-resistant (XDR) bacterial infections [10–12]. However, the double and triple combined antibiotic therapies suggested by the researchers were all colistin-based [13]. Presently, colistin is a last-line therapeutic option in the treatment of difficult bacterial infections. Besides the toxicity of the drug, there is a growing resistance to this last-line drug, as reported globally [14–17]. These reports necessitate the continued search for alternative antibiotic combinations that will exclude colistin in combined therapeutic measures [18]. There are also suggestions that such antibiotic synergistic combinations might not necessarily be the optimal options because it is thought that, as treatment progresses, there will be diminishing strength in antibiotic synergism [19]. However, as the problem of difficult-to-treat bacterial superbugs persists, the attention of researchers is currently focused on the use of herbal derivatives with antimicrobial properties, with suggestions that such plants could be synergistic enhancers [20,21]. It is thought that such combined therapy can help with expanding the spectrum of antibiotics as well as being less toxic while preventing the emergence of resistant bacteria strains [22].

Due to the expected significant advantages associated with phytotherapy, several researchers are now looking into the effectiveness of combinations of conventional antimicrobials and plant derivatives with antimicrobial properties [22–24]. This is expected to provide less toxic antimicrobial herbal alternatives that could be used as combined therapies in the treatment of XDR bacterial infections. One such plant reported by researchers in different regions of the world due to its impressive antimicrobial properties is *Nigella sativa* (NS), or black cumin [25–27]. In our previous study, we combined *N. sativa* with chloroquine in the treatment of malaria induced in mice with *Plasmodium berghei* [28]. The obtained results showed significant parasite clearance over a significant period, indicating that NS potentiated the effect of chloroquine when compared with chloroquine alone. Middle Eastern and Far Eastern countries have used *Nigella sativa* oil as a natural remedy or as a condiment/spice in food and food products from ancient times. As documented earlier, there is abundant evidence that *Nigella sativa* oil has been used in combination with synthetic medicines to treat various diseases due to its strong anti-inflammatory and antioxidant properties [28]. Studies have shown that *Nigella sativa* essential oil contains both volatile and nonvolatile bioactive compounds. It also contains alkaloids, saponins, and terpenoids, which are reported to possess antimicrobial activity [27]. Thymoquinone and thymol are the most reported active volatile constituents, possessing antitumor, antihistaminic, antidiabetic, antihypertensive, anti-inflammatory, and antimicrobial abilities. Numerous studies have reported the antimicrobial and antiparasitic activities [28].

The present work therefore looks at a possible synergistic effect of *N. sativa* with common antibiotics that show treatment failures with bacterial infections due to resistance to these drugs. The use of *N. sativa* with the aforementioned antibiotics could enhance their antimicrobial efficacy. This study aims at evaluating the synergistic effect of combining *N. sativa* with oxacillin (OXA), augmentin (AUG), and cefuroxime (CEF) on different XDR MRSA isolates, as well as looking into the possible mechanism of action of *N. sativa* on the isolates.

2. Materials and Methods

2.1. Ethical Considerations

Approval for the research was given by the Deanship of Scientific Research (approval number: 186388). MRSA clinical isolates were from routine hospital diagnoses for care of patients. They were from the microbial bank at the College of Medicine, Medical Microbiology division, of King Faisal University.

2.2. Bacterial Isolates and Antimicrobial Susceptibility Determination

Six non-replicate clinical MRSA isolates from specimens of blood, sputum, pus, and wound swaps were used for the investigation. They had been stored in the Microbank of the Microbiology division of the College of Medicine, King Faisal University at a temperature of −80 °C. They were cultured on blood agar and incubated aerobically at 37 °C for 24 h. Isolates were identified with a Vitek compact 2 automated system (BioMerieux, Marcy L'Etoile, France) using the Gram-positive ID cards according to the guidelines of the manufacturer. The antimicrobial susceptibility and minimum inhibitory concentrations were determined using the AST-GN cards of the Vitek 2 compact automated system (BioMerieux, Marcy L'Etoile, France). They were against the following antibiotics: augmentin (AUG), benzyl penicillin (BENZ), oxacillin (OXA), cefuroxime (CEF), cefuroxime/axetil (CEF/AXE), clindamycin (CLD), amikacin (AK), imipenem (IMP), ciprofloxacin (CIP), levofloxacin (LEVO), erythromycin (ERY), sulfamethoxazole/trimethoprim (SXT), tigecycline (TG), tetracycline (TET), rifampicin (RIF), and gentamicin (GEN). Confirmation of resistance against imipenem (IMP), tigecycline (TG), and amikacin was by disc diffusion method (Oxoid Ltd., Basingstoke UK). All of the MRSA isolates had been confirmed by the presence of the *mecA* gene.

2.3. Nigella sativa and MRSA Susceptibility Test

Nigella sativa (NS) black seed oil, a product of Al Hussan Food Products Factory, Riyadh was purchased from a local herbal medicine shop in Al-Ahsa, Saudi Arabia. According to the manufacturer, it is 100% pure organic cold pressed oil. Undiluted and diluted forms of the oil extract were used for the investigation. Oil extract was diluted in 0.2% dimethyl sulfoxide (DMSO) to obtain concentrations of 1000 µg/mL, 750 µg/mL, 500 µg/mL, 250 µg/mL, and 100 µg/mL dilutions, representing 100%, 75%, 50%, 25%, and 10% concentrations. In these, 0.01 mL of each concentration was used to make the actual concentrations 10, 7.5, 5.0, 2.5, and 1.0 µg/mL. The susceptibility of the isolates was tested against these dilutions of NS by the well diffusion method. Mueller-Hinton agar (MHA) was seeded with each bacterial isolate and spread out to cover the entire surface of the agar using sterile cotton swabs, moistened with the bacterial suspension [29,30]. Seven evenly distributed wells were punched into the MHA using a sterile cork borer of 6 mm diameter. The six NS dilutions were introduced into the wells aseptically, while the seventh well, serving as the control, was filled with an equal volume of 0.2% DMSO. All plates were allowed to diffuse under room temperature for 1 h according to the recommendations of the National Committee for Clinical Laboratory standards (NCCLS). All plates were incubated aerobically at 37 °C for 24 h in an upright position. Experiments were carried out in three replicates with zones of inhibition measured in millimeters (mm) 24 h post-incubation, and the results are presented as means ± standard deviation.

2.4. Determination of Time–Kill Assay

The CLSI guidelines were used for the determination of the time–kill assay using a nutrient broth (NB) [31]. MRSA bacteria strains 1, 4, and 5, which were randomly selected from six phenotypically different isolates, were inoculated into tubes containing NB to form a 5×10^5 CFU/mL bacteria suspension. They were each tested against combinations of NS, OXA, AUG, and CEF and for the time–kill assay. Tubes contained NB, a bacterial strain, and NS, while a second set had the bacterial strain, NB, NS, and one antibiotic. According to the McFarland standard, all bacterial suspensions were diluted to about 10^6 CFU/mL and incubated aerobically at 37 °C in an orbital shaker for 48 h. At hours 0, 1, 3, 6, 24, and 48, 2 mL of each suspension were drawn out from each tube and inoculated into blood agar. The inoculum was spread out using sterile inoculating loops, with all plates incubated aerobically at 37 °C for 24 h. The viability of the MRSA isolates was evaluated by counting the bacterial colonies or noting the lack of microbial growth [3], while time–kill analysis curves were plotted with synergism, defined as described earlier [32,33].

2.5. Antimicrobial Synergistic NS and β-Lactam Antibiotics Assay

Bacterial strains were tested against the two concentrations of NS (7.5 µg/mL and 5.0 µg/mL) and each with the combination of the three β-lactam antibiotics to evaluate the synergistic activity with oxacillin (OXA), augmentin (AUG), and cefuroxime (CEF). The antimicrobial agents were used at their break points (OXA: 1 mg; AUG: 20/10 mg; CEF: 30 mg). Synergistic assay on MRSA strains 1, 4, and 5 was accessed using a spectrophotometer (BOECO, Hamburg Germany) with the additive/synergy effect calculated as earlier described [32,34,35]. Accordingly, the fractional inhibitory concentration (FIC) of each agent was calculated using the following formula:

OD_{600} of wells of agent in combination with the drug.
OD_{600} of wells of agent alone.

2.6. Molecular Assay by SEM and TEM Microscopy

SEM and TEM imaging were performed to evaluate the treatment effects on both the bacterial surface and within bacterial cells. The previously described method was used for the preparation of MRSA bacterial samples for scanning electron microscopy (SEM) [36]. Treated bacterial cultures as well as untreated samples that served as controls were incubated in a shaker incubator at 37 °C for 24 h. The resulting samples were centrifuged and prefixed in a 2.5% glutaraldehyde solution at 4 °C for 24 h, after which they were rinsed in PBS and post-fixed with 100% acetone applied at the last stage. Gold sputtering was used to obtain a layer 20 nm thick. The images were obtained with SEM (JSM 6390 LA, JEOL, Tokyo, Japan) at a 15 KV accelerating voltage.

Preparation and observation of TEM microscopy samples is as described previously, but with modifications [37,38]. Slices of selected MRSA bacterial samples were fixed by immersion in 2.5% glutaraldehyde (GA) in a 0.1 M sodium cacodylate buffer with pH 7.4 at a temperature of 4 °C for 1 h, then washed in cacodylate buffer. All bacterial samples were double-fixed in 1% osmium tetroxide (OsO_4) in a cacodylate buffer at room temperature for 90 min. They were then dehydrated in acetone and embedded in Epon-Araldite (502 kit, Pelco, CA, USA). Then, 500–1000 nm sections of bacteria samples were obtained in a Leica EM UC6 (Wetzlar, Germany), ultra-microtome mounted on glass slides, stained with 1% toluidine blue stain. For light microscopy observations, bacterial samples were further dissected to 50-70 nm [37]. Staining of Epon-sectioned samples was carried out with the Leica automated EM stain (0.5% uranyl acetate and 3% lead citrate). All samples' sections were scanned and examined using JEM 1011 (JEOL) electron microscope at 80 kv.

2.7. Gas Chromatography/Mass Spectrometry (GC/MS) Analysis

The extract of 100% pure organic cold pressed oil of *Nigella sativa* was analyzed by gas chromatography/mass spectrometry (GC/MS), and data were recorded on a GCMS-QP2010 Plus (Shimadzu Corporation, Kyoto, Japan). The column used was a RTX-5MS® fused silica capillary (30 m × 0.25 mm i.d and 0.25 µm film thickness); the oven temperature initially was held at 45 °C for 2 min and then increased to 280 °C at 4 °C/min. The carrier gas was helium with a flow rate of 2.0 mL/min; the temperature of the injector and detector were 250 and 300 °C, respectively, the split ratio was 1:30, and the injection volume was 1 µL. The ionization energy for the mass spectrometer was 70 eV. Identification of components was confirmed from the mass spectra library.

2.8. Statistical Analysis

Data are presented as the mean ± SD and the susceptibility analysis is presented in percentages. GraphPad Prism version 8.0 (San Diego, CA, USA) statistical software was used for statistical interpretation of the results. Two-way ANOVA, applying Tukey's multiple comparison test, was used to assess the statistical significance of zones of inhibition of various concentrations of NS on the different MRSA isolates. Additionally, one-way ANOVA, multiple comparison was used to compare the time–kill assay results and to determine the existence of any significant differences. Significance was taken to be $p < 0.05$ and p-values were calculated between groups.

3. Results

3.1. Antimicrobial Susceptibility of the MRSA Isolates

The MRSA isolates in this investigation were highly resistant to other antibiotics, with the exception of tigecycline and gentamicin, with resistance of 17% and 33%, respectively (Figure 1). The minimum inhibitory concentration (MIC) results are shown in Table 1. Differences in antimicrobial susceptibility and MIC values show that the isolates differ phenotypically. This difference is also seen in the antimicrobial susceptibility to the dilutions of NS, as shown in Figure 2 for all the MRSA isolates. All the isolates were inhibited by the various concentrations of NS, including the lowest concentration of 0.1 µg/mL, as shown in Figure 2. The least effective of the NS concentrations against the MRSA isolates was 0.1 µg/mL, which exhibited the lowest inhibitory effect among the isolates, with the exception of MRSA 2. Overall, there was no specific pattern in antimicrobial inhibition, as all the isolates responded differently to the NS dilutions. The mean zone of inhibition for MRSA 5 and 6 was more with the 10 µg/mL NS concentration, while MRSA 2 and 3 were inhibited more by the 7.5 and 5.0 µg/mL NS concentrations. For all the isolates, a comparison of differences in mean zones of inhibition between 10.0 µg/mL NS and 7.5, 5.0, and 2.5 µg/mL was not found to be statistically significant.

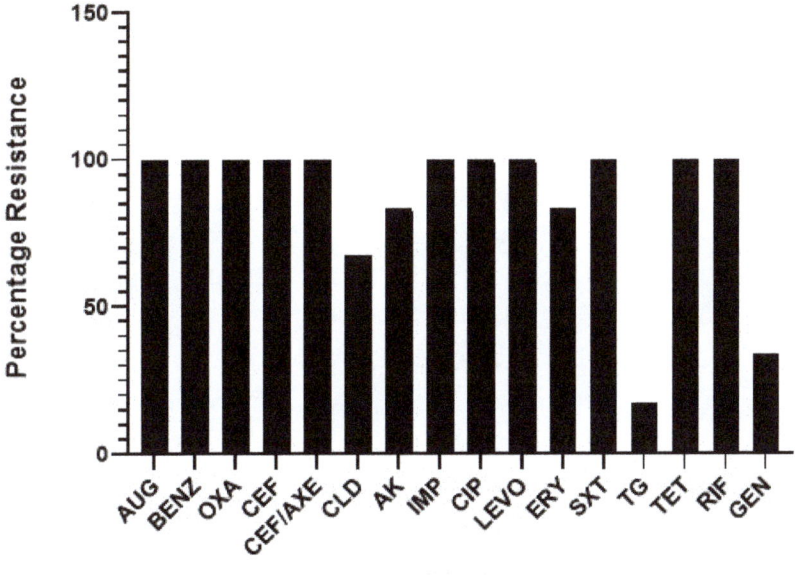

Figure 1. Antimicrobial resistance of methicillin-resistant *Staphylococcus aureus*. Augmentin (AUG), benzyl penicillin (BENZ), oxacillin (OXA), cefuroxime (CEF), cefuroxime/axetil (CEF/AXE), clindamycin (CLD), amikacin (AK), imipenem (IMP), ciprofloxacin (CIP), levofloxacin (LEVO), erythromycin (ERY), sulfamethoxazole/trimethoprim (SXT), tigecycline (TG), tetracycline (TET), rifampicin (RIF), and gentamicin (GEN).

However, comparisons of the mean zones of inhibition for all the isolates with a 10 µg/mL NS concentration and with 1.0 µg/mL as well as 0.1 µg/mL showed statistically significant differences, with p-values of 0.034 and 0.0001, respectively. Additionally, comparisons of the mean zones of inhibition resulting from 7.5 µg/mL, when compared with those resulting from the lower NS concentrations, were statistically similar to those at

10.0 µg/mL NS. Differences in zones of inhibition between this 7.5 µg/mL NS concentration and the 1.0 µg/mL were significant (p-value: 0.0012).

Table 1. Minimum inhibitory concentration of the MRSA isolates against tested antibiotics.

Antibiotic	MRSA 1	MRSA 2	MRSA 3	MRSA 4	MRSA 5	MRSA 6
Augmentin	≤2	≤2	≤2	≤2	≤2	≤2
Benzyl penicillin	≤0.25	≤0.25	≤0.25	≤0.25	≤0.25	≤0.25
Oxacillin	≥4	≥8	≥8	≥4	≥8	≥4
Cefuroxime	≤1	8	2	8	≤1	≤1
Cefuroxime/Axetil	8	≤1	≥64	8	≥64	2
Clindamycin	≤0.5	2	≤0.5	≥4	≥4	≥4
Amikacin	≥16	8	≤4	≥16	≥16	≥16
Imipenem	≤1	≤1	≤1	≤1	≤1	≤1
Ciprofloxacin	≥8	≥8	≥8	≥8	≥8	≥8
Levofloxacin	≥8	≥8	4	≥4	≥8	≥8
Erythromycin	≤0.25	≥8	≥8	≥8	1	≥8
Sulfamethoxazole/trimethoprim	8	16	16	8	16	16
Tigecycline	≤0.12	≤0.12	≤0.12	≤0.12	≤0.12	256
Tetracycline	≥32	≥32	≥32	≥32	≥32	≥320
Rifampicin	≤1	≤0.5	≥4	2	≥4	≥4
Gentamicin	≥16	≤4	≤4	≤4	≤4	8

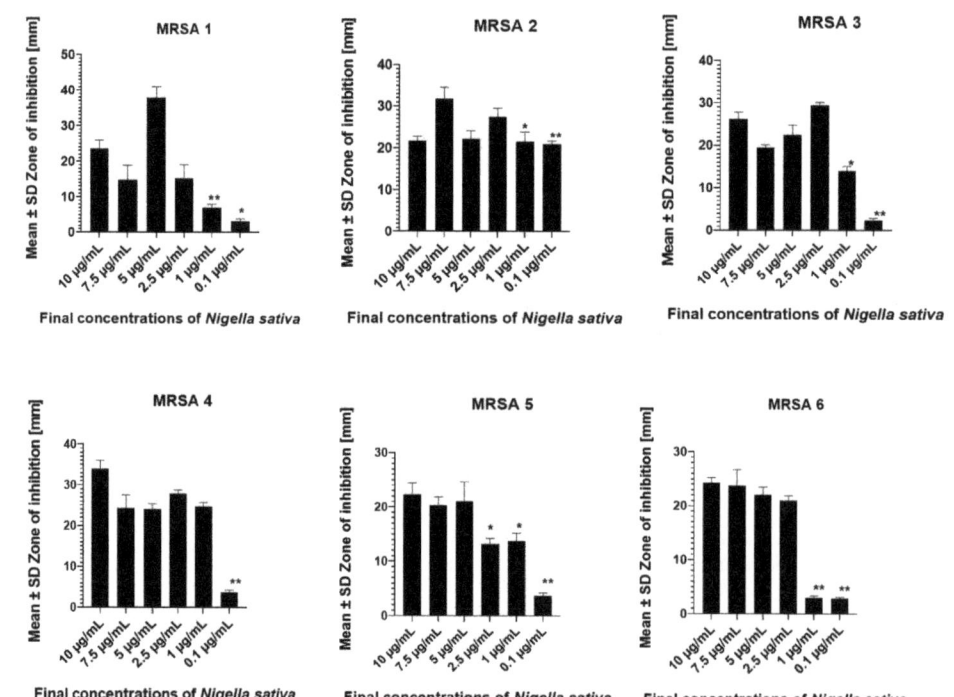

Figure 2. Showing the zones of mean ± SD inhibition of methicillin-resistant *Staphylococcus aureus* (MRSA), MRSA 1–6 bacterial isolates against *Nigella sativa* (NS) dilutions. Comparison of 10 µg/mL and other concentrations. * p-value: 0.034; ** p-value: 0.0001.

MRSA 1 was the isolate that was most inhibited by the 5.0 µg/mL NS dilution. As with the higher NS concentrations, differences in mean zones of inhibition were significant when compared with those of the 1.0 and 0.1 µg/mL NS, with *p*-values of 0.045 and 0.0002, respectively. For the 2.5 µg/mL NS concentration, statistical differences in inhibition zones were significant when compared to the lower NS dilutions (Figure 2).

3.2. Time–Kill Kinetics

Results on the effect of NS alone, and NS in combination with oxacillin (OXA), augmentin (AUG), and/or cefuroxime (CEF) are shown in Figure 3A-F. There were variations in antimicrobial effects based on strains of MRSA, as well as the type of antibiotic tested. A rapid rate of killing was seen more often with combinations of NS and antibiotics than with NS alone.

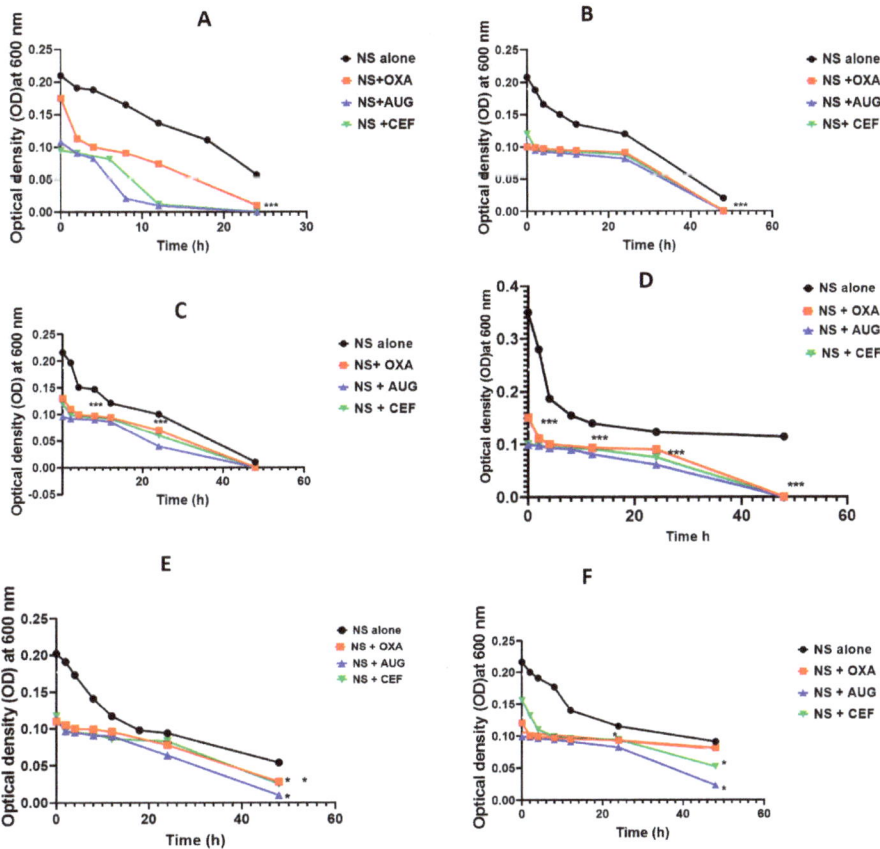

Figure 3. Time–kill assay curves of 7.5 µg/mL concentration of *Nigella sativa* (NS) alone and in combination with antibiotics against (**A**) MRSA 1, (**B**) MRSA 4, and (**C**) MRSA 5 bacterial isolates. (**A**) *** Represents significant values at $p < 0.0039$ for NS + OXA, $p < 0.0016$ for NS + AUG and $p < 0.0142$ for NS + CEF; (**B**) *** Represents significant values at $p < 0.0113$ for NS + OXA, $p < 0.0061$ for NS + AUG and $p < 0.0053$ for NS + CEF; (**C**) *** Represents significant values at $p < 0.0179$ for NS + OXA, $p < 0.0336$ for NS + AUG and $p < 0.0180$ for NS + CEF. Time–kill assay curves of 5.0 µg/mL concentration of *Nigella sativa* (NS) alone and in combination with antibiotics against (**D**) MRSA 1, (**E**) MRSA 4, and (**F**) MRSA 5 bacteria isolates. (**D**) *** Represents significant values at $p < 0.0408$ for NS + OXA, $p < 0.0200$ for NS + AUG and $p < 0.0494$ for NS + CEF; (**b**) * Represents significant values at $p < 0.0331$ for NS + OXA, $p < 0.0083$ for NS + AUG, and $p < 0.0254$ for NS + CEF; (**F**) * Represents significant values at $p < 0.0161$ for NS + OXA, $p < 0.0019$ for NS + AUG and $p < 0.0022$ for NS + CEF.

In the combination of AUG with 7.5 µg/mL NS, the killing rate for MRSA 1 was more rapid than in combinations of NS with CEF and OXA in a time-dependent fashion, as shown in Figure 3A-C. Additionally, differences in these killing times were statistically significant when compared with the control (7.5 µg/mL NS alone). However, for the MRSA 1 time–kill kinetics, although antibiotic combinations with NS displayed a significantly difference in killing time, the time–kill kinetic curve between AUG and OXA did show a statistically significant difference, indicating that time–kill with AUG was more rapid. The results of the MRSA 5 time–kill assay showed significant differences between the NS and antibiotic combinations and NS alone. The killing times for 0-24 h were markedly different from those for 48 h. Additionally, AUG displayed more rapid killing with respect to CEF and OXA. For this group of 7.5 µg/mL NS with antibiotic combination total killing was seen within 24 h for MRSA 1 and 48 h for MRSA 4 and 5 (Figure 3A–C).

The time–kill assay of the 5 µg/mL NS and antibiotic combination is shown in Figure 3D–F for the MRSA isolates 1, 4, and 5. The results showed complete killing for MRSA 1 at 48 h with combinations as compared with the effect of NS alone. The killing was rapid and statistically significant, with AUG showing a more rapid effect as compared to the control. In MRSA 4, the killing was not total but again AUG displayed rapid killing kinetics with CEF, with OXA showing similar rates of killing (Figure 3E). Additionally, for MRSA 5, there was no total killing after 48 h. However, AUG displayed more rapid killing compared to CEF and OXA. In addition, the antibiotic combinations' time–kill kinetics were statistically significant compared to NS alone.

3.3. Synergistic Effect of NS and β-Lactams with FIC Index Analysis

The results presented in Table 2 are those of the FIC index interpretation that defines the time–kill assay synergistically for antibiotics and NS combinations. Combinations of 5.0 µg/mL NS with antibiotics on MRSA 1 displayed synergism. The best effect was with AUG, while the worst was with OXA. Synergism was observed within 4 h on isolates that exhibited extensive resistance to antibiotics. In MRSA 4, a similar pattern was observed, except that synergistic effects were seen for AUG and CEF within 4 h, while with OXA, an additive effect was mostly displayed. For MRSA 5, the combination of NS with CEF had an additive effect compared with AUG and OXA, which displayed synergism within 8 h. Overall, the study with 5 µg/mL combinations clearly indicates a synergistic effect.

Table 2. Fractional inhibitory concentration index synergy interpretation of different MRSA isolates measured at time intervals for combinations of 5.0 µg/mL N. sativa and antibiotics.

Bacterial Isolate/MRSA Type	Antibiotic Combination	Fractional Inhibitory Concentration Index Time (h)				Outcome
		2	4	8	12	
MRSA 1						
	NS + OXA	0.4	0.5	0.7	0.7	Synergism/Additive Effect
	NS + AUG	0.3	0.5	0.6	0.5	Synergism/Additive Effect
	NS + CEF	0.4	0.5	0.7	0.6	Synergism/Additive Effect
MRSA 4						
	NS + OXA	0.5	0.6	0.7	0.8	Synergism/Additive Effect
	NS + AUG	0.5	0.5	0.6	0.8	Synergism/Additive Effect
	NS + CEF	0.5	0.5	0.7	0.7	Synergism/Additive Effect
MRSA 5						
	NS + OXA	0.5	0.5	0.5	0.8	Synergism/Additive Effect
	NS + AUG	0.5	0.5	0.5	0.7	Synergism/Additive Effect
	NS + CEF	0.7	0.6	0.6	0.7	Additive Effect

NS = *Nigella sativa*, OXA = oxacillin; AUG = augmentin; CEF = cefuroxime. The interaction was defined as synergistic if the FIC index was less than or equal to 0.5, additive if the FIC index was greater than 0.5 and less than or equal to 1.0, indifferent if the FIC index was greater than 1.0 and less than or equal to 2.0, and antagonistic if the FIC index was greater than 2.0.

The synergistic time–kill assay, as interpreted with the FIC index for a 7.5 µg/mL NS combination with antibiotics, is shown in Table 2. The combination of OXA, AUG, and CEF antibiotics all displayed synergism, with AUG and CEF exhibiting the best synergism up to 12 h. The pattern of synergistic effect on MRSA 4 was different, however. AUG had the best effect, but only for 4 h, which was then followed by additive effects. In MRSA 5, NS OXA combinations only produced additive effects. However, synergism was only observed for 2 h, as indicated in Table 2 for AUG and CEF combination. The overall FIC index ranged from 0.05 to 0.7, indicating synergism and additive effects.

3.4. SEM and TEM Assay on Effect of Combined NS, Antibiotic Treatment

The structural appearance of MRSA treated with concentrations of NS and in combination with antibiotics was analyzed using SEM. Figure 4A shows MRSA 4 clusters displaying well-formed shapes, while bacterial cell surface disruption is seen in 4B after treatment with 5.0 µg/mL NS. In Figure 4C,D, cellular aggregation of bacteria and cell destruction is seen in combined treatments of NS with oxacillin and augmentin. In Figure 4E,F, similar destruction of bacteria cell surface and cellular aggregation were observed in the combined treatment of MRSA 5 with 7.5 µg/mL NS, augmentin, and cefuroxime. Figure 5A–F represent TEM monograph analysis of the different MRSA isolates with NS 5 and 7.5 µg/mL concentrations. Figure 5A shows altered MRSA 5 cell membrane and dead bacterial cells after exposure to 5.0 µg/mL NS. The figure also shows disruption of bacterial cell division. Figure 5B also shows MRSA 4 cell wall damage after exposure to 7.5 µg/mL NS with oxacillin, as well as vacuoles created in the cytoplasm and perhaps the accumulation of NS within the cell. Figure 5C shows dead bacteria cells and a damaged cell wall in MRSA 4 treated with 7.5 µg/mL and augmentin, while Figure 5D displays MRSA 4 isolates treated with a combination of 7.5 µg/mL and cefuroxime. Figure 5E shows the effects of MRSA 1 treated with 5.0 µg/mL NS plus oxacillin and Figure 5F shows the effect on MRSA 1 treated with 5.0 µg/mL NS plus augmentin, showing cell wall destruction (black arrows). These micrographs show that NS disrupts the MRSA bacterial cell wall, thereby causing cell death. In combination with β-lactam antibiotics, these effects were potentiated and can be described as a bactericidal effect.

TEM interpretation of combined treatment of NS and antibiotics is shown in Figure 6A–F. The figure gives TEM monographs of the different MRSA bacterial isolates treated with a combination of 7.5 µg/mL NS concentrations and antibiotics. Figure 6A shows damaged MRSA 4 cell walls, disrupted bacterial replication, and cell death with oxacillin. The figure also shows more cell death due to fewer cells, with similar observations seen with MRSA 5 in Figure 6B. In combination treatments with augmentin on MRSA 1, Figure 6C shows more cell deaths, while Figure 6D also displays cell death and the disruption of cell division in MRSA 5. Additionally, the TEM images in Figure 6E show the effect of treatments with 7.5 µg/mL NS in combination with cefuroxime led to MRSA 1 complete and incomplete cell wall disrupted and bacterial cell death. Figure 6F shows complete destruction by 7.5 µg/mL NS plus cefuroxime in MRSA 5. These effects clearly indicate that the combinations were bactericidal.

3.5. Results of GC-MS Analysis

The GC-MS analysis of volatile compounds contained in *N. sativa* oil used in this study showed that the major components were thymoquinone at 7.85%, *p*-cymene at 5.18%, trans-anethole at 1.52%, and linalool at 1.12%, as presented in Table 3 and Figure 7.

Table 3. GC-MS data.

Com Pound Name	Rt	Area (%)
p-Cymene	9.841	5.18
Linalool	13.498	1.12
Thymoquinone	18.018	7.85
trans-Anethole	19.023	1.52
m-Thymol	19.872	0.71

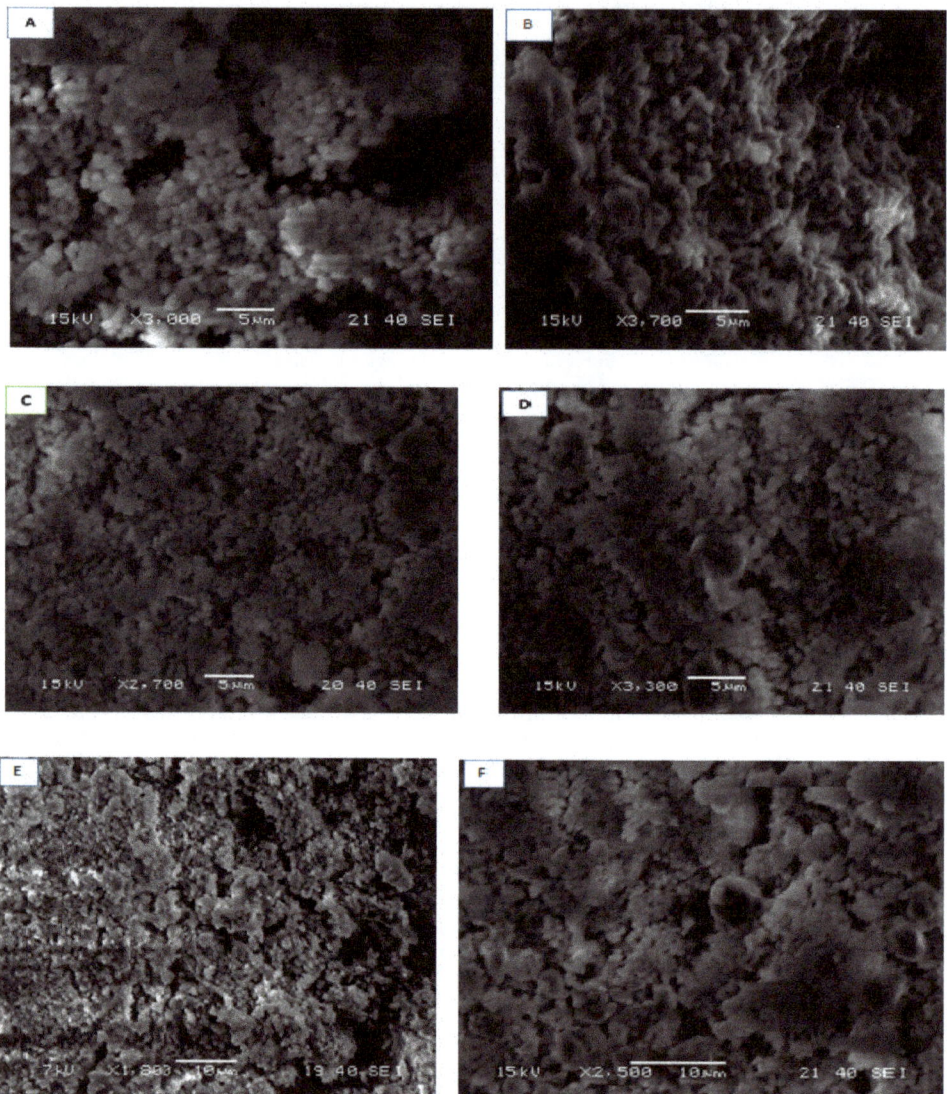

Figure 4. SEM micrographs of untreated, NS, and NS plus β-lactam antibiotics treated methicillin-resistant *S. aureus* isolates. (**A**) Control methicillin-resistant *Staphylococcus aureus* (MRSA 4) without any treatment, showing clusters of bacteria. (**B**) MRSA 4 treatment with 5.0 µg/mL *Nigella sativa* (NS), displaying surface alterations and destruction. (**C**) SEM of MRSA 4 treated with a combination of 5.0 µg/mL NS and oxacillin. (**D**) Augmentin combination with the same concentration of NS, showing surface destruction of *S. aureus*. (**E**) MRSA 5 at 2700× magnification showing 7.5 µg/mL NS treatment in combination with augmentin. (**F**) Combination treatment with cefuroxime and 7.5 µg/mL NS at 1800× showing MRSA 5 bacteria cluster surface destruction.

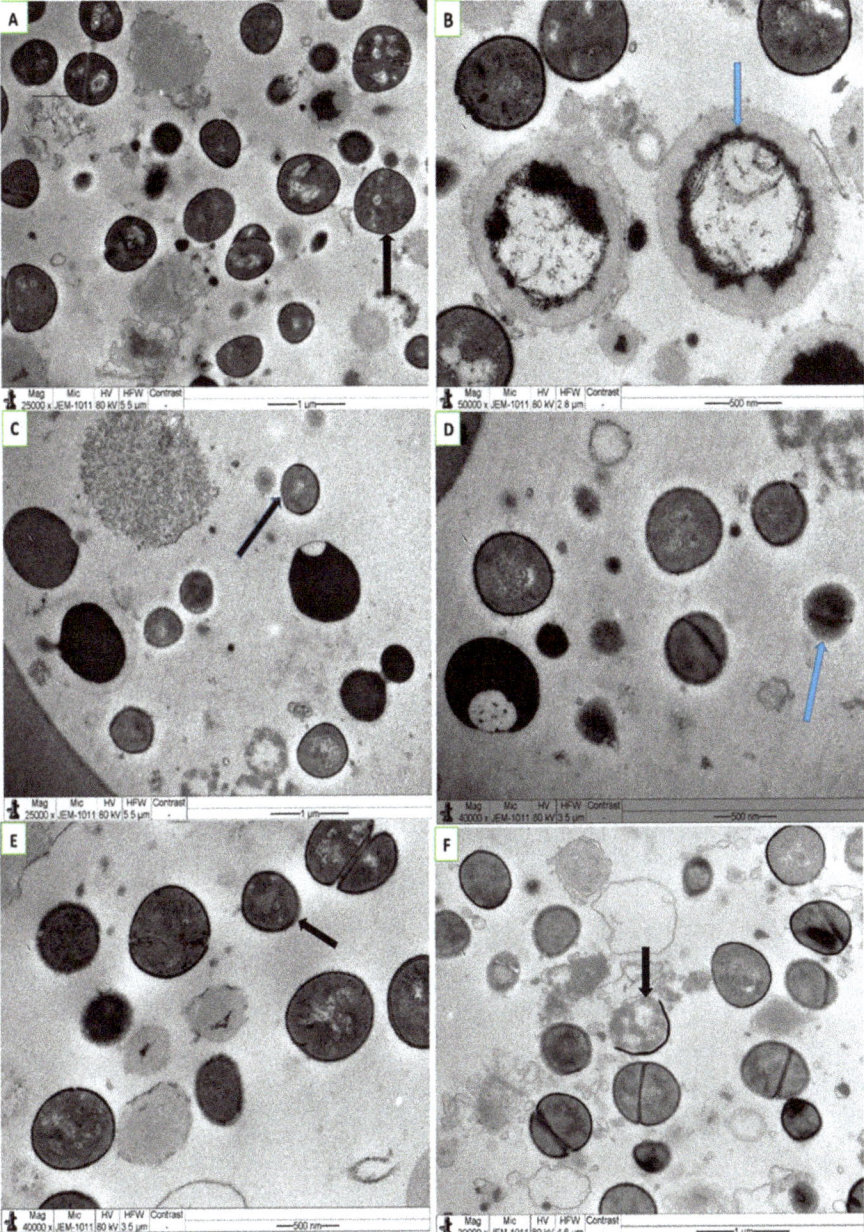

Figure 5. TEM micrographs of methicillin-resistant *Staphylococcus aureus* (MRSA) treated with NS and NS plus β-lactam antibiotics. (**A**) 5.0 µg/mL of NS at 25,000× showing MRSA 5 cell wall destruction (black arrow). (**B**) 5.0 µg/mL NS plus oxacillin showing MRSA 4 cell death at 50,000× magnification (blue arrow). (**C**) MRSA 5 treated with NS 5.0 µg/mL plus augmentin at 25,000× showing incomplete cell wall destruction (black arrow) and (**D**) MRSA 4 treated with 5.0 µg/mL NS plus cefuroxime showing cell death (blue arrow) at 40,000× magnifications. (**E**) MRSA 1 treated with 5.0 µg/mL NS plus oxacillin and (**F**) MRSA 1 treated with 5.0 µg/mL NS plus augmentin, showing cell wall destruction (black arrows) at a magnification of 30,000×.

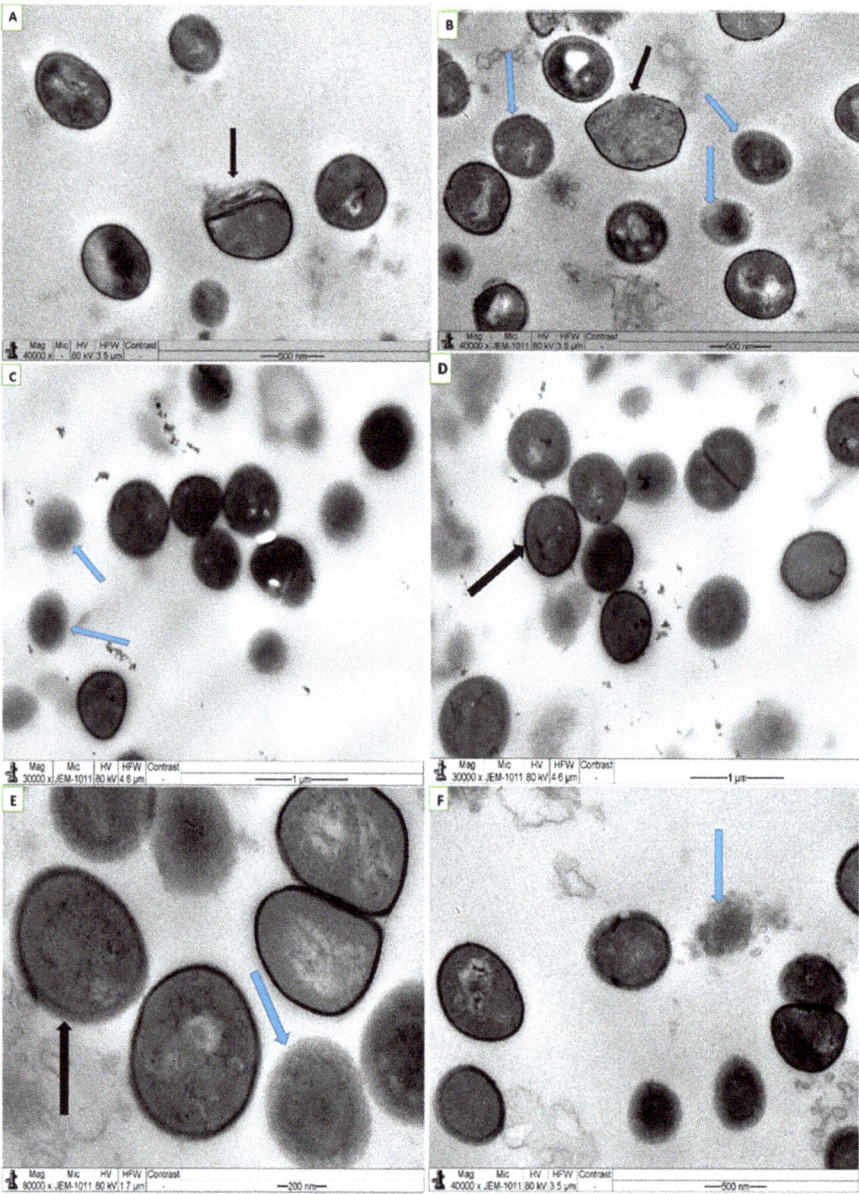

Figure 6. TEM micrographs of methicillin-resistant *Staphylococcus aureus* (MRSA) treated with NS and NS plus β-lactam antibiotics. (**A**) 7.5 µg/mL NS plus oxacillin at a magnification of 40,000×, showing incomplete destruction of MRSA 4 cell wall (black arrow) and (**B**) 7.5 µg/mL NS plus oxacillin, showing incomplete of destruction of MRSA 5 cell wall (blue arrow). (**C**) MRSA 1 treated with 7.5 µg/mL NS plus augmentin, showing dead bacterial cells at a magnification of 30,000× (blue arrow). (**D**) MRSA 5 treated with 7.5 µg/mL NS plus augmentin, showing complete cell wall destruction. (**E**) 7.5 µg/mL NS plus cefuroxime, showing incomplete (black arrow) and complete (blue arrow) destruction of MRSA 1 cell wall at a magnification of 80,000×. (**F**) Complete destruction by 7.5 µg/mL NS plus cefuroxime of MRSA 5 cell wall at a magnification of 40,000× (blue arrow).

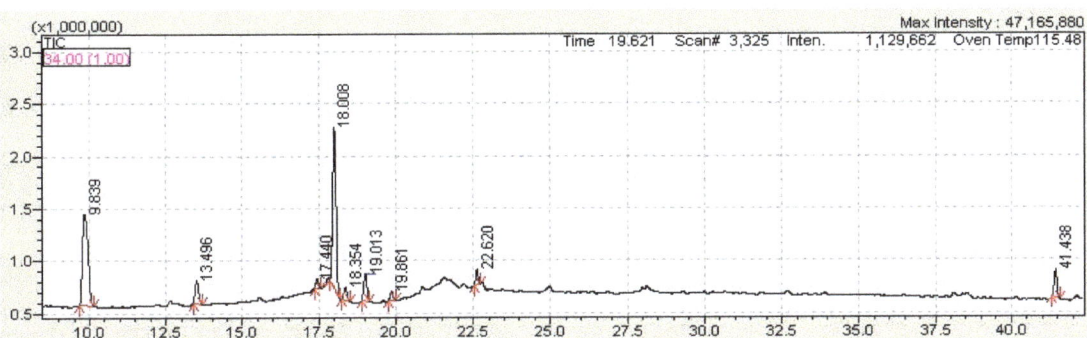

Figure 7. Chromatogram of *N. Sativa* oil characterized by GC-MS analysis.

4. Discussion

The MRSA isolates examined here were extremely drug-resistant and fit into the classification of XDR, as they were resistant to aminoglycosides, β-lactams, fluoroquinolones, macrolides, and tetracycline [39–11]. However, this study has shown that *Nigella sativa* (NS), a naturally derived herbal product, inhibits the growth of these XDR MRSA isolates, thereby confirming earlier findings. This suggests that NS derivatives could serve as possible alternatives in the management of extreme drug-resistant (XDR) MRSA isolates. The inherent antimicrobial potential of NS derivatives had been reported as equally effective as that of clinically available antibiotics [26,32,42]. All these reports demonstrated better inhibition of MRSA isolates by NS as compared to commonly used antibiotics, as also seen in the present study.

In this investigation, the isolates responded differently to various concentrations of NS, as seen in the exhibited zones of inhibition. Additionally, although there were differences among the isolates in zones of inhibition, all NS concentrations, including the lowest concentration of 0.1 μg/mL, were able to hinder bacterial growth, a finding that is similar to earlier reports [32,43]. Differences in zones of inhibition could be attributed to phenotypic differences in the MRSA strains. However, that the lowest concentration of NS exhibited growth inhibition against the isolates in this study points to its effectiveness as a potential antimicrobial.

The study also shows the time–kill kinetics for the MRSA strains used in this study to be more rapid in NS and β-lactam combined therapies than with NS alone. This suggests the possibility of a combined additive effect or potentiation of NS to those of the antibiotics that the MRSA isolates had previously been resistant to. These findings are in agreement with earlier suggestions for the need to develop a synergistic herbal drug product that could be suitable for use in combined therapeutic measures to combat the scourge of bacterial resistance [44–46]. Phytotherapy combinations with proven synergistic efficacy would not only have a multi-targeted mechanism of action but could be a main tool in delaying, alleviating, or reducing resistance to existing antimicrobials [32,44]. Additionally, our findings show NS synergistic activity in combination with OXA, AUG, and CEF against XDR MRSA isolates, with the best effect seen in the NS-AUG combination as opposed to NS-OXA and NS-CEF, similar to an earlier report [32]. This reported that, in NS β-lactam synergism, there was a reversal in resistance to augmentin by MRSA, findings that are similar to those of this investigation. An earlier report on the synergistic effects of combining the by-products contained in the plant with conventional antimicrobial drugs found improved effects compared to antimicrobials alone [47]. This might explain why all NS β-lactam combinations were more effective than NS or the antibiotic alone. On the other hand, that the combination of 0.5 mg/mL NS and β-lactam showed varying results (Figure 3D-F), with complete killing seen with MRSA 1, suggests that differences in bacterial strains could be a contributory factor, as had been reported previously [25].

However, that there was better killing against the same MRSA 4 and 5 isolates (Figure 3E,F) in the 7.5 µg/mL NS and antibiotic combinations could point to a dose-dependent NS concentration, a view expressed earlier [32]. Molecular insight was gained by examining the probable mechanism of action of NS alone and with β-lactam antibiotic combinations using SEM and TEM techniques. A SEM micrograph analysis showed bacterial cell aggregation without the usual well-defined clustering of S. aureus. This finding is consistent with previous studies that reported the effect of antibiotics on bacterial cells [48,49]. NS alone disrupted the bacterial cell surface and therefore caused destruction, which was evident in the bacterial growth inhibition. However, in the combinations of NS with OXA and AUG, where there was marked cellular aggregation/cell destruction, we can point to the possible synergistic/additive effects of NS, as shown in the FIC results in Tables 2 and 3, all of which created significant changes in the molecular ultrastructure that Gram-positive bacteria such as MRSA use for survival. It could also mean that binding of β-lactam antibiotics to penicillin binding protein (PBP) sites was significantly enhanced. Note that the isolates used in this study exhibited marked antimicrobial resistance. The TEM micrograph analysis also confirmed this view. It showed cell death and cell surface disruption, similar to the ultrastructural changes in the MRSA isolates from a previous study with NS alone [32]. The molecular structural changes seen in the TEM micrographs could also be due to interference in the transportation or the synthesis of PBP by NS. Such cell wall destruction, either by NS or in combination with β-lactam antibiotics, would be expected to remove the bacterial protective barriers, thus leading to cell lysis, as shown by the TEM micrograph results.

Generally, the mode of action of augmentin as a β-lactam is that it leads to the inhibition of bacterial cell wall peptidoglycan by binding and inhibiting PBPs [50]. It is documented that antimicrobial resistance results from the activation of the Mec A gene and its variants, which leads to the formation of penicillin-binding protein 2A (PBP2a), which binds to β-lactams, thus creating resistance [50]. However, we noted that alkaloid plant components, alone or when combined with conventional antibiotics, could have an effect on bacterial acquired resistance, which could explain the NS and antibiotic combined effects seen in this investigation [3].

N. sativa oil is rich in diverse volatile compounds involved in various biological activities [51]. The GC-MS results confirmed that N. sativa essential oil is a good source of bioactive components such as p-cymene, linalool, thymoquinone, transanethole, and m-thymol, which have been evaluated by various reports and are considered to possess good antimicrobial activity [51–54]. Earlier reports documented synergistic effects of the extracts of black cumin with streptomycin and gentamicin against antibiotic sensitive S. aureus and other bacterial isolates [55,56]. Thymoquinone was indicated to exert synergism with the antibiotics against S. aureus [56]. Thus, thymoquinone an abundant component of N. sativa is reported to be the bioactive compound with multiple pharmacological actions including being a strong antimicrobial [55,57]. Additionally, as other reports show synergistic effects when thymoquinone is combined with synthetic and natural compound, the present study further confirms that the contents of N. sativa essential oil are potent at inhibiting bacterial activity [54,58].

5. Conclusions

Our findings indicate that N. sativa had a bactericidal effect against XDR methicillin-resistant Staphylococcus aureus, even at low concentration. NS synergistically improved the efficacy of β-lactam antibiotics to which, ab initio, they had been resistant. The study also showed, by SEM and TEM molecular analysis, that NS used bacterial cell wall disruption as a possible mechanism of action. This appeared to have improved the binding of β-lactam antibiotics to PBP, as evident in the destruction of the MRSA cell wall and lysis shown in TEM micrographs. However, further studies will be needed to evaluate in detail the nature of this binding and to what type of membrane protein in rapidly emerging resistant bacterial strains.

Author Contributions: Conceptualization, methodology, formal analysis, and writing—original draft preparation, L.I.B.-E. and P.M.E.; software, P.M.E. and H.I.M.I.; validation, investigation, resources, data curation, and writing—review and editing, L.I.B.-E., P.M.E. and H.I.M.I.; funding acquisition, L.I.B.-E. All authors have read and agreed to the published version of the manuscript.

Funding: The Deanship of Scientific Research, King Faisal University (grant No. 186388) funded the research under Nasher Track.

Institutional Review Board Statement: Not required as isolates were routine diagnostic specimen.

Informed Consent Statement: Not applicable.

Data Availability Statement: Data is contained within the article and correspondence author can be contacted for more information.

Acknowledgments: The authors acknowledge the Deanship of Scientific Research, King Faisal University for the financial support. The authors would like to thank Maged El-Sayed Mohamed, Hani Al-Rasasi, Hajer Salman Al-Dehailan, Fatimah Mohammed Alquaimy, and Fatimah Ahmad AlJaafari for their technical assistance.

Conflicts of Interest: The authors declare no conflict of interest with respect to the research, authorship nor in the article publication.

References

1. Ippolito, G.; Leone, S.; Lauria, F.N.; Nicastri, E.; Wenzel, R.P. Methicillin-resistant Staphylococcus aureus: The superbug. *Int. J. Infect. Dis.* **2010**, *14*, S7–S11. [CrossRef]
2. Papp-Wallace, K.M.; Endimiani, A.; Taracila, M.A.; Bonomo, R.A. Carbapenems: Past, Present, and Future. *Antimicrob. Agents Chemother.* **2011**, *55*, 4943–4960. [CrossRef] [PubMed]
3. Konaté, K.; Mavoungou, J.F.; Lepengué, A.N.; Aworet-Samseny, R.R.; Hilou, A.; Souza, A.; Dicko, M.H.; M'Batchi, B. Antibacterial activity against β- lactamase producing Methicillin and Ampicillin-resistants Staphylococcus aureus: Fractional Inhibitory Concentration Index (FICI) determination. *Ann. Clin. Microbiol. Antimicrob.* **2012**, *11*, 18. [CrossRef] [PubMed]
4. Bæk, K.T.; Gründling, A.; Mogensen, R.G.; Thøgersen, L.; Petersen, A.; Paulander, W.; Frees, D. β-Lactam Resistance in Methicillin-Resistant Staphylococcus aureus USA300 Is Increased by Inactivation of the ClpXP Protease. *Antimicrob. Agents Chemother.* **2014**, *58*, 4593–4603. [CrossRef]
5. McGuinness, W.A.; Malachowa, N.; DeLeo, F.R. Vancomycin Resistance in Staphylococcus aureus. *Yale J. Biol. Med.* **2017**, *90*, 269–281. [PubMed]
6. Lesho, E.; Yoon, E.-J.; McGann, P.; Snesrud, E.; Kwak, Y.; Milillo, M.; Onmus-Leone, F.; Preston, L.; Clair, K.S.; Nikolich, M.; et al. Emergence of Colistin-Resistance in Extremely Drug-Resistant Acinetobacter baumannii Containing a Novel pmrCAB Operon During Colistin Therapy of Wound Infections. *J. Infect. Dis.* **2013**, *208*, 1142–1151. [CrossRef]
7. Kaur, M.; Rai, J.; Randhawa, G.K. Recent advances in antibacterial drugs. *Int. J. Appl. Basic Med. Res.* **2013**, *3*, 3–10. [CrossRef] [PubMed]
8. Aslam, B.; Wang, W.; Arshad, M.I.; Khurshid, M.; Muzammil, S.; Rasool, M.H.; Nisar, M.A.; Alvi, R.F.; Aslam, M.A.; Qamar, M.U.; et al. Antibiotic resistance: A rundown of a global crisis. *Infect. Drug Resist.* **2018**, *11*, 1645–1658. [CrossRef]
9. Lee, K.; Yong, D.; Jeong, S.H.; Chong, Y. Multidrug-ResistantAcinetobacterspp.: Increasingly Problematic Nosocomial Pathogens. *Yonsei Med. J.* **2011**, *52*, 879–891. [CrossRef]
10. Lim, T.-P.; Tan, T.-Y.; Lee, W.; Sasikala, S.; Tan, T.-T.; Hsu, L.-Y.; Kwa, A.L. In-Vitro Activity of Polymyxin B, Rifampicin, Tigecycline Alone and in Combination against Carbapenem-Resistant Acinetobacter baumannii in Singapore. *PLoS ONE* **2011**, *6*, e18485. [CrossRef]
11. Albur, M.; Noel, A.; Bowker, K.; MacGowan, A. Bactericidal Activity of Multiple Combinations of Tigecycline and Colistin against NDM-1-Producing Enterobacteriaceae. *Antimicrob. Agents Chemother.* **2012**, *56*, 3441–3443. [CrossRef]
12. Urban, C.; Mariano, N.; Rahal, J.J. In Vitro Double and Triple Bactericidal Activities of Doripenem, Polymyxin B, and Rifampin against Multidrug-Resistant Acinetobacter baumannii, Pseudomonas aeruginosa, Klebsiella pneumoniae, and Escherichia coli. *Antimicrob. Agents Chemother.* **2010**, *54*, 2732–2734. [CrossRef] [PubMed]
13. Cai, Y.; Chai, D.; Wang, R.; Liang, B.; Bai, N. Colistin resistance of Acinetobacter baumannii: Clinical reports, mechanisms and antimicrobial strategies. *J. Antimicrob. Chemother.* **2012**, *67*, 1607–1615. [CrossRef] [PubMed]
14. Gharaibeh, M.H.; Shatnawi, S.Q. An overview of colistin resistance, mobilized colistin resistance genes dissemination, global responses, and the alternatives to colistin: A review. *Veter. World* **2019**, *12*, 1735–1746. [CrossRef] [PubMed]
15. Rhouma, M.; Beaudry, F.; Letellier, A. Resistance to colistin: What is the fate for this antibiotic in pig production? *Int. J. Antimicrob. Agents* **2016**, *48*, 119–126. [CrossRef] [PubMed]
16. Liu, Y.-Y.; Wang, Y.; Walsh, T.R.; Yi, L.-X.; Zhang, R.; Spencer, J.; Doi, Y.; Tian, G.; Dong, B.; Huang, X.; et al. Emergence of plasmid-mediated colistin resistance mechanism MCR-1 in animals and human beings in China: A microbiological and molecular biological study. *Lancet Infect. Dis.* **2016**, *16*, 161–168. [CrossRef]

17. Barbieri, N.L.; Nielsen, D.W.; Wannemuehler, Y.; Cavender, T.; Hussein, A.; Yan, S.-G.; Nolan, L.K.; Logue, C.M. mcr-1 identified in Avian Pathogenic Escherichia coli (APEC). *PLoS ONE* **2017**, *12*, e0172997. [CrossRef] [PubMed]
18. Elsayed, A.; Abdulrahman, A.A.; Aboulmagd, E.; Alsultan, A.A. Synergic bactericidal activity of novel antibiotic combinations against extreme drug resistant Pseudomonas aeruginosa and Acinetobacter baumannii. *Afr. J. Microbiol. Res.* **2014**, *8*, 856–861. [CrossRef]
19. Pena-Miller, R.; Laehnemann, D.; Jansen, G.; Fuentes-Hernandez, A.; Rosenstiel, P.; Schulenburg, H.; Beardmore, R. When the Most Potent Combination of Antibiotics Selects for the Greatest Bacterial Load: The Smile-Frown Transition. *PLoS Biol.* **2013**, *11*, e1001540. [CrossRef] [PubMed]
20. Sibanda, T.; Okoh, A.I. The challenges of overcoming antibiotic resistance: Plant extracts as potential sources of antimicrobial and resistance modifying agents. *Afr. J. Biotechnol.* **2007**, *6*, 2886–2896.
21. Hübsch, Z.; Van Zyl, R.; Cock, I.; Van Vuuren, S. Interactive antimicrobial and toxicity profiles of conventional antimicrobials with Southern African medicinal plants. *S. Afr. J. Bot.* **2014**, *93*, 185–197. [CrossRef]
22. Aiyegoro, O.A.; Okoh, A.I. Use of bioactive plant products in combination with standard antibiotics: Implications in antimicrobial chemotherapy. *J. Med. Plant Res.* **2009**, *3*, 1147–1152.
23. Haroun, M.F.; Al-Kayali, R.S. Synergistic effect of Thymbra spicata L. extracts with antibiotics against multidrug-resistant Staphylococcus aureus and Klebsiella pneumoniae strains. *Iran. J. Basic Med. Sci.* **2016**, *19*, 1193–1200. [PubMed]
24. Teow, S.-Y.; Liew, K.; Ali, S.A.; Khoo, A.S.-B.; Peh, S.-C. Antibacterial Action of Curcumin against Staphylococcus aureus: A Brief Review. *J. Trop. Med.* **2016**, *2016*, 1–10. [CrossRef]
25. Emeka, L.B.; Emeka, P.M.; Khan, T.M. Antimicrobial activity of Nigella sativa L. seed oil against multi-drug resistant Staphylococcus aureus isolated from diabetic wounds. *Pak. J. Pharm. Sci.* **2015**, *28*, 1985–1990. [PubMed]
26. Ugur, A.R.; Dagi, H.T.; Ozturk, B.; Tekin, G.; Findik, D. Assessment of In vitro antibacterial activity and cytotoxicity effect of Nigella sativa oil. *Pharmacogn. Mag.* **2016**, *12*, 471–S474. [CrossRef] [PubMed]
27. Utami, A.T.; Pratomo, B.; Noorhamdani. Study of Antimicrobial Activity of Black Cumin Seeds (Nigella sativa L.) Against Salmonella typhi In Vitro. *J. Med. Surg. Pathol.* **2016**, *1*, 3. [CrossRef]
28. Emeka, P.M.; Badger-Emeka, L.I.; Eneh, C.M.; Khan, T.M. Dietary supplementation of chloroquine with nigella sativa seed and oil extracts in the treatment of malaria induced in mice with plasmodium berghei. *Pharmacogn. Mag.* **2014**, *10*, S357–S362. [CrossRef] [PubMed]
29. Magaldi, S.; Mata-Essayag, S.; de Capriles, C.H.; Perez, C.; Colella, M.; Olaizola, C.; Ontiveros, Y. Well diffusion for antifungal susceptibility testing. *Int. J. Infect. Dis.* **2004**, *8*, 39–45. [CrossRef]
30. Balouiri, M.; Sadiki, M.; Ibnsouda, S.K. Methods for in vitro evaluating antimicrobial activity: A review. *J. Pharm. Anal.* **2016**, *6*, 71–79. [CrossRef] [PubMed]
31. CLSI. *Methods for Determining Bactericidal Activity of Antimicrobial Agents*; Approved Guideline, CLSI document M26-A; Clinical and Laboratory Standards Institute: Wayne, PA, USA, 1998.
32. Uzair, B.; Hameed, A.; Nazir, S.; Khan, B.A.; Fasim, F.; Khan, S.; Menaa, F. Synergism Between Nigella sativa Seeds Extract and Synthetic Antibiotics Against Mec A Gene Positive Human Strains of Staphylococcus aureus. *Int. J. Pharmacol.* **2017**, *13*, 958–968. [CrossRef]
33. Sopirala, M.M.; Mangino, J.E.; Gebreyes, W.A.; Biller, B.; Bannerman, T.; Balada-Llasat, J.-M.; Pancholi, P. Synergy Testing by Etest, Microdilution Checkerboard, and Time-Kill Methods for Pan-Drug-Resistant Acinetobacter baumannii. *Antimicrob. Agents Chemother.* **2010**, *54*, 4678–4683. [CrossRef] [PubMed]
34. Meletiadis, J.; Pournaras, S.; Roilides, E.; Walsh, T.J. Defining fractional inhibitory concentration index cut offs for additive interactions based on self-drug additive combinations, Monte Carlo simulation analysis, and in vitro-in vivo correlation data for antifungal drug combinations against Aspergillus fumigatus. *Antimicrob. Agents Chemother.* **2010**, *54*, 602–609. [CrossRef]
35. Meletiadis, J.; Mouton, J.W.; Meis, J.F.G.M.; Bouman, B.A.; Donnelly, P.J.; Verweij, P.E.; Eurofung Network. Comparison of Spectrophotometric and Visual Readings of NCCLS Method and Evaluation of a Colorimetric Method Based on Reduction of a Soluble Tetrazolium Salt, 2,3-Bis {2-Methoxy-4-Nitro-5-[(Sulfenylamino) Carbonyl]-2H- Tetrazolium-Hydroxide}, for Antifungal Susceptibility Testing of Aspergillus Species. *J. Clin. Microbiol.* **2001**, *39*, 4256–4263. [CrossRef] [PubMed]
36. Thammawat, S.; Sangdee, K. Time-kill profiles and cell-surface morphological effects of crude Polycephalomyces nipponicus Cod-MK1201 mycelial extract against antibiotic-sensitive and -resistant Staphylococcus aureus. *Trop. J. Pharm. Res.* **2017**, *16*, 407. [CrossRef]
37. Thomas, P.; Reddy, K.M. Microscopic elucidation of abundant endophytic bacteria colonizing the cell wall–plasma membrane peri-space in the shoot-tip tissue of banana. *AoB Plants* **2013**, *5*, 11. [CrossRef]
38. Ran, Y.; Hu, W.; Zhuang, K.; Lu, M.; Huang, J.; Xu, F.; Xu, X.; Hua, X.; Lama, J.; Ran, X.; et al. Observation of Viruses, Bacteria, and Fungi in Clinical Skin Samples under Transmission Electron Microscopy. In *The Transmission Electron Microscope—Theory and Applications*; Khan Maaz; IntechOpen: Rijeka, Croatia, 2015. [CrossRef]
39. Falagas, M.E.; Karageorgopoulos, D.E. Pandrug Resistance (PDR), Extensive Drug Resistance (XDR), and Multidrug Resistance (MDR) among Gram-Negative Bacilli: Need for International Harmonization in Terminology. *Clin. Infect. Dis.* **2008**, *46*, 1121–1122. [CrossRef] [PubMed]
40. Basak, S.; Singh, P.; Rajurkar, M. Multidrug Resistant and Extensively Drug Resistant Bacteria: A Study. *J. Pathog.* **2016**, *2016*, 1–5. [CrossRef] [PubMed]

41. Sweeney, M.T.; Lubbers, B.V.; Schwarz, S.; Watts, J.L. Applying definitions for multidrug resistance, extensive drug resistance and pandrug resistance to clinically significant livestock and companion animal bacterial pathogens. *J. Antimicrob. Chemother.* **2018**, *73*, 1460–1463. [CrossRef] [PubMed]
42. Naz, H. Nigella sativa: The miraculous herb. *Pak. J. Biochem. Mol. Biol.* **2011**, *44*, 44–48. Available online: http://pjbmb.org.pk/images/PJBMBArchive/2011/PJBMB_44_1_Mar_2011/10.pdf (accessed on 26 March 2021).
43. Chaieb, K.; Kouidhi, B.; Jrah, H.; Mahdouani, K.; Bakhrouf, A. Antibacterial activity of Thymoquinone, an active principle of Nigella sativa and its potency to prevent bacterial biofilm formation. *BMC Complement. Altern. Med.* **2011**, *11*, 29. [CrossRef] [PubMed]
44. Wagner, H. Synergy research: Approaching a new generation of phytopharmaceuticals. *Fitoterapia* **2011**, *82*, 34–37. [CrossRef] [PubMed]
45. Ventola, C.L. The antibiotic resistance crisis: Part 1: Causes and threats. *Pharm. Ther.* **2015**, *40*, 277–283. Available online: https://www.ncbi.nlm.nih.gov/pubmed/25859123 (accessed on 26 March 2021).
46. Thakur, P.; Chawla, R.; Goel, R.; Narula, A.; Arora, R.; Sharma, R.K. Augmenting the potency of third-line antibiotics with Berberis aristata: In vitro synergistic activity against carbapenem-resistant Escherichia coli. *J. Glob. Antimicrob. Resist.* **2016**, *6*, 10–16. [CrossRef] [PubMed]
47. Rosato, A.; Vitali, C.; De Laurentis, N.; Armenise, D.; Milillo, M.A. Antibacterial effect of some essential oils administered alone or in combination with Norfloxacin. *Phytomedicine* **2007**, *14*, 727–732. [CrossRef]
48. Ozkaya, G.U.; Durak, M.Z.; Akyar, I.; Karatuna, O. Antimicrobial Susceptibility Test for the Determination of Resistant and Susceptible S. aureus and Enterococcus spp. Using a Multi-Channel Surface Plasmon Resonance Device. *Diagnostics* **2019**, *9*, 191. [CrossRef]
49. Park, H.; Jang, C.-H.; Cho, Y.B.; Choi, C.-H. Antibacterial effect of tea-tree oil on methicillin-resistant Staphylococcus aureus biofilm formation of the tympanostomy tube: An in vitro study. *In Vivo* **2008**, *21*, 1027–1030.
50. Pinho, M.G.; Filipe, S.R.; De Lencastre, H.; Tomasz, A. Complementation of the Essential Peptidoglycan Transpeptidase Function of Penicillin-Binding Protein 2 (PBP2) by the Drug Resistance Protein PBP2A in Staphylococcus aureus. *J. Bacteriol.* **2001**, *183*, 6525–6531. [CrossRef] [PubMed]
51. Kazemi, M. Phytochemical Composition, Antioxidant, Anti-inflammatory and Antimicrobial Activity ofNigella sativaL. Essential Oil. *J. Essent. Oil Bear. Plants* **2014**, *17*, 1002–1011. [CrossRef]
52. Herman, A.; Tambor, K.; Herman, A. Linalool Affects the Antimicrobial Efficacy of Essential Oils. *Curr. Microbiol.* **2015**, *72*, 165–172. [CrossRef]
53. Forouzanfar, F.; Bazzaz, B.S.F.; Hosseinzadeh, H. Black cumin (Nigella sativa) and its constituent (thymoquinone): A review on antimicrobial effects. *Iran. J. Basic Med. Sci.* **2014**, *17*, 929–938. [PubMed]
54. Kwiatkowski, P.; Pruss, A.; Masiuk, H.; Mnichowska-Polanowska, M.; Kaczmarek, M.; Giedrys-Kalemba, S.; Dołęgowska, B.; Zielińska-Bliźniewska, H.; Olszewski, J.; Sienkiewicz, M. The effect of fennel essential oil and trans-anethole on antibacterial activity of mupirocin against Staphylococcus aureus isolated from asymptomatic carriers. *Adv. Dermatol. Allergol.* **2019**, *36*, 308–314. [CrossRef] [PubMed]
55. Halawani, E. Antibacterial activity of thymoquinone and thymohydroquinone of Nigella sativa L. and their interaction with some antibiotics. *Adv. Biol. Res.* **2009**, *3*, 148–152.
56. Elnour, S.A.; Abdelsalam, E.B. Some Biological and Pharmacological Effects of the Black Cumin (Nigella sativa): A Concise Review. *Am. J. Res. Commun.* **2018**, *6*, 10–35. Available online: http://www.usa-journals.com/wp-content/uploads/2018/02/Elnour_Vol63.pdf (accessed on 26 March 2021).
57. Sahak, M.K.A.; Kabir, N.; Abbas, G.; Draman, S.; Hashim, N.H.; Adli, D.S.H. The Role ofNigella sativaand Its Active Constituents in Learning and Memory. *Evid. Based Complement. Altern. Med.* **2016**, *2016*, 1–6. [CrossRef]
58. Dera, A.A.; Ahmad, I.; Rajagopalan, P.; Al Shahrani, M.; Saif, A.; Alshahrani, M.Y.; Alraey, Y.; Alamri, A.M.; Alasmari, S.; Makkawi, M.; et al. Synergistic efficacies of thymoquinone and standard antibiotics against multi-drug resistant isolates. *Saudi. Med. J.* **2021**, *42*, 196–204. [CrossRef] [PubMed]

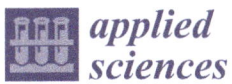

Review

Potential Role of Plant Extracts and Phytochemicals Against Foodborne Pathogens

Farhat Ullah [1], Muhammad Ayaz [1,*], Abdul Sadiq [1], Farman Ullah [2], Ishtiaq Hussain [3], Muhammad Shahid [4], Zhanibek Yessimbekov [5], Anjana Adhikari-Devkota [6] and Hari Prasad Devkota [6,7,*]

1. Department of Pharmacy, University of Malakand, Khyber Pakhtunkhwa (KP) 18000, Pakistan; drfarhatullah@uom.edu.pk (F.U.); a.sadiq@uom.edu.pk (A.S.)
2. Department of Pharmacy, Kohat University of Science and Technology (KUST), Kohat 26000, Khyber Pakhtunkhwa, Pakistan; farmanullah@kust.edu.pk
3. Department of Pharmaceutical Sciences, Abbottabad University of Science and Technology, Abbottabad 22010, Pakistan; ishtiaqdr025@gmail.com
4. Department of Pharmacy, Sarhad University of Science and Information Technology, Peshawar KPK 25000, Pakistan; Shahidsalim_2002@hotmail.com
5. Shakarim State University of Semey, Semey 071412, Kazakhstan; zyessimbekov@semgu.kz
6. Graduate School of Pharmaceutical Sciences, Kumamoto University, 5-1 Oe-honmachi, Kumamoto 862-0973, Japan; anjana@kumamoto-u.ac.jp
7. Program for Leading Graduate Schools, Health Life Sciences: Interdisciplinary and Glocal Oriendted (HIGO) Program, Kumamoto University, 5-1 Oe-honmachi, Kumamoto 862-0973, Japan
* Correspondence: mayaz@uom.edu.pk (M.A.); devkotah@kumamoto-u.ac.jp (H.P.D.)

Received: 26 May 2020; Accepted: 29 June 2020; Published: 2 July 2020

Abstract: Foodborne diseases are one of the major causes of morbidity and mortality, especially in low-income countries with poor sanitation and inadequate healthcare facilities. The foremost bacterial pathogens responsible for global outbreaks include *Salmonella* species, *Campylobacter jejuni*, *Escherichia coli*, *Shigella* sp., *Vibrio*, *Listeria monocytogenes* and *Clostridium botulinum*. Among the viral and parasitic pathogens, norovirus, hepatitis A virus, *Giardia lamblia*, *Trichinella spiralis*, *Toxoplasma* and *Entamoeba histolytica* are commonly associated with foodborne diseases. The toxins produced by *Staphylococcus aureus*, *Bacillus cereus* and *Clostridium perfringens* also cause these infections. The currently available therapies for these infections are associated with various limited efficacy, high cost and side-effects. There is an urgent need for effective alternative therapies for the prevention and treatment of foodborne diseases. Several plant extracts and phytochemicals were found to be highly effective to control the growth of these pathogens causing foodborne infections in in vitro systems. The present review attempts to provide comprehensive scientific information on major foodborne pathogens and the potential role of phytochemicals in the prevention and treatment of these infections. Further detailed studies are necessary to evaluate the activities of these extracts and phytochemicals along with their mechanism of action using in vivo models.

Keywords: foodborne diseases; giardiasis; herbal drugs; ethnobotany; toxoplasmosis

1. Introduction

Foodborne diseases are caused by consumption of microbial contaminated foods, herbs and beverages as well as hazardous chemicals including heavy metals, mycotoxins, bacterial toxins as well as fermentation byproducts like biogenic amines and ethyl carbamate [1–3]. Most these foodborne diseases are caused by pathogenic bacteria, viruses and parasites and are of global public health concern [4]. Each year about 600 million people are affected by foodborne diseases worldwide and about 420,000 people die due to these illnesses [5–8]. The most common symptoms associated with pathogens-induced foodborne diseases are vomiting, abdominal pain, diarrhea, fever and chills that may progress to severe complications such as life-threatening dehydration and hemolytic uremic syndrome (HUS) [9]. The bacterial-induced foodborne diseases are caused by infections with *Salmonella*, *Campylobacter* spp., *Escherichia coli*, *Shigella*, *Vibrio*, *Listeria monocytogenes* and *Clostridium botulinum* and *Clostridium perfringens* [4]. The commonly reported viruses are Norovirus and Hepatitis A, while the parasites involved are *Cryptosporidium* spp, *Giardia lamblia*, *Trichinella spiralis*, *Cyclospora* spp, *Toxoplasma canis* and *Entamoeba histolytica* [10,11] The toxins produced by *Staphylococcus aureus*, *Bacillus cereus* and *Clostridium perfringens* also prompt this debilitating disease [12]. Recently, there is a dramatic increase in the outbreak of foodborne disease, part of which is due to the emergence of pathogens resistance against current therapies and decontamination strategies [13]. Theses pathogens use food stuff as carrier to get transferred from one host to another one [14]. The diseases caused by these pathogens are a major public health concern and globally produce a social and economic impact.

The proper handling, use of cold chain and addition of chemical preservatives are currently the mainstay to ensure the preservation and safety of food materials. However, the use of synthetic preservatives is associated with a high occurrence of side-effects, thereby raising the demand for the use of natural preservatives [15,16]. The main treatment options for foodborne diseases are systematic treatments like antidiarrheal and antiemetic medications, use of oral rehydration salts and the use of antibiotics [17]. However, the emergence of multi drug-resistant (MDR pathogens) is another global issue that requires the discovery of alternative antimicrobial agents [18–20].

Medicinal plants play a vital role in the treatment and prevention of various diseases and their promotion and there is growing interest in the search for new drugs from natural resources [21–26]. People living in many developing countries in Asia and Africa are mostly dependent on traditional medicines for healing purposes due to their limited access to modern medical facilities. They also have more cases of foodborne diseases because of their poor hygiene and exposure to contaminated drinking water and food materials [27,28]. Various studies have regularly reported the antimicrobial activities of traditional medicines from this part of the world. Medicinal plants offer a substantial opportunity as they contain various bioactive chemical constituents (phytochemicals) that can act as antimicrobial agents. Natural products are also reported to act as synergists along with many modern drugs to combat MDR pathogens [29]. Thus, the exploration of these natural antimicrobials is a hope to curtail foodborne diseases. Traditional medicines have long been used for treating diseases caused by foodborne pathogens and various studies have shown their efficacy in the management of foodborne diseases [30]. Recently, there is a greater interest in the naturally occurring preservatives due to the side-effects associated with the use of artificial preservatives in foodstuffs. Crude plant materials including extracts, essential oils and isolated components have been extensively evaluated to prevent the invasion of pathogens responsible for food spoilage and therefore may limit the spread of foodborne infections [31].

Plants/plant-derived products inhibit/modify the growth of bacteria by several mechanisms. These may include, inhibiting the adherence of the pathogen to host cells [32], causing loss of osmoregulation of microbe and loss of transmembrane electrochemical gradient, increasing NO production thus causing lethal action [33], inhibition of synthesis of the cell wall, proteins and nucleic acids of the pathogen [34]. This review summarizes the therapeutic effectiveness of medicinal plants and isolated natural compounds against pathogens implicated in foodborne infections.

2. Materials and Methods

Published literature related to the role of phytochemicals in foodborne infections was collected using different search engines like PubMed, Google Scholar, SciFinder, Scopus, Web of Science, EBSCO, PROTA and JSTOR. Only in-depth, well designed (having control groups) studies reporting mechanistic results and published in journals of good quality were included in the manuscript.

3. Plant Extracts and Phytochemicals against Bacteria Causing Foodborne Diseases

3.1. Campylobacter Species

Campylobacter jejuni is a Gram-negative, non-spore-forming and non-fermenting bacteria. It is one of the most common causes of foodborne diseases in the US and Europe. Humans are usually infected by the ingestion of contaminated food, milk, water or interaction with animals [35]. Globally, about 9.6 million people are infected by *C. jejuni* annually [36]. For the treatment of *C. jejuni* infection, tetracyclines and fluoroquinolones are the drugs of choice; however, these days they are associated with a high degree of antibiotic-resistance [37,38]. Alternatively, phytochemicals can be utilized as they have the potential to combat foodborne diseases caused by *C. jejuni*. Dholvitayakhun et al. reported the inhibitory activity of extracts of *Adenanthera pavonina* L., *Moringa oleifera* Lam. and *Annona squamosa* L. against *C. jejuni* [39]. In these plants, among the flavonoids, kaempferol, quercetin and rutin are present which possess strong antimicrobial properties [40]. *Mammea africana* Sabine is used traditionally for the treatment of infections, stomach pain and skin ailments in Africa [41]. A coumarin, mammea A/AA was isolated by Canning et al. from *Mammea africana* and evaluated its activity against *C. jejuni*. It was found to be very potent with a minimum inhibitory concentration (MIC) value of 0.25 µg/mL [42]. Castillo et al. evaluated 28 plants against *C. jejuni*, out of which 21 were active. Of these 21 active plants, 4 plants including *Artemisia ludoviciana* Nutt , *Acacia farnesiana* (L.) Willd. *Opuntia ficus-indica* (L.) Mill. and *Cynara scolymus* L. were most potent having minimal bactericidal concentration (MBC) values of 0.5, 0.3, 0.4 and 2 mg/mL, respectively. They also tested the anti-adherence activity of these 4 plants against *C. jejuni*, as adherence of the microbe to mucosal cells is important for its virulence. The results proved that extracts were able to inhibit the attachment of *C. jejuni* [32]. Another mechanism of *C. jejuni* pathogenicity is cell lysis, entry into the host cell and production of a virulent cytotoxin, cytolethal distending toxin (CDT) [43]. Extracts of *A. ludoviciana* and *A. farnesiana* were shown to prevent the production of CDT along with a decrease in cytoplasmic pH and cellular ATP concentration and damages the bacterial cell membrane [44]. Moreover, motility also contributes to the virulence of *C. jejuni*. The subinhibitory concentrations of natural compounds, i.e., carvacrol (0.002%), *trans*-cinnamaldehyde (0.01%) and eugenol 0.01%) prominently decrease the motility of *C. jejuni*. Furthermore, these natural compounds also reduce other virulence potentials of this pathogen [45].

Several researchers have reported the potential antibacterial activity of essential oils (EO) of various plants against *C. jejuni* that are commonly used in the traditional system of medicine. These plants include *Syzygium aromaticum* (L.) Merr. & L.M.Perry [46,47], *Citrus limon* (L.) Osbeck and *Citrus bergamia* Risso [48], tea tree oil, Leptospermum oil [49], coriander (*Coriandrum sativum* L.) [50], *Daucus carota* L. [51], *Cuminum cyminum* L. [52], garlic (*Allium sativum* L.) [53], clove (*Syzygium aromaticum*), thyme (*Thymus vulgaris* L.) [54], eucalyptus (*Eucalyptus globulus* Labill.), sage (*Salvia officinalis* L.), rosemary (*Rosmarinus officinalis* L.), juniper (*Juniperus communis* L.), lavender (*Lavandula officinalis* Chaix), *Myrtus communis* L., *Laurus nobilis* L., pine oil (*Pinus brutia*) [55], *Juniperus excelsa* M.Bieb. [56], *Inula helenium* L [52], marigold (*Calendula officinalis* L.), ginger (*Zingiber officinale* L.), patchouli (*Pogostemon cablin*), gardenia (*Gardenia jasminoides* (Blanco) Benth.), cedarwood (*Cedrus atlantica* (Endl.) Manetti ex Carrière), carrot seed (*Daucus carota* L.), celery seed (*Apium graveolens* L.), mugwort (*Artemisia vulgaris* L.), spikenard (*Nardostachys jatamansi* (D.Don) DC.), orange bitter oils (*Citrus* x *aurantium* subsp. *amara* (Link) Engl.), etc [47].

Terminalia macroptera Guill. & Perr. has been used for treating various infectious diseases in West Africa. Silva et al. subjected 100 clinical isolates of *C. jejuni* to the ethanolic extract of *T. macroptera* and recorded a MIC value as low as 6.25 µg/mL, which was similar to that of co-trimoxazole, used as the positive control, therefore suggests a therapeutic potential of *T. macroptera* in foodborne disease caused by *C. jejuni* [57]. In South Africa, Samie et al. conducted a study on clinically isolated *C. jejuni* from stool samples ($n = 110$) to find a complementary therapeutic remedy for this infection. They tested extracts of 18 plants i.e., *Annona* sp., *Bauhinia galpinii* N.E.Br., *Bridelia micrantha* (Hochst.) Baill.,

Carissa edulis (Forssk.) Vahl, *Cissampelos torulosa* E.Mey. ex Harv. & Sond., *Elaeodendron transvaalensis* (Burtt Davy) R.H.Archer, *Ficus sycomorus* L., *Lippia javanica* (Burm.f.) Spreng., *Momordica balsamina* L., *Mucuna coriacea* Baker, *Peltophorum africanum* Sond., *Pouzolzia mixta* Solms, *Pterocarpus angolensis* DC, *Rhoicissus tridentate* (L.f.) Wild & R.B.Drumm., *Sida alba* L., *Syzygium cordatum* Hochst. ex Krauss, *Ximenia caffra* Sond. and *Zornia milneana* Mohlenbr. on these isolated bacterial strain. All the extracts were active, but potent activity was observed with the extracts of *P. angolensis* and *L. javanica* having an MIC of 90 µg/mL [58]. The extract of *Cryptolepis sanguinolenta* (Lindl.) is used traditionally for treating different infections in Guinea Bissau. An alkaloid cryptolepine has been isolated from this plant. When tested on a collection of 106 clinical strains of *C. jejuni* by Paulo et al. in Portugal, it was found to be very effective. They recorded MIC$_{50}$ of this alkaloid was equal to that of ampicillin in their study [59]. Jarriyawattanachaikul et al. in Thailand, evaluated 26 Thai plants against *C. jejuni* in search of complementary therapy for infection caused by this bacterium. They found 7 active plants, i.e., taew kaao (*Cratoxylum formosum* (Jacq.) Benth. & Hook.f. ex Dyer), golden shower (*Cassia fistula* L.), mangosteen (*Garcinia mangostana* L.), ginger (*Zingiber officinale* Roscoe), garlic (*Allium sativum* L.), onion (*Allium cepa* L.) and shallot (*Allium ascalonicum* L.), among which *C. formosum* possesses the strongest antibacterial activity as observed from its MIC of 0.3 mg/mL [60]. A traditional beverage, kombucha, showed strong activity against *C. jejuni* [61]. Black and green tea, which are the most widely consumed beverages in the world also have confirmed antibacterial propensity against *C. jejuni* [62]. Aslim et al. have obtained convincing results of the essential oil of *Origanum minutiflorum* O.Schwarz & P.H.Davis against a ciprofloxacin-resistant strain of *C. jejuni*. [63]. Many Australians plants possess antimicrobial properties and have been utilized by the native populations for centuries as traditional medicines for GIT diseases. In a study by Kurekci et al., 109 plants from Australia were tested against *C. jejuni*. Most of these plants were active as their MICs fall between 32 and 1024 µg/mL. *Eucalyptus occidentalis* Endl. was the most active plant reported with MIC of 32 µg/mL [64].

3.2. Salmonella

Salmonella is a rod-shaped, Gram-negative, motile, non-spore-forming bacteria belonging to family Enterobacteriaceae. Members of this genus are facultative anaerobes, oxidase negative and catalase-positive bacteria [65]. *Salmonella* species exist everywhere in nature, however, the gastrointestinal tracts of mammals, reptiles, birds and insects and environment polluted with humans or animals' excreta are the main reservoirs [66]. Their characteristic to survive and grow over a wide range of temperature (2–54 °C) and pH (3.6–9.6) makes them difficult to control [67]. Salmonellosis, which is an infection caused by *Salmonella* species is one of the leading causes of foodborne diseases [68]. Transmission to humans occurs via consumption of contaminated food, mostly of animal origins such as milk, eggs and meat. The antibiotics ampicillin, chloramphenicol and co-trimoxazole were once considered as the mainstay treatments for *Salmonella* infection but are largely replaced by fluoroquinolones due to bacterial resistance to antibiotics. Recently, resistance to fluoroquinolones has also emerged [69], thus necessitating the use of traditional medicines for *Salmonella* infections.

Extracts of *Acacia nilotica* L. have been tested against *Salmonella* species in which the extract disrupted the cell wall of bacteria with consequent release of electrolytes and cellular constituents [70]. Another study conducted by Khan et al. in India has also confirmed the potential use of *A. nilotica* against *Salmonella*. They recorded MIC as 9.75 µg/mL in their study [71]. Sugarcane bagasse has also been tested for anti-*Salmonella* activity. It was found to be bacteriostatic and caused leakage of electrolytes [72]. In South Africa, herbs are used as traditional medicine for the treatment of GIT disorders, e.g., stomach pain, diarrhea, etc. Bisi-Johnson et al. conducted a comprehensive study to scientifically prove the effectiveness of traditional plants for treating Salmonella infection. These plants include *Aloe arborescens* Mill., *Acacia mearnsii* De Wild., *Aloe striata* Haw., *Eucomis autumnalis* (Mill.) Chitt., *E. comosa* (Houtt.) Wehrh., *Cyathula uncinulata* (Schrad.) Schinz, *Hydnora africana* Thunb., *Hermbstaedtia odorata* (Bur ch. ex Moq.) T. Cooke, *Hypoxis latifolia* Wight, *Psidium guajava* L., *Pelargonium sidoides* DC., *Schizocarphus nervosus* (Burch.) van der Merwe. Although most of the studied plants were active in the study, but *A. arborescens*, *A. striata*, *C. uncinulata*, *E. autumnalis*, *E. comosa* and *P. guajava* were particularly potent. The *Salmonella* species used in this study was extended spectrum beta-lactamase positive (ESBL) [73]. In another study from South Africa, the potent antibacterial activity of medicinal was been reported which include *Hypericum roeperianum* Schimp. ex A.Rich., *Cremaspora triflora* (Thonn.) K.Schum., *Heteromorpha arborescens* (Spreng.) Cham. & Schltdl., *Pittosporum viridiflorum* Sims, *Bolusanthus speciosus* (Bolus) Harms, *Calpurnia aurea* (Aiton) Benth., *Maesa lanceolata* Forssk., *Elaeodendron croceum* (Thunb.) DC. and *Morus mesozygia* Stapf. All the plant extracts used were active against *Salmonella* isolates, but *Cremaspora triflora* and *Maesa lanceolata* were very potent having MIC of 0.12 and 0.13 mg/mL, respectively [74]. *Entada abyssinica* A.Rich. is traditionally used in bacterial infections of the gastrointestinal tract (GIT). A total of 8 compounds were isolated from this plant including flavonoids and terpenoids and tested for anti-*Salmonella* activity. Entadanin was found to be the most potent compound having a MIC of 1.56 µg/mL [75]. *Leea indica* (Burm. f.) Merr. from Saudi Arabia [76], *Leea indica, Sclerocarya birrea* (A.Rich.) Hochst. from South Africa [77,78], *Lawsonia inermis* L. from Pakistan [79], *Rhus succedanea* L. from India [80], *Achillea clavennae* L., *Achillea holosericea* Sm., *Achillea lingulata* Waldst. & Kit. and *Achillea millefolium* L. from Japan [81], *Butomus umbellatus* L., *Polygonum amphibium* L. and two species of the genus *Sparganium* (*S. erectum* L. and *S. emersum* Rehmann) from Turkey [82], *Spathodea campanulata* P.Beauv., *Ficus bubu* Warb., *Carica papaya* L., *Cissus aralioides* (Welw. ex Baker) Planch., *Piptadeniastrum africana* (Hook.f.) Brenan, *Hilleria latifolia* (Lam.) H.Walter, *Gladiolus gregarious* Welw. ex Baker and *Phyllanthus muellerianus* (Kuntze) Exell from Cameroon [83,84], persimmon (*Diospyros lotus* L.), guava (*Psidium guajava* L.), sweetsop (*Annona squamosal* Linn.) and *Cichorium intybus* L. from China [85,86], *Anisophyllea laurina* R. Br ex Sabine from Guinea [87], *Sambucus australis* Cham. & Schltdl. from Brazil [88], *Terminalia avicennioides* Guill. & Perr., *Momordica balsamina, Combretum paniculatum* Vent., *Trema guineensis* (Schum. & Thonn.) Ficalho, *Morinda lucida* Benth. and *Ocimum gratissimum* L. from Nigeria [89] were reported to have strong antibacterial activity against *Salmonella* species. It has been observed that EO disrupt and increase the permeability of bacterial cell walls, therefore causing the release of intracellular organelles and proteins. The end result is inactivation and death of the microbes as reviewed by Franklyne et al. [90]. Most of the spices contain EO and consumption of spices has additional health benefits. The common spice ingredients like black pepper, fennel, coriander, cardamom are rich in EO [91].

Biosynthesized nanoparticles of metals (metals + natural materials) are frequently reported to have enhanced pharmacological activities. A newly emerged concept is nano-antibiotics [92], which use plants mediated biogenic nanoparticles with improved antimicrobial, chemotherapeutic and biologic properties [93,94]. Using this approach, several metals are reduced using aqueous extracts of medicinal plants [95] and then used as antimicrobial agents with advanced drug delivery and therapeutic outcomes [96]. Silver (Ag) nanoparticles of aqueous leaf extract of *Eupatorium odoratum* L. were shown to have high anti-*Salmonella* activities than the aqueous leaf extract of *E. odoratum* and also $AgNO_3$ [97]. Silver nanoparticles using the aqueous leaf extracts of *Lippia citriodora* (Palau) Kunth have also been proved to be active against *Salmonella* species [98]. Other authors have also applied nanoparticles of phytoconstituents against *Salmonella* and obtained potent antibacterial activity [99–101].

3.3. Escherichia coli

Escherichia coli (*E. coli*), Gram-negative rods, belongs to *Enterobacteriaceae* family. They represent a vital part of human intestinal normal flora [102]. Enterohemorrhagic *E. coli* (EHEC) produces verotoxin which causes gastrointestinal cramps and diarrhea [103]. The most prevalent serotype O157:H7 which can lead to HUS followed by neurological disorders and kidney failure. Consumption of unhygienic foods including meat, unprocessed milk, fruits, vegetables can transmit the microbes [104]. This important pathogen involved in foodborne diseases was once highly responsive to fluoroquinolones and beta-lactams, but now is resistant to these antibiotics [105]. Therefore, alternative strategies, e.g., traditional medicines as such and compounds derived from such sources are used to treat foodborne diseases caused by *E. coli*. *Acacia nilotica* (L.) Del has been found to disintegrate the cell wall of *E. coli* and release nucleic acids, proteins with a reduction in viable cell growth [70]. In an in vitro study by Elisha et al., nine plants (*Hypericum roeperianum* Schimp. ex A.Rich., *Cremaspora triflora* (Thonn.) K.Schum., *Heteromorpha arborescens* (Spreng.) Cham. & Schltdl., *Pittosporum viridiflorum* Sims, *Bolusanthus speciosus* (Bolus) Harms, *Calpurnia aurea* (Aiton) Benth., *Maesa lanceolata* Forssk., *Elaeodendron croceum* (Thunb.) DC. and *Morus mesozygia* Stapf) were selected for antibacterial activity against *E. coli*. All were found to be active against *E. coli* and thus could be used in the therapeutic management of *E. coli* infection. The lowest MIC was observed for *Maesa lanceolata* as 0.04 mg/mL [74]. *Wasabia japonica* (Miq.) Matsum. is an edible plant that grows at shady, humid and cool places in Japan, China, New Zealand and Korea, and possesses many medicinal properties. This plant inhibits *E. coli* strain O157:H7 which is widely responsible for diarrhea in foodborne diseases [106]. *Punica granatum* L. (pomegranate) is a well-known fruit and is abundantly used throughout the world. It is widely used in traditional medicine for a variety of indications including anti-angiogenic, anti-cancer and antimicrobial [107,108]. Pomegranate contains a variety of phytochemicals (ellagitannins and gallotannins, catechins, procyanidins, flavonoids, anthocyanins and anthocyanidins) [109]. Its antimicrobial activity against *E. coli* has been reported by several researchers [110–112]. Traditional healers of the Limpopo province of South Africa use a variety of medicinal plants for treating diarrhea [113]. Mathabe et al. performed antibacterial experiments to scientifically validate the traditional use of plants against diarrhea/foodborne disease-causing bacteria, i.e; *E. coli*. Their findings confirmed the potential action of *Gymnosporia senegalensis* (Lam.) Loes., *Indigofera daleoides* Harv., *Ozoroa insignis* Delile, *Punica granatum* L., *Spirostachys africana* Sond. and *Syzygium cordatum* Hochst. ex Krauss in limiting *E. coli* infection [114]. Similarly, in Puerto Rico, traditional medicines are used as an alternative therapy for GIT infections. *Tamarindus indica* L., *Phyllanthus acidus* (L.), *Punica granatum* L., *Citrus aurantifolia* (Chrism.) Swingle, *Citrus aurantium* L. were active against *E. coli* [115].

3.4. Staphylococcus aureus

Staphylococcus aureus (*S. aureus*), a Gram-positive, coagulase producing facultative anaerobe is a major cause of foodborne diseases and hospitalization [104]. In addition to causing clinical infections, *S. aureus* also causes food poisoning (a foodborne disease). Individuals suffering from *Staphylococcal* food poisoning are presented with diarrhea, abdominal cramps, nausea and profuse vomiting usually between 1–8 h after food consumption [116]. This pathogen produces exoproteins that are heat stable and are known as *Staphylococcal* enterotoxins (SEs). These toxins act as virulence factors [117] and are mostly responsible for food poisoning and are grouped into five toxin groups designated classically as SEA to SEE. Other *Staphylococcal* enterotoxins (SEG to SER and SEU) have also been described recently [118–120]. *Staphylococcal* foodborne disease outbreak without harboring enterotoxins has also been reported [121]. Traditional medicine is widely practiced in South Africa for treating GIT problems. Bisi-Johnson et al. evaluated the anti–staphylococcal activity of plants used in traditional medicine for GIT related problems including diarrhea and vomiting which are indication of food poisoning. They found that the medicinal plants including *Aloe arborescens* Mill., *Aloe striata* Haw., *Cyathula uncinulata* (Schrad.) Schinz, *Eucomis autumnalis* (Mill.) Chitt., *Eucomis comosa* (Houtt.) Wehrh., *Hypoxis latifolia* Wight, *Hermbstaedtia odorata* (Burch. ex Moq.) T.Cooke, *Scilla nervosa* (Burch.) J.P.Jessop, *Pelargonium sidoides* DC., *Psidium guajava* L. and *Hydnora africana* Thunb. possess strong antibacterial potential towards *S. aureus* and validates the scientific evidence of the use of these plants for food poisoning caused by *S. aureus* [73]. The plant extracts of *Aristolochia indica*, *Cuscuta pedicellata*, *Melilotus indicus* and *Tribulus terrestris* fruit which are traditionally used in Pakistan for various ailments including diarrhea have anti–staphylococcal activity [122]. From Togo, anti–staphylococcal activity has been reported for *Holarrhena floribunda* (G.Don) T.Durand & Schinz [123], from Cameroon, for *Vismia rubescens* Oliv., *Vismia laurentii* De Wild [124,125], from South Africa, *Chrysophyllum albidum* G. Don-Holl., *Terminalia ivorensis* A.Chev. [126,127], from Sudan, *Combretum hartmannianum* Schweinf., *Combretum pentagonum* M.A.Lawson, *Anogeissus schimperi* Hochst. ex Hutch. & Dalziel and *Terminalia arjuna* (Roxb. ex DC.) Wight & Arn. [128], from Egypt, clove (*Syzygium aromaticum*), cress (*Lepidium sativum* L.), lemongrass

(*Cymbopogon citratus* (DC.) Stapf.), Oregano (*Origanum vulgare* L.), rosemary (*Rosmarinus officinalis* L.), sage (*Salvia officinalis* L.) [129], from Algeria, *Stachys guyoniana* Noë ex Batt. and *Mentha aquatic* L., *Centaurea diluta* Ait. subsp. *algeriensis*, *Ferula vesceritensis* Coss. & Durieu ex Trab., *Genista saharae* Coss. & Durieu and *Zilla macroptera* Coss. [130–132] and *Clerodendrum myricoides* (Hochst.) R. Br. ex Vatke from Kenya, [133].

Juglone is a natural compound occurring in plants such as black walnut (*Juglans nigra* L.). This compound has antibacterial property and inhibits *S. aureus* by binding to DNA and disrupts cell wall synthesis, thus stressing the bacterial cells to increasing peroxidative environment [134]. Tetrandrine is an alkaloid isolated from the radix of *Stephania tetrandra* S. Moore. It inhibits *S. aureus* by binding to the peptidoglycan [135]. *Fraxinus rhynchophylla* Hance and its active constituent fraxetin is antibacterial to *S. aureus* via inhibition of essential proteins synthesis. It also decreases the activity of topoisomerase I and topoisomerase II [136]. Several researchers have reported active compounds from medicinal plants that are active against staphylococcal bacteria [137–139]. Essential oils are also utilized against *S. aureus* and studies have shown potential benefits of essential oils derived from *Petroselinum crispum* (Mill.) Fuss, *Cuminum cyminum* L, white mustard (*Sinapis alba* L.), *Chamaecyparis obtusa* (Siebold & Zucc.) Endl. [140–143].

3.5. Shigella

Shigella is a genus of Gram-negative bacteria. It has four species, *S. flexneri*, *S. sonnei*, *S. dysenteriae* and *S. boydii*. These are rod-shaped, non-motile, non-spore forming and facultative anaerobic bacteria [144]. They cause diseases commonly known as shigellosis, characterized by profuse watery diarrhea, fever, abdominal cramps and also bloody dysentery. Ingestion of as low as 100 numbers of these bacteria can cause foodborne disease. These bacteria attack the epithelial cells of the colon of primates only. The resultant inflammation causes high intestinal motility and diarrhea which even leads to dysentery [145]. The virulence of Shiga toxin is like that of verotoxin of *E. coli*, which halts protein synthesis in the host cells [104,146]. In Iran, pomegranate (*Punica granatum*) is commonly used to treat diarrhea. Mahboubi et al. reported that the the extracts of pomegranate were active against *Shigella* [147]. Another study has reported the anti-*Shigella* activity of five plants, e.g., *Thymus vulgaris* L., *Thymus carmanicus* Jalas, *Zataria multiflora* Boiss., *Ziziphora clinopodioides* Lam. and *Ziziphora tenuior* L. Among these *Thymus caramanicus* and *Zataria multiflora* were found comparatively more active having MIC values of 0.78 and 1.56 mg/mL, respectively [148]. In a study by Vuuren et al. 23 traditionally used plants for various ailments including diarrhea, were subjected to antibacterial activity against *Shigella* bateria. Although, all the plants had antibacterial property, *Acacia burkei* Benth. (MIC 0.25 mg/mL), *Acanthospermum glabratum* (DC.) Wild (0.44 mg/mL), *Brachylaena transvaalensis* Hutch. ex E.Phillips & Schweick. (0.5 mg/mL), *Catharanthus roseus* (L.) G.Don (0.41 mg/mL), *Chenopodium ambrosioides* L. (0.5 mg/mL), *Cissampelos hirta* Klotzsch (0.38 mg/mL), *Gymnosporia senegalensis* (Lam.) Loes. (0.63 mg/mL), *Lippia javanica* (0.5 mg/mL), *Mangifera indica* L. (0.25 mg/mL), *Melia azedarach* L. (0.57 mg/mL), *Psidium guajava* L. (0.33 mg/mL), *Sarcostemma viminale* (L.) R.Br. (0.5 mg/mL), *Schotia brachypetala* Sond. (0.58 mg/mL), *Sclerocarya birrea* (A.Rich.) Hochst. (0.34 mg/mL), *Syzygium cordatum* Hochst. ex Krauss (0.43 mg/mL) and *Terminalia sericea* Burch. ex DC. (0.04 mg/mL) were particularly potent [149]. Essential oils are also utilized for foodborne infections caused by *Shigella* [150,151].

3.6. Listeria monocytogenes

Listeria monocytogenes (*L. monocytogenes*), a Gram-positive, non-spore-forming, facultative anaerobe widely affecting food, meat, poultry and seafood [152]. This pathogen grows between 0.4 and 50 °C [104]. The virulence factors of *L. monocytogenes* include the production of beta hemolysin, catalase and superoxide dismutase. It has been implicated in foodborne outbreaks [153]. This microbe can survive refrigeration, high salt content and low pH [154]. These properties enable *L. monocytogenes* to contaminate food even after food postprocessing [155]; *L. monocytogenes* being a foodborne pathogen is challenged with extracts and compounds derived from medicinal plants. In a study by Yoon et al. in South Korea, 69 herbal extracts were tested for inhibition of *L. monocytogenes*. Psoraleae Semen and Sophorae Radix extracts were found potent in their study [156]. Attachment of *L. monocytogenes* to the human intestinal epithelium and its subsequent invasion results in listeriosis. Motility, lecithinase and hemolysin production are the major virulence factors of this pathogen. The virulence factors, i.e., motility, lecithinase and hemolysin production were also decreased. Furthermore, the expression of the virulence genes was downregulated by cinnamaldehyde, carvacrol and thymol more than 3-folds [157,158]. The essential oils are reported to possess antilisterial activity. Essential oils of *Zataria multiflora* Boiss. from Turkey [159], *Carum copticum* (L.) Benth. & Hook.f. ex C.B.Clarke from Iran [160], *Thymus capitatus* (L.) Hoffmanns. & Link from Tunisia [161], *Cymbopogon citratus* D.C. Stapf. from Brazil [162], *Eryngium foetidum* L. from Italy [163] have been reported to have the potential of inhibiting *L. monocytogenes*.

3.7. Clostridium spp.

Clostridium botulinum (*C. botulinum*) is a Gram-positive, rod-shaped, motile, obligate anaerobe [164]. It is a spore-forming bacterium and produces a neurotoxin known as botulinum [165]. It causes a foodborne disease known as foodborne botulism. This happens after ingestion of the preformed toxin produced by *C. botulinum*. The major virulence factor is toxin production [166]. Seven types of toxins have been identified. These are named as A–G. Among these, A, B and E toxin types are associated with foodborne illness. The symptoms of foodborne botulinum are blurred vision, dry mouth, nausea, vomiting, abdominal cramps and difficulty in swallowing [167,168]. Toosendanin, a natural compound, prevents botulinum in animals [169].

C. perfringens, a Gram-positive, spore-forming bacteria has a widespread anaerobic environmental distribution including soil, foodstuff and is part of human flora [170]. Extracts from traditionally important medicinal plants including *Psidium guajava* L., *Haematoxylum brasiletto* H.Karst. and *Euphorbia prostrata* Aiton were found highly effective against *C. perfringens* type A [171]. Likewise, essential oils from *Satureja montana* L. tested against *C. perfringens* type A at a concentration of 1.56%, showed inhibitory activity causing structural damage and cell lysis. Moreover, a synergistic effect between $NaNO_2$ and *Satureja montana* EOs was observed and the findings suggest the potential combined use of savory essential oil and minimal amounts of the synthetic additive, $NaNO_2$ to control *C. perfringens* [172]. The natural product, berberine demonstrated efficacy towards the *C. perfringens* disease based on significantly decreased mortality and lesion scores at 1.0 mL/L, in vitro [173]. Extracts from several plants *Pueraria thunbergiana* (Siebold & Zucc.) Benth., *Astragalus membranaceus* (Fisch.) Bunge, *Eucommia ulmoides* Oliv., *Coptis japonica* (Thunb.) Makino, *Akebia quinata* (Houtt.) Decne. and *Rhus chinensis* Mill. exhibited considerable activity against *C. perfringens* [174].

3.8. Bacillus cereus

B. cereus, a Gram-positive spore-forming bacterium, is frequently implicated in foodborne infections. Among the pathogenic aspects of the bacterium is the production of tissue-damaging exo-enzymes. The bacterium secretes toxins including hemolysins, phospholipases, emesis-inducing toxins and proteases [175]. In the in vitro antibacterial assay against *B. cereus*, the extract of *Dryopteris erythrosora* (D.C. Eaton) Kuntze exhibited an MIC of 0.0156 mg/mL, followed by *Siegesbeckia glabrescens* (SG) Makino leaf (0.0313 mg/mL), *Morus alba* L. bark (0.0313 mg/mL), *Carex pumila* Thunb. root (0.0625 mg/mL) and *Citrus paradisi* Macfad. seed (0.0625 mg/mL) extracts. The combined inhibitory effects of extracts against *B. cereus* were also determined. A combination of *D. erythrosora* and *C. pumila* extracts showed a partial synergistic inhibition, with a fractional inhibitory concentration index of 0.75. The single and combined inhibitory activities of selected plant extracts against *B. cereus* in reconstituted infant rice cereal were also investigated and showed the MICs of *S. glabrescens*, *M. alba*, *D. erythrosora* and *C. pumila* extracts against *B. cereus* as 1.0, 2.0, 2.0 and 8.0 mg/mL, respectively [176]. The plant extracts of *Rhus coriaria* L. and *Hipiscus sabdariffa* L. were investigated against six presumptive *Bacillus cereus* isolates that were isolated from 49 samples of food, soil, manure and eggshells in Amman, Jordan. It was observed that the inhibition of the growth of bacteria was proportional to the increase in extract concentrations. Complete inhibition of the growth was demonstrated at the highest concentrations. The authors concluded that *Rhus coriaria* and *Hibiscus sabdariffa* have the potential to be used as food preservatives against wider spectra of spoilage microorganisms in food [177].

3.9. Vibrio cholerae

V. cholerae, a Gram-negative curved rod from family *Vibrionaceae* has two major virulence factors including cholera toxin, causing profuse rice-watery diarrhea and toxin-coregulated pilus that is mediated in intestinal colonization [178]. Cholera caused by toxigenic *V. cholerae* is a major public health problem particularly in less developed regions of the world with poor sanitation facilities [179]. The extracts of *Ocimum basilicum* L., *Opuntia ficus-indica* (L.) Mill., *Acacia farnesiana* (L.) Willd. and *Artemisia ludoviciana* Nutt. were found active against *V. cholera*, with MBCs values ranging from 0.5–3.0-mg/mL [180]. Recently, solvent-based extracts from red chili, sweet fennel and white pepper were reported to inhibit cholera toxin production. Further, capsaicin the active ingredient of chili prevented the synthesis of cholera toxin in different strains of *V. cholerae*. Capsaicin declined the expression of virulent genes (*ctxA, tcpA* and *toxT*) yet increased the expression of *hns* gene that transcribes a global prokaryotic gene regulator (H-NS) [181]. Solvents based extracts from 32 Mexician plants were evaluated for their inhibitory effects against *V. cholera* strains (O1, O139). Among these, *Acacia farnesiana* and *Artemisia ludoviciana* ethanolic extracts were more effective with minimum Bactericidal Concentrations of 4.0–7.0 and 4.0–6.0-mg/mL respectively [182]. In another study, the extracts of *Terminalia chebula* Retz. and *Syzygium cumini* (L.) Skeels exhibited considerable activity against *V. cholerae*, *Aeromonas hydrophila* and *Bacillus subtilis*, with MBCs (0.25–4 mg/mL). These results favor the use of ethnopharmacological important plants in the management of diarrhea, especially those associated with cholera [183].

4. Plant Extracts and Phytochemicals against Viruses Causing Foodborne Diseases

4.1. Norovirus

Norovirus is single-stranded, positive-sense RNA and non-enveloped virus which is also known as winter vomiting bug [184]. It is a major cause of acute gastroenteritis affecting people of all ages. The transmission of the virus occurs via contaminated food. After entry into the body, the virus replicates in the intestines. It takes one to two days for symptoms to appear. The major symptom reported is gastroenteritis [185]. Other symptoms include watery diarrhea, abdominal cramps, nausea and vomiting. The infection is self-limiting, and recovery occurs within two to three days. There is no specific treatment for norovirus infection. Supportive therapy includes maintaining fluid and electrolyte balance [186]. A combination of juice and polyphenols from pomegranate is effective for eradicating norovirus infection [187]. Chinese galls and pomegranate significantly reduces the attachment of norovirus P protein to their receptors (human histo-blood group antigens) which is an important step for this pathogen virulence. Along with other phytochemicals, tannic acid is responsible for this blocking action [188]. Similarly, grape (*Vitis vinifera* L.) seed extract is used in GIT diseases and has been proved to have potential anti-norovirus activity [189]. Allspice oil and lemongrass oil can reduce viral infection by degrading the capsid of the virus [190]. Curcumin, a natural compound from *Curcuma longa* L. and juice of mulberry (*Morus alba* L.) were tested for anti-noroviral activity and were found to have good inhibitory activity on norovirus.

4.2. Astrovirus

Astroviruses are non-enveloped, positive-sense single-stranded RNA viruses causing GIT disorders particularly pediatric diarrhea. The astrovirus capsid acts as enterotoxin and thus disrupts gut epithelial barrier [191]; *Achyrocline bogotensis* (Kunth) DC. extracts were evaluated for their antirotavirus (RRV) and anti-astrovirus (Yuc8) activities. The nontoxic concentrations displayed considerable antiviral potentials against both viruses. The activity can be attributed to the presence of steroids, sterols, terpenes, phenols, flavonoids and sesquiterpene lactones [192]. *Spirulina platensis* ethanolic extract was tested and revealed a considerable decline in vitro for infectious units of various types of viruses including adenovirus (type 7), astrovirus (type 1), Coxsackievirus B4, rotavirus (Wa strain) and adenovirus (type 40) [193]. Northern Nigerian plants have been investigated against poliovirus, astrovirus, herpes simplex viruses and parvovirus. The obtained results showed that the test samples showed considerable activity against viruses at 100–400 mg/100 mL dose [194].

4.3. Hepatitis-A Virus

The hepatitis A virus (HAV), a picornavirus is a widespread cause of hepatitis and is transmitted via oral intake of contaminated food, water and blood transfusion [195]. Medicinal plants including *Alnus japonica* (Thunb.) Steud. have revealed significant virucidal activity against HAV and at a concentration of 50-µg/mL has reduced HAV titer by 3.43 ± 0.24 logs. Similarly, *Artemisia annua* L., *Allium sativum* L., *Allium fistulosum* L. and *Agrimonia pilosa* Ledeb. extracts exhibited 2.33 ± 0.43, 2.10 ± 0.41, 2.07 ± 0.60 and 2.03 ± 0.26-log reductions, respectively [196]. It has been observed that green tea extract has a strong anti-HAV activity with a direct effect on the viral particles. Supplementing tap water with the extract with continuous shaking every 15 min for 1 h caused a significant reduction in the percentage of HAV plaque counts. There is a strong recommendation of supplementing water with a small concentration of green tea extract that does not cause an observed change in its color and taste for 1 h with persistent shaking before usage in endemic areas for HAV infections [197].

4.4. Rotavirus

Rotavirus infections represent the leading cause of dehydrating gastroenteritis among children less than 5 years of age. Despite the worldwide vaccinations against rotavirus, it is still a major cause of fatality (>200,000 deaths annually) especially in low-income countries [198]. These viruses usually infect enterocytes, thus induce diarrhea via the decline in the absorptive capacity of enterocytes, increase intestinal secretion stimulated by viral non-structural protein 4 and activation of the enteric nervous system [199]. It has been observed that supplementation *Nelumbo nucifera* Gaertn., *Aspalathus linearis* (Burm.f.) R.Dahlgren, *Urtica dioica* L., *Glycyrrhiza glabra* L. and *Olea europaea* L. extracts are effective in the managment of rotavirus induced diarrhea [200,201]. Moreover, aqueous extracts from *Nelumbo nucifera*, *Urtica dioica*, *Aspalathus linearis*, *Glycyrrhiza glabra* and *Olea europaea* leaves were reported to exhibit substantial antiviral potentials with IC_{50} of <300 µg/mL. Likewise, 18β-glycyrrhetinic acid and luteolin isolated from *G. glabra* and *A. linearis* exhibited IC_{50} of 46 µm and 116 µm, respectively [201]. *Rubia cordifolia* L. extracts, isolated compounds including xanthopurpurin and vanillic acid were quite effective against rotavirus and inhibited its multiplication by augmenting virus-mediated apoptosis in MA-104 cells [202]. The antirotavirus activity of *Bauhinia variegata* L. was examined, which showed antiviral activity against rotavirus in vitro with therapeutic index ranged from 0.2 to 23 and a reduction in virus titers ranged from 0.25 $\log_{10}$ to 4.75 $\log_{10}$. These results demonstrated that *B. variegata* has a potential for the pharmacotherapeutic management of rotavirus induced gastroenteritis [203]. The antiviral activity of different extracts from *Calliandra haematocephala* Hassk. leaves against rotavirus (RV) infection was evaluated both in vitro and in vivo. *C. hematocephala* at non-cytotoxic concentrations exhibited antirotavirus activities at a different magnitude of potency with therapeutic index ranging from 1.3 to 32 and a reduction in virus titer ranging from 0.25 $\log_{10}$ to 5.75 $\log_{10}$. In the in vivo study, oral administration of the methanol extract at 50 mg and 100 mg/kg/day significantly reduced mortality, virus titers, duration and severity of diarrhea, as well as alleviation of lesion in the small intestine in rotavirus infected mice [204]. The leaf of Japanese big-leaf magnolia (*Magnolia obovate* Thunb.) has long been used as a natural packaging material for traditional foods in Japan. The extract significantly inhibited cytopathic effects and mRNA expression of rotaviral proteins in SA11-infected MA104 cells and thus can be used as a medicine or food additive to prevent and ameliorate rotavirus-induced diarrhea in individuals that may have difficulty in benefitting from the rotavirus vaccines [205].

5. Plant Extracts and Phytochemicals against Parasites Causing Foodborne Diseases

5.1. Giardia lambia

Giardiasis is a human parasitic infection most commonly transmitted through the ingestion of infected food and is associated with significant morbidity [206]. The most common cause of giardiasis is the protozoan, *Giardia lamblia* commonly called *G. intestinalis* and *G. duodenalis*. Several treatment strategies are devised for its eradication which includes nutritional intervention, ingestion of probiotics and phytotherapeutic agents [207]. Several natural products including *Allium sativum*, berberine and flavonoid-rich herbs, *Piper longum* L., *Butea monosperma* (Lam.) Taub. and various isolated compounds have been found effective in the eradication of giardiasis [208,209].

Natural products based therapeutics play a significant role in the treatment and management of giardiasis, mediated through eradication of parasite and thus relieving the unwanted symptoms of infection. Several herbs are extensively reported for their effectiveness in *Giardia* infections; *Allium sativum* is a well-known household remedy against numerous human diseases including microbial and parasitic infections [210]. In a study, Harris et al. reported the anti-giardial potentials of crude *A. sativum* and its isolated compounds; *A. sativum* crude extract exhibited IC_{50} of 0.3-mg/mL against *Giardia intestinalis*, whereas, the isolated compounds allyl mercaptan, diallyl disulfide, diallyl sulfide, allyl alcohol and dimethyl disulfide showed IC_{50} values of 0.037, 0.1, 1.3, 0.007 and 0.2 mg/mL, respectively [33].

Furthermore, the incubation of *Giardia* trophozoites in the presence of whole *A. sativa* exhibited considerable decline in the parasite motility, flagellar movement and ultimate swelling of the trophozoite. The mechanisms underlying these events involve the loss of osmoregulation of parasite and loss of transmembrane electrochemical gradient. Microscopic studies revealed morphologic changes in the ventral disc of the parasite which can be responsible for its inability to attached to its host cell [33]. In another clinical study, Soffar and Mokhtar administered fresh *A. sativum* distilled water extract (5 mL) or 0.6 mg commercially available capsules to 26 children infected with *G. lamblia* for three days and observed its beneficial effects against giardiasis [211]. The symptoms of giardiasis were effectively subsided in all the groups of children with thirty-six hours of therapy and the stool examination revealed complete eradication of parasite [211]. Allicin isolated from *A. sativum* is reported to mediate its action against the parasite via inhibition of giardia's cysteine proteases and inhibition of products responsible for unwanted symptoms of giardiasis [212,213]. Moreover, *A. sativa* also increases the mucosal nitric oxide (NO) production via stimulation of nitric oxide synthase, which subsequently increases the liberation of NO from enterocytes and exhibits direct giardicidal effects [33].

Piper longum L. is a well-known folk medicine for the treatment of gastrointestinal disorders and helminthesis [214]. In a study, Tripathi et al. investigated the giardicidal actions of crude extracts of *P. longum*. Treatment with crude ethanolic extract (125 µg/mL) and aqueous extracts (250 µg/mL) showed 100% lethality against *Giardia lamblia*. In an animal model of giardiasis, *P. longum* crude ethanolic extract, aqueous extract and fruit powder at doses of 250, 450 and 900 mg/kg, respectively significantly (75%) diminished the live trophozoites count in the intestinal mouse aspirates after five days of therapy [215]. The two important gastroprotective herbs including *Piper longum* and *Butea monosperma* have been combined in a traditional herbal formulation called Pippali rasayana (PR). This formulation is very famous in folk medicine for the treatment of helminthesis and chronic dysentery. In a study, Agarwal et al. reported the anti-giardial effects of PR formulation in an animal model. The in vivo study revealed that PR administration in doses of 225, 450 and 900 mg/kg exhibited 62%, 79% and 98% parasitic clearance, respectively. Moreover, PR significantly augmented the macrophage phagocytic activity and macrophage migration index at all the tested doses. As the PR formulation is inactive against the parasite in vitro, so it was proposed that the formulation may mediate its anti-giardial activity through boosting of host immune system and thereby increasing clearance mechanisms [216]. To further explore the clinical significance of PR formulation, Agarwal et al. extended the study and included fifty human subjects with all signs and symptoms of giardiasis including cysts and Giardia trophozoites in the stool samples. The subjects were divided into two groups; the treated group was maintained on PR (1 g T.D.S) for fifteen days, whereas the second group served as a placebo control. After the completion of therapy, stool samples were analyzed for *G. lamblia*, frequency of diarrhea and mucous content of the stool. In the treated group, 92% inhibition of *Giardia* and a significant decline in diarrhea and mucous were observed. A boost in the cell-mediated immune system indicated by a decline in leukocyte migration was also observed [217].

In a study, Miyares et al. evaluated the giardicidal potential of propolis in 136 subjects with well-known symptoms of giardiasis. In the five days' trials, propolis was administered in 20, 30% solutions (adults) and 10% solution (children) and duodenal aspirates were evaluated for giardicidal activity. Results of the study revealed 60% giardicidal activity for 30% solution and 40% giardicidal activity for 20% solution in adults whereas, 52% giardicidal activity was observed in children after administration of 10% solution. The standard drug, tinidazole exhibited a 40% efficacy [218]. Several studies have confirmed the efficacy of berberine and berberine rich plants including *Coptis chinensis* Franch., *Berberis vulgaris* L., *Berberis aquifolium* Pursh, *Berberis aristata* DC. and *Hydrastis canadensis* L. in the management of gastrointestinal disorders like parasitic infestation and diarrhea [219,220]. Berberine is highly effective against Giardia trophozoites and mediates its beneficial effects via morphologic changes in the trophozoites including changes in the shape of vacuoles, trophozoites swelling and deposition of glycogen deposits [221]. Berberine hydrochloride at a dose of 5 mg/kg showed a 68% decline in the stool–*Giardia* content and a significant decline in giardiasis symptoms in a clinical study [222]. In a clinical trial, berberine administered in doses of 5, 10 mg/kg for 5–10 days showed a 47%, 55%, 68% and 90% decline in the Giardia content in all the treated groups of children. The standard drugs, furazolidone and metronidazole exhibited a 92% and 95% efficiency against *Giardia* [223]. In vitro studies have revealed high efficacy of crude extracts from these plants in comparison to pure berberine, which can be attributed to the synergistic interactions of berberine with other isoquinoline alkaloids present in these plants [224]. Natural flavonoids including epicatechin, quercetin, epigallocatechin, apigenin and kempferol, which are abundant in several natural products like *Quercus robur* L., *Hamamelis virginiana* L. and *Croton lechleri* Müll.Arg. are extensively reported for giardicidal potentials [225–227]. In a study, flavonoids and tannins rich plants including *Origanum vulgare* L., *Psidium guajava* L., *Mangifera indica* L. and *Plantago major* L. showed high anti-giardial activity in comparison to the standard drug, tinidazole [228]. Barbosa E et al. reported the antigiardial activity of flavonoids isolated from *Geranium mexicanum* Kunth, *Helianthemum glomeratum* (Lag.) Lag. ex Dunal, *Cuphea pinetorum* Benth. and *Rubus coriifolius* Liebm. Among the isolated compounds, kempferol, tiliroside and epicatechin exhibited IC_{50} values of 2.057, 1.429 and 0.072 µmol/kg, respectively against *G. lambia* [229].

5.2. Entamoeba histolytica

Amoebiasis is a ubiquitous gastrointestinal disorder most prevalent in less developed countries with poor sanitation and socioeconomic status, affecting about 12% of global population [230]. It is known to be the third leading cause of mortality [231–233]. The causative agent of amoebiasis is *Entamoeba histolytica*, which is associated with typical symptoms of amoebic dysentery, abdominal cramps, bloating or tenderness and stomachache [234,235]. Among the currently available chemotherapeutics, metronidazole is an effective amoebicide, but is associated with unwanted side-effects like carcinogenesis, mutagenesis, nausea and vomiting [236,237]. The stratagem of utilizing natural drugs in antiamoebic therapy traces back to the pre-historic era. For instance, emetine isolated from *Cephaelis ipecacuanha* (Brot.) A.Rich. is used as a front line anti-amoebic drug [238]. Currently, a large population is dependent on traditional therapeutics for the management of various diseases [18,25,239]. Medicinal plant and herbal drugs represent an indispensable part of the traditional medicine practiced in many countries owing to low costs, frequent availability, biosafety and ancestral knowledge [240–242]. Hence, in search of more effective drugs, traditionally used natural products are of great importance. Several natural products and isolated compounds have been scientifically validated for effective eradication of *Entamoeba histolytica*, for potential drug development. For instance, bruceantin, a potent amoebicide from *Brucea antidysenterica* J.F.Mill. exhibited IC$_{50}$ of 0.018 µg/mL [243], parthenin from *Parthenium hysterophorus* L. [244], extracts and isolated compounds from *Brucea javanica* (L.) Merr. fruits and *Simarouba amara* Aubl. [245] and alkaloids from *Alstonia angustifolia* Wall. ex A.DC. roots [246] were extensively studied against *E. histolytica*. Cimanga et al. investigated the effect of *Morinda morindoides* (Baker) Milne-Redh. leaves extracts and isolated compounds against *E. histolytica* [247]. The crude methanolic extract and aqueous decoction showed significant anti-amoebic action with IC$_{50}$ values of 1.7 and 3.1 µg/mL, respectively. Among the isolated compounds, kempferol, apigenin, luteolin, apigenin-7-*O*-glucoside and luteolin-7-*O*-glucoside exhibited IC$_{50}$ values of 10.3, 12.7, 17.8, 22.3 and 37.4 µg/mL, respectively against *E. histolytica*.

Tona et al. evaluated forty-five Congolese plant extracts used in traditional medicine against *E. histolytica*. Among the tested samples, *Mangifera indica* L., *Rauwolfia obscura* K.Schm., *Carica papaya* L., *Euphorbia hirta* L., *Hymenocardia acida* Tull., *Jatropha curcas* L., *Maprounea africana* Mull. Arg., *Paropsia brazzeana* Baill., *Psidium guajava* L., *Cryptolepis sanguinolenta* (Lindl.) Schltr. and *Quassia africana* (Baill.) Baill. were highly active with IC$_{50}$ values of 7.81, 31.5, 7.81, 31.25, 31.25, 31.25, 31.25, 7.81, 7.81, 7.81 and 31.5 µg/mL, respectively [248]. In another study, Sohni et al. investigated the antiamoebic potentials of an herbal formulation containing *Zingiber officinale*, *Berberis aristata*, *Boerhavia diffusa* L., *Tinospora cordifolia* (Willd.) Miers and *Terminalia chebula* extracts. Among these plant extracts, *Berberis aristata* and *Tinospora cordifolia* showed IC$_{50}$ values of 100 and 1000 µg/mL, respectively. All these plants in a combined formulation exhibited an IC$_{50}$ of 1000 µg/mL. The herbal formulation was also tested against some enzymes of *E. histolytica* including DNase, RNase, aldolase, alkaline, acid phosphatases and α-amylase that are known to play a significant role in the virulence and invasiveness of the parasite. Results confirmed various degrees of inhibition of these enzymes [249]. Owing to the traditional use of *Salvia polystachya* Cav. for the treatment of dysentery in the Mexican traditional medicine, Calzada et al. investigated various isolated compounds from *Salvia polystachya* against *E. histolytica* and *G. lamblia* trophozoites. Among the tested compounds, Linearolactone was most active showing IC$_{50}$ value of 22.9 and 28.2 mM against *E. histolytica* and *G. lamblia*, respectively. Whereas, polystachynes A, B and D, exhibited modest antiprotozoal potentials with IC$_{50}$ values ranging from 117.0–160.6 mM against *E. histolytica* and 107.5–134.7 mM against *G. lamblia* [250].

In the search for new antiprotozoal drugs from natural products, Calzada et al. studied the inhibitory effects of twenty-six traditional Mexican drugs against *E. histolytica* and *G. lamblia*. Among the tested samples, *Chiranthodendron pentadactylon* Larreat., *Annona cherimola* Mill., *Punica granatum*, *Dichondra argentea* Humb. & Bonpl. ex Willd., *Chenopodium ambrosioides* L. and *Chrysactinia mexicana* A.Gray were most active showing IC$_{50}$ values of 2.5, 14.8, 29.5, 38.3, 45.2, 45.3 µg/mL, respectively against *E. histolytica*. Whereas, *Dorstenia contrajerva* L., *Senna villosa* (Mill.) H.S. Irwin & Barneby, *Ruta chalepensis* L., *Cocos nucifera* L. and *Chiranthodendron pentadactylon* Larreat. exhibited IC$_{50}$ values of 23.3, 32.1, 37.8, 44.1, 44.2 µg/mL, respectively against *G. lamblia* [251]. In another study, the same group investigated the antiprotozoal efficiency of crude extracts and isolated compounds from the roots of *Geranium mexicanum* against *E. histolytica* and *G. lamblia*. Among the crude samples, dichloromethane–methanol, ethyl acetate, fraction 13 (from ethyl acetate) and aqueous fractions showed IC$_{50}$ values of 79.2, 66.7, 51.5 and 221.6 µg/mL, respectively against *E. histolytica* and 100.4, 63.7, 59.7 and 215.9 µg/mL, respectively against *G. lamblia*. Among the isolated compounds, epicatechin, catechin, β-sitosterol 3-*O*-β-D-glucopyranoside and tyramine revealed IC$_{50}$ values of 1.9, 65.6, 82.2 and 54.2 µg/mL, respectively against *E. histolytica* and 1.6, 33.9, 61.5 and 68.9 µg/mL, respectively against *G. lamblia* [252]. The antiprotozoal potential of another traditional plant, *Rubus coriifolius* and its isolated compounds were investigated by Alanís et al. against *E. histolytica* and *G. lambia*. In the crude fractions, dichloromethane–methanol was most active with IC$_{50}$ values of 11.6 and 55.6 µg/mL, respectively against *E. histolytica* and *G. lamblia*. Whereas, the isolated compounds including epicatechin, catechin, nigaichigoside, β-sitosterol-3-O-β-D-glucopyranoside, hyperin, gallic acid and ellagic acid exhibited IC$_{50}$ value of 1.9, 65.5, 111.9, 82.16, 143.6, 220 and 56.5 µg/mL, respectively against *E. histolytica* and 1.6, 34.0, 123.6, 61.5, 49.2, 70.3 and 24.9 µg/mL, respectively against *G. lamblia* [253].

5.3. Toxoplasma gondii

Toxoplasmosis is a parasitic infection caused by *Toxoplasma gondii* and transmitted from infected pregnant women and contaminated food and is a major cause of foodborne hospitalization and death [254]. Meat from various sources including pork, cattle, wild game meat, poultry meat, lamb if not properly cooked and vegetables contaminated with oocysts, infected water and feces can cause transmission of toxoplama infection [255]. Proper cleansing, cooking of meat and washing of fruits and vegetables can significantly reduce the risk of toxoplasmosis. Immunocompromised and organ transplant individuals are at more risk to develop this infection. Several toxoplasmosis outbreaks in Korea are reported to be linked with the use of uncooked pork [256]. Toxoplasmosis is reported as a major cause of neurologic infections in HIV infected individuals [257]. Toxoplasmosis is reported as the second major cause of foodborne infections and the fourth major cause of hospitalization and deaths in the United States [4]. In Greece, toxoplasmosis has been reported among the top five contributors of foodborne infections, leading to major disabilities and deaths [258].

Several studies regarding the efficacy of natural products against toxoplasmosis have been reported. In a study, Youn et al. reported the antiparasitic potentials of traditionally used plant extracts against *Toxoplasma gondii* and *Neospora caninum* [259]. Solvent extracts of *Sophora flavescens* Aiton, *Torilis japonica* (Houtt.) DC., *Ulmus macrocarpa* Hance, *Sinomenium acutum* (Thunb.) Rehder & E.H.Wilson and *Pulsatilla koreana* (Yabe ex Nakai) Nakai ex T. Mori collected from South Korea were tested. Among the tested herbs, *T. japonica* exhibited significant inhibitory potential against *T. gondii* by inhibiting parasite proliferation from 54% to 99% at 19.5–156 ng/mL; *S. flavescens* extracts restrain *T. gondii* growth by 27.2–98.7% at a concentration ranging from 39-ng/mL to 156 ng/mL. Extracts from other plants including *Pulsatilla koreana*, *U. macrocarpa* and *S. acutum* showed moderate antiparasitic activity against *T. gondii*. Wright et al. tested the effectiveness of isolated compounds from *Simarouba amara* and *Brucea javanica* fruits against *Toxoplasma gondii*, *E. histolytica* and *Giardia intestinalis*. Among the tested compounds, ailanthinone, bruceantin, bruceine B, bruceine C, bruceine D, brusatol, glaucarubinone and quassin exhibited IC$_{50}$ values of 0.0251, 0.0115, 0.75, 0.842, 7.56, 0.179, 0.374 and 111 µM, respectively [260].

In a study, Choi et al. tested methanolic extracts from fifteen traditional herbs against *T. gondii*. Among the tested samples, *Sophora flavescens*, *Zingiber officinale*, Meliae Cortex, *Acorus gramineus* Aiton, *Dryopteris crassirhizoma* Nakai and *Glycyrrhiza glabra* were potent and exhibited EC$_{50}$ values of 0.20, 0.18, 0.77, 0.11, 0.15 and 0.13 mg/mL, respectively against *Toxoplasma gondii* [261].

5.4. Cryptosporidium

Cryptosporidium spp. belongs to the family, *Cryptosporidiidae*. The most common species that cause human infection are the *Cryptosporidium parvum* and *Cryptosporidium hominis*. They can be transmitted from animals, human-to-human, water, food, and tend to cause waterborne outbreaks. The clinical manifestation in immunocompetent patients is self-limiting when compared to immunocompromised individuals where it causes chronic diarrhea not responding to treatment [262]. *Cryptosporidium* spp. are well recognized as causes of diarrheal disease and is increasingly identified as an important cause of morbidity and mortality worldwide [263]. The ethanolic extract from olive (*Olea europaea*) pomace, after oil pressing and phenol recovery, reproducibly inhibited *Cryptosporidium parvum* development (MIC = 250–500 µg/mL, IC$_{50}$ = 361 (279–438) µg/mL, IC$_{90}$ = 467 (398–615) µg/mL) [264]. In an in vivo study, the extract of *Curcuma longa* L. had the highest effect on *Cryptosporidium* oocysts shedding. The inhibitory effect was observed at a rate of 100% on the 7th day of treatment at 750 mg/kg and on the 5th day at 1000 mg/kg in the watery extracts. At a rate of 100% on the 4th day at 1000 mg/kg in alcoholic extracts [265]. Potential cryptosporicidal effects have been observed for blueberry with its polyphenolic compounds, cinnamon with its phenolic compounds and onion with its flavonoids and sulfide compounds, garlic with its allicin, mango with its mangiferin, olive pomace with its oleuropein, pomegranate with its polyphenols and tannins and oregano with its carvacrol especially against *Cryptosporidium parvum* and *Cryptosporidium hominis* [266]. The anti-*Cryptosporidium* efficacies of various plant extracts were evaluated in four groups of age-matched neonatal Swiss albino mice. There was a 100% reduction in *Cryptosporidium* oocyst excretion in stool and copro-DNA of *O. europaea*-treated infected mice after 2 weeks. Thus, the plant of *O. europaea* is a promising natural therapeutic for cryptosporidiosis [267].

A detailed list of antiprotozoal activity of important medicinal plant extract and phytochemicals against foodborne parasites is provided in Table 1. Chemical structures of some of the plants derived bioactive compounds are given in Figure 1.

Table 1. Summary of effects of plant extracts and phytochemicals against foodborne parasites.

Plant Source	Part Used	Effective against	Mechanism/IC$_{50}$	Reference
Allium sativum	Crude methanolic eextract	G. intestinalis	300 µg/mL ↓ Parasite motility ↓ Flagellar movement ↑Trophozoite swelling ↓Transmembrane electrochemical gradient ↓ Osmoregulation ↑ Morphologic changes in the ventral disc	[33]
	Allyl mercaptan Diallyl disulfide Diallyl sulfide Allyl alcohol Dimethyl disulfide	G. intestinalis	37 µg/mL 100 µg/mL 1300 µg/mL 7 µg/mL 200 µg/mL	[33]
	Aqueous extract commercial capsule	G. lamblia	↓Giardiasis symptoms ↓Giardia stool content	[211]
	Allicin	G. lamblia	↓ Cysteine proteases ↓ Giardia waste products	[212,213]
Piper longum	Crude ethanolic extract and aqueous extract of fruit powder	G. lamblia	100% Lethality ↓ Trophozoites count	[215]
Piper longum and Butea monosperma	Pippali Rasayana Formulation at 225, 450, 900 mg/kg	G. lamblia	62%, 79%, 98% Parasite clearance ↑ Macrophage phagocytic action ↑Macrophage migration index ↑Host immune system ↑Clearance of parasite wastes	[216]
	Pippali Rasayana Formulation 1 g T.D.S	G. lamblia	↑Giardia inhibition (92%) ↓Diarrhea frequency ↓Stool mucous content ↓Leukocyte migration	[217]
Coptis chinensis, Berberis vulgaris, Berberis aristata, Berberis aquifolium, Hydrastis canadensis	Crude extracts, Berberine	G. lamblia	↑Morphologic changes in trophozoites ↑ Trophozoites Swelling ↑Glycogen deposition ↓Giardia stool content	[221–224]
Quercus robur, Hamamelis virginiana, Croton lechleri	Epicatechin, Quercetin, Epigallocatechin, Apigenin, Kempferol	G. lamblia	↑Giardia inhibition	[225–227]
Origanum vulgare, Psidium guajava, Mangifera indica, Plantago major	Flavonoids and tannins rich crude extracts	G. lamblia	↑Antigiardial activity	[228]

Table 1. Cont.

Plant Source	Part Used	Effective Against	Mechanism/IC$_{50}$	Reference
Geranium mexicanum, Helianthemum glomeratum, Cuphea pinetorum and Rubus coriifolius	Kempferol Tiliroside Epicatechin	G. lamblia	2.05 µmol/kg 1.42 µmol/kg 0.07 µmol/kg	[229]
Geranium mexicanum	Dichloromethane-methanol extract	E. histolytica G. lamblia	79.2 µg/mL 100.4 µg/mL	[252]
	Ethyl acetate extract	E. histolytica G. lamblia	66.7 µg/mL 63.7 µg/mL	
	Aqueous extract	E. histolytica G. lamblia	221.6 µg/mL 215.9 µg/mL	
	Epicatechin	E. histolytica G. lamblia	1.9 µg/mL 1.6 µg/mL	
	Catechin	E. histolytica G. lamblia	65.6 µg/mL 33.9 µg/mL	
	β-Sitosterol 3-O-β-D-glucopyranoside	E. histolytica G. lamblia	82.2 µg/mL 61.5 µg/mL	
	Tyramine	E. histolytica G. lamblia	54.2 µg/mL 68.9 µg/mL	
Rubus coriifolius	Dichloromethane-methanol extract	E. histolytica G. lamblia	11.6 µg/mL 55.6 µg/mL	[253]
	Epicatechin	E. histolytica G. lamblia	1.9 µg/mL 1.6 µg/mL	
	Catechin	E. histolytica G. lamblia	65.5 µg/mL 34.0 µg/mL	
	Nigaichigoside	E. histolytica G. lamblia	111.9 µg/mL 123.6 µg/mL	
	β-Sitosterol 3-O-β-D-glucopyranoside	E. histolytica G. lamblia	82.16 µg/mL 61.5 µg/mL	
	Hyperin	E. histolytica G. lamblia	143.6 µg/mL 49.2 µg/mL	
	Gallic acid	E. histolytica G. lamblia	220.1 µg/mL 70.3 µg/mL	
	Ellagic acid	E. histolytica G. lamblia	56.5 µg/mL 24.9 µg/mL	
Allium sativum	Methanolic extract	E. histolytica G. lamblia	61.8 µg/mL 64.9 µg/mL	[251]
Aloysia triphylla	Methanolic extract	E. histolytica G. lamblia	113.4 µg/mL 106.9 µg/mL	
Annona cherimola	Methanolic extract	E. histolytica G. lamblia	14.8 µg/mL 146.0 µg/mL	
Artemisia absinthium	Methanolic extract	E. histolytica G. lamblia	72.3 µg/mL 135.4 µg/mL	
Artemisia ludoviciana	Methanolic extract	E. histolytica G. lamblia	82.2 µg/mL 95.1 µg/mL	
Bocconia frutescens	Methanolic extract	E. histolytica G. lamblia	96.4 µg/mL 79.3 µg/mL	
Cesalpinia pulcherrima	Methanolic extract	E. histolytica G. lamblia	182.2 µg/mL 49.9 µg/mL	
Carica papaya	Methanolic extract	E. histolytica G. lamblia	153.0 µg/mL 128.8 µg/mL	
Cocos nucifera	Methanolic extract	E. histolytica G. lamblia	59.6 µg/mL 44.1 µg/mL	
Chenopodium ambrosioides	Methanolic extract (Green plant)	E. histolytica	45.2 µg/mL	
	Methanolic extract (Red Plant)	G. lamblia	106.5 µg/mL	
Chenopodium murale	Methanolic extract	E. histolytica G. lamblia	90.3 µg/mL 99.8 µg/mL	
Chiranthodendron pentadactylon	Methanolic extract	E. histolytica G. lamblia	2.5 µg/mL 44.2 µg/mL	
Chrysactinia mexicana	Methanolic extract	E. histolytica G. lamblia	45.3 µg/mL 106.5 µg/mL	

Table 1. Cont.

Plant Source	Part Used	Effective Against	Mechanism/IC$_{50}$	Reference
Dorstenia contrajerva	Methanolic extract	E. histolytica	47.1 µg/mL	
		G. lamblia	23.3 µg/mL	
Dichondra argentea	Methanolic extract	E. histolytica	38.3 µg/mL	
		G. lamblia	284.7 µg/mL	
Geranium mexicanum	Methanolic extract	E. histolytica	139.9 µg/mL	
		G. lamblia	267.1 µg/mL	
Hippocratea excelsa	Methanolic extract	E. histolytica	233.2 µg/mL	
		G. lamblia	72.7 µg/mL	
Lippia alba	Methanolic extract	E. histolytica	58.1 µg/mL	
		G. lamblia	109.4 µg/mL	
Lygodium venustum	Methanolic extract	E. histolytica	178.4 µg/mL	
		G. lamblia	74.3 µg/mL	
Matricaria recutita	Methanolic extract	E. histolytica	102.1 µg/mL	
		G. lamblia	67.1 µg/mL	
Ocimum basilicum	Methanolic extract	E. histolytica	41.7 µg/mL	
		G. lamblia	79.4 µg/mL	
Punica granatum	Methanolic extract	E. histolytica	29.5 µg/mL	
		G. lamblia	198.5 µg/mL	
Ruta chalepensis	Methanolic extract	E. histolytica	61.9 µg/mL	
		G. lamblia	37.8 µg/mL	
Schinus molle	Methanolic extract	E. histolytica	82.4 µg/mL	
		G. lamblia	154.7 µg/mL	
Senna villosa	Methanolic extract	E. histolytica	133.1 µg/mL	
		G. lamblia	32.1 µg/mL	
Thymus vulgaris	Methanolic extract	E. histolytica	90.9 µg/mL	
		G. lamblia	68.7 µg/mL	
Sophora flavescens Torilis japonica, Ulmus macrocarpa, Sinomenium acutum	Alcoholic extracts	T. gondii	99.7%	[259]
			99.9%	
			99.8%	
			99.7%	
Pulsatilla koreana			99.6%	
Sophora flavescens			0.20	
Meliae cortex			0.77	
Acorus gramineus	Methanolic extracts	T. gondii	0.11	[261]
Dryopteris crassirhizoma			0.15	
Glycyrrhiza glabra			0.13	
Zingiber officinale			0.18	
	Ailanthinone		0.02 µM	
	Bruceantin		0.01 µM	
	Bruceine A		NT	
	Bruceine B		0.75 µM	
	Bruceine C	T. gondii	0.84 µM	[260]
	Bruceine D		7.56 µM	
	Brusatol		0.17 µM	
	Glaucarubinone		0.37 µM	
	Quassin		11 µM	
	Ailanthinone		0.13 µM	
	Bruceantin		0.03 µM	
	Bruceine A		0.22 µM	
Brucea javanica	Bruceine B		0.63 µM	[260]
Simarouba amara	Bruceine C	E. histolytica	0.49 µM	
	Bruceine D		0.06 µM	
	Brusatol		0.32 µM	
	Glaucarubinone		1130 µM	
	Ailanthinone		45.44 µM	
	Bruceantin		1.20 µM	
	Bruceine A		8.84 µM	
	Bruceine B		NT	
	Bruceine C	G. intestinalis	NA	[260]
	Bruceine D		NA	
	Brusatol		6.17 µM	
	Glaucarubinone		12.42 µM	
Brucea antidysenterica	Bruceantin	E. histolytica	0.01 µg/mL	[243]
Brucea javanica, Simarouba amara	Bruceantin	E. histolytica	0.01 µg/mL	[245]
	Glaucarubol		5 µg/mL	

Table 1. Cont.

Plant Source	Part Used	Effective Against	Mechanism/IC$_{50}$	Reference
	Quercetin		105.2 µg/mL	
	Quercetin-7,4-dimethylether		70.3 µg/mL	
	Quercetin-3-O-rutinoside		120.7 µg/mL	
	Quercetin-3-O-rhamnoside		93.2 µg/mL	
	Kempferol-3-O-rhamnoside		64.7 µg/mL	
	Kempferol-3-O-rutinoside		72.5 µg/mL	
	Kempferol-7-O-rhamnosyl-sophoroside		>125 µg/mL	
Morinda morindoides	Chrysoeriol-7-O-neohesperidoside	E. histolytica	>125 µg/mL	[247]
	Apigenin-7-O-glucoside		22.3 µg/mL	
	Luteolin-7-O-glucoside		37.4 µg/mL	
	Kempferol		10.3 µg/mL	
	Apigenin		12.7 µg/mL	
	Luteolin		17.8 µg/mL	
	Gaertneroside		4.3 µg/mL	
	Gaertneric acid		7.1 µg/mL	
	Methoxygaertneroside		2.3 µg/mL	
	Epoxygaertneroside		1.3 µg/mL	
Justicia insularis	Leaves water extract	E. histolytica	>500 µg/mL	
Draceana reflexa	Leaves water extract	E. histolytica	62.5 µg/mL	
Costus afer	Juice	E. histolytica	125 µg/mL	
Vitex madiensis	Leaves water extract	E. histolytica	>500 µg/mL	
Cissius areloides	Leaves water extract	E. histolytica	>500 µg/mL	
Datura arborea	Leaves water extract	E. histolytica	125 µg/mL	
Morinda morindoides	Leaves water extract	E. histolytica	15.62 µg/mL	
Nauclea latifolia	Root-bark water extract	E. histolytica	125 µg/mL	
	Laves water extract		>500 µg/mL	
Heinsia pulchella	Root-bark water extract	E. histolytica	15.62 µg/mL	
Crossopteryx febrifuga	Laves water extract	E. histolytica	125 µg/mL	
Pteridium aquilinum	Twigs water extract	E. histolytica	>500 µg/mL	
Phytollaca dodecandra	Laves water extract	E. histolytica	>500 µg/mL	
Mangifera indica	Stem-bark water extract	E. histolytica	7.81 µg/mL	
Rauwolfia obstura	Root-bark water extract	E. histolytica	31.5 µg/mL	
Voacanga africana	Root-bark water extract	E. histolytica	62.5 µg/mL	
Tithonia diversifolia	Leaves water extract	E. histolytica	62.5 µg/mL	
Ceiba pentandra	Stem-bark water extract	E. histolytica	125 µg/mL	[248]
Dialum englerianum	Stem-bark water extract	E. histolytica	62.5 µg/mL	
Carica papaya	Immature seeds water extract	E. histolytica	62.5 µg/mL	
	Mature seeds water extract		<7.81 µg/mL	
Garcinia kola	Stem-bark water extract	E. histolytica	125 µg/mL	
Tetracera poggei	Leaves water extract	E. histolytica	>500 µg/mL	
Alchornea cordifolia	Leaves water extract	E. histolytica	125 µg/mL	
Bridelia ferruginea	Root-bark water extract	E. histolytica	62.5 µg/mL	
Euphorbia hirta	Leaves water extract	E. histolytica	250 µg/mL	
Hymenocardia acida	Stem-bark water extract	E. histolytica	31.25 µg/mL	
	Root-bark water extract		250 µg/mL	
Jatropha curcas	Leaves water extract	E. histolytica	31.25 µg/mL	
Maprounea africana	Leaves water extract	E. histolytica	62.5 µg/mL	
	Root-bark water extract		31.25 µg/mL	
Cajanus cajan	Leaves water extract	E. histolytica	>500 µg/mL	
Paropsia brazzeana	Root-bark water extract	E. histolytica	<7.81 µg/mL	
Harungana madagascariensis	Stem-bark water extract	E. histolytica	62.25 µg/mL	
Sida rhombifolia	Leaves water extract	E. histolytica	62.5 µg/mL	
Pentacletra macrophylla	Stem-bark water extract	E. histolytica	250 µg/mL	
Myrianthus arboreus	Leaves extract	E. histolytica	>500 µg/mL	
Psidium guajava	Leaves extract	E. histolytica	62.5 µg/mL	
	Stem-bark water extract		<7.815 µg/mL	
Ongokea gore	Stem-bark water extract	E. histolytica	>500 µg/mL	
Ryptolepis sanguinolenta	Root-Bark water extract	E. histolytica	<7.815 µg/mL	
Zingiber officinale	Ethanolic extract	E. histolytica	>1000 µg/mL	
Boerhavia diffusa	Ethanolic extract	E. histolytica	>1000 µg/mL	
Tinospora cordifolia	Ethanolic extract	E. histolytica	1000 µg/mL	[249]
Terminalia chebula	Ethanolic extract	E. histolytica	>1000 µg/mL	
Berberis aristata	Ethanolic extract	E. histolytica	100 µg/mL	

Table 1. Cont.

Plant Source	Part Used	Effective Against	Mechanism/IC$_{50}$	Reference
Salvia polystachya	Polystachyne A	E. histolytica	153.8 µg/mL	[250]
		G. lamblia	134.7 µg/mL	
	Polystachyne B	E. histolytica	117.0 µg/mL	
		G. lamblia	107.8 µg/mL	
	Polystachyne D	E. histolytica	160.6 µg/mL	
		G. lamblia	107.5 µg/mL	
	Linearolactone	E. histolytica	22.9 µg/mL	
		Giardia lamblia	28.2 µg/mL	
	Kaempferol	E. histolytica	27.7 µg/mL	
		G. lamblia	30.5 µg/mL	

NT: not tested, **NA:** not active, ↑: Increase/activate, ↓: decrease/inhibit, ↔: no effect/not modulate, **CDT:** cytolethal distending toxin, **EO:** essential oils.

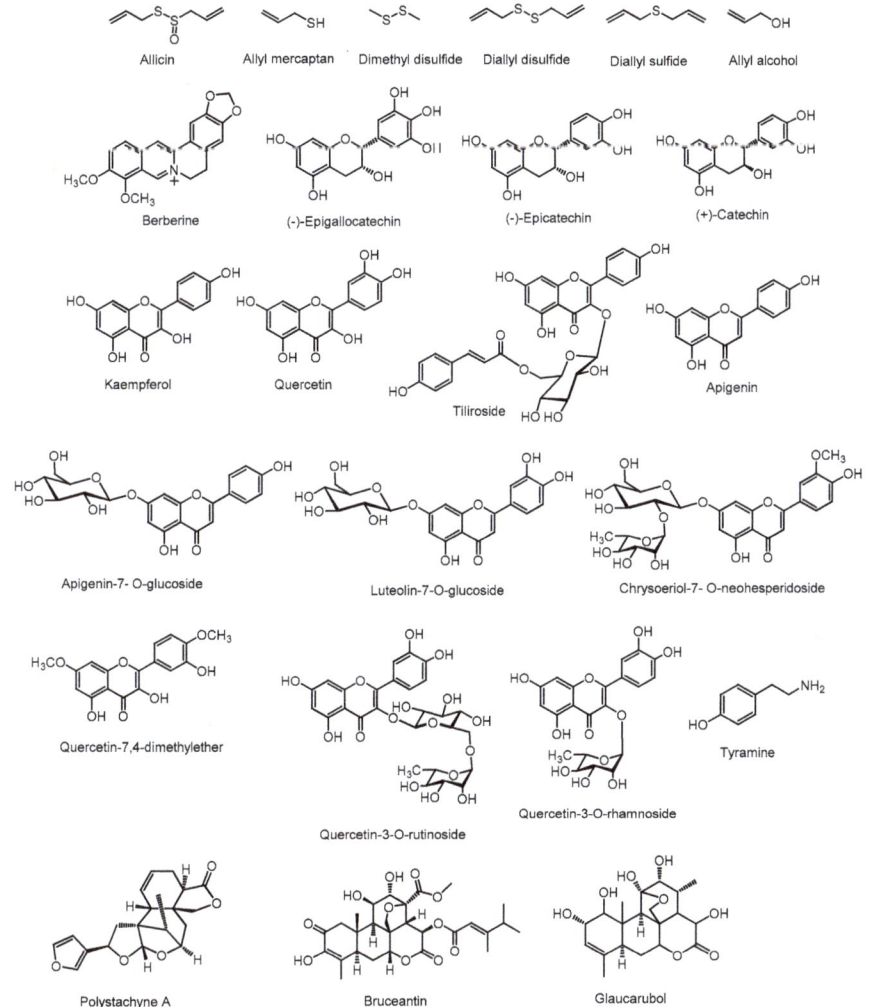

Figure 1. Chemical structures of some of the phytochemicals discussed in this manuscript.

6. Mechanisms of Antimicrobial Activity

Various mechanisms have been reported for the antimicrobial activities of medicinal plants and isolated natural antimicrobials. These natural products affect those pathways of macromolecular metabolism which are proven targets for antibiotic intervention. Among the existing antibacterial agents, it is clear that protein and cell wall biosynthesis are the targets of the widest variety of natural products [34]. The pathways of macromolecular metabolism as antimicrobial targets of natural products include inhibition of protein synthesis, inhibition of cell wall synthesis, disruption of membrane integrity, inhibition of RNA synthesis, inhibition of DNA synthesis, dysfunction of microtubules, inhibition of lipid synthesis, inhibition of cell division, dysfunction in ion uptake, reduction in protein secretion, dysfunction of RNA processing and inhibition of DNA methylation. These mechanisms have been investigated for the antimicrobial properties of medicinal plants and natural products including *Hemidesmus indicus* (L.) R. Br. ex Schult., *Leucas aspera* (Willd.) Link, *Plumbago zeylanica* L., *Tridax procumbens* (L.) L. [268], *Syzygium cumini* (L.) Skeels [269], *Combretum albidum* G.Don, *Hibiscus acetosella* Welw. ex Hiern, *Hibiscus cannabinus* L., *Hibiscus furcatus* Willd., *Punica granatum* L. and *Tamarindus indica* L. [270], 5,6,7-trihydroxyflavone (baicalein) [271], flavones [272], *Hibiscus sabdariffa*, *Rosmarinus officinalis*, *Syzygium aromaticum*, *Thymus vulgaris* [273], linalyl acetate, (+)menthol, thymol [274], *Origanum vulgare* [275], essential oils [276], caffeine [277], allspice oil, lemongrass oil, citral [278], alkaloids [279], *Boerhaavia diffusa* [280], paeonol (PA) and 1,2,3,4,6-penta-O-galloyl-β-D-glucopyranose (PGG) from *Paeonia lactiflora* Pall. [281], *Aristolochia bracteolata* Lam. [282], *Rhizophora apiculate* Blume, *Phyllanthus niruri* L., *Scutellaria baicalensis* Georgi, *Geum japonicum* L. and *Momordica charantia* L. [283]. Plants being mixture of numerous compounds can act on several targets like, inhibition of bacterial cell wall synthesis, protein synthesis and interference with microbial metabolic pathways. Hence, as a whole, the activity of crude extracts may be due to more than one antibacterial mechanism. Further, different compounds in the extract can act synergistically as well as can antagonize the effect of each other depending upon their respective concentrations. Considering the presence of large number of chemical compounds present in the extracts of medicinal plants, it is most likely that their antimicrobial activity can be attributed to more than a single specific antimicrobial mechanism.

7. Persisting Challenges

However, many plant extracts and their isolated phytochemicals have been reported to show potent activity against foodborne illness causing agents, there have not been detailed studies about their mechanism using in vivo studies. As the systematic treatment, use of oral rehydration salts and antibiotics are also of great concern for their use in foodborne illness in children and their efficacies [17], alternative therapies like herbal extracts and compounds should be used with proper caution and with the support of scientific evidence regarding the other dosage forms of these herbal products. Human gut microbiota plays a vital role in sustaining gastrointestinal health via inhibition of pathogenic microbes. The use of broad-spectrum antibiotics causes inhibition of normal flora beside pathogenic bacteria, thus provide the opportunity to other pathogens and secondary infections emerge [284,285]. On the other hand, herbal products like tea and many herbs and vegetables are also reported to be the source of foodborne microorganisms [286,287]. Herbal products contaminated with mycotoxins, bacterial toxins, as well as bacterial strains are reported to cause foodborne infections. For instance, herbs contaminated with *Salmonella* is a major cause of foodborne infections in North America and Europe [286]. Subsequently, several approaches were adopted to decontaminate these products including irradiation which effectively eradicate *Salmonella, S. aureus, Comphylobacter* sp., *Listeria* and *E. coli* without affecting nutritional properties of these products [288].

Natural product research has broadly emerged into two major fields including ethnopharmacology and toxicology. However, both strategies were successful regarding the discovery of numerous drugs against several diseases, yet the development of antimicrobial agents from these sources is limited [289]. To augment the development of antimicrobial agents from the herbal source it is important to elucidate exact molecular antimicrobial mechanisms of these products. This information will enable researchers not only to have better control of these microbes but will use modern technologies to synthesize more potent and effective derivatives. Moreover, studies regarding the efficacy of these agents in combination with other herbs and drugs is limited. For instance, a combination of several EOs in combined form does not produce the synergistic antimicrobial effect and subsequently their use as a food preservative is limited. These agents can also interact with food ingredients which significantly affect their quality. Like, EOs beside their great beneficial effects has limited efficacy as a food preservative due to the intense aroma and toxicity issues. EOs used as preservatives in food are reported to change organoleptic properties of foodstuff and their higher doses can produce severe toxicological responses [290,291].

8. Conclusions

Foodborne diseases are one of the main causes of morbidity and mortality, especially in low-income countries having poor sanitation and inadequate healthcare facilities. Several plant extracts and phytochemicals including catechin, epigallocatechin, apigenin, kempferol, berberine, tiliroside and quercetin were found to be highly effective to control the growth of these foodborne pathogens causing infections in in vitro systems. Various mechanisms have been reported for the antimicrobial activities of medicinal plants and they affect those pathways of macromolecular metabolism which are the proven targets for antibiotic intervention. Medicinal plants can impact more than a single specific antimicrobial target as they contain a large number of biochemical phytoconstituents. Once utilized, natural products with antimicrobial properties can be effective for the prevention and treatment of foodborne diseases and can increase the shelf life of food products. However, most of the studies covered in this review are performed using in vitro assays. Further detailed in vivo studies for exploration of effectiveness and mechanism of their activities are necessary. Along with that, most of these studies were performed in the in vitro systems without the addition of food, simulated gastric and/or intestinal juice. Various such factors may alter the activity of these extracts and compounds when used in complex biologic systems such as in vivo and human studies. Future studies should also focus on the pharmacokinetic and toxicological aspects of plant extracts and phytochemicals.

Author Contributions: F.U. (Farhat Ullah), F.U. (Farman Ullah), M.A., A.A.-D., A.S., I.H. conceived the idea, performed literature review, data collection, interpretation and manuscript preparation. M.S., Z.Y., A.A.-D. and H.P.D. revised the manuscript. All authors have read and agreed to the published version of the manuscript.

Funding: There is no particular funding to support this research.

Conflicts of Interest: The authors declare no conflicts of interest.

References

1. Rane, S. Street vended food in developing world: Hazard analyses. *Indian J. Microbiol.* **2011**, *51*, 100–106. [CrossRef]
2. Nout, M. Fermented foods and food safety. *Food Res. Int.* **1994**, *27*, 291–298. [CrossRef]
3. Ayaz, M.; Junaid, M.; Subhan, F.; Ullah, F.; Sadiq, A.; Ahmad, S.; Imran, M.; Kamal, Z.; Hussain, S.; Shah, S.M. Heavy metals analysis, phytochemical, phytotoxic and anthelmintic investigations of crude methanolic extract, subsequent fractions and crude saponins from *Polygonum hydropiper* L. *BMC Complement. Altern. Med.* **2014**, *14*, 465. [CrossRef] [PubMed]
4. Scallan, E.; Hoekstra, R.M.; Angulo, F.J.; Tauxe, R.V.; Widdowson, M.-A.; Roy, S.L.; Jones, J.L.; Griffin, P.M. Foodborne illness acquired in the United States—Major pathogens. *Emerg. Infect. Dis.* **2011**, *17*, 7. [CrossRef] [PubMed]
5. Kumagai, Y.; Gilmour, S.; Ota, E.; Momose, Y.; Onishi, T.; Bilano, F.; Luanni, V.; Kasuga, F.; Sekizaki, T.; Shibuya, K. Estimating the burden of foodborne diseases in Japan. *Bull. World Health Organ.* **2015**, *93*, 540–549. [CrossRef]
6. Olsen, S.J.; MacKinon, L.C.; Goulding, J.S.; Bean, N.H.; Slutsker, L. Surveillance for Foodborne-Disease Outbreaks, United States, 1993–1997. *MMWR CDC Surveill. Summ.* **2000**, *49*, 1–62. [PubMed]
7. Park, M.S.; Kim, Y.S.; Lee, S.H.; Kim, S.H.; Park, K.H.; Bahk, G.J. Estimating the burden of foodborne disease, South Korea, 2008–2012. *Foodborne Pathog. Dis.* **2015**, *12*, 207–213. [CrossRef]

8. Available online: https://www.who.int/activities/estimating-the-burden-of-foodborne-diseases (accessed on 26 May 2020).
9. Buchanan, R.L.; Smith, J.L.; Long, W. Microbial risk assessment: Dose-response relations and risk characterization. *Int. J. Food Microbiol.* **2000**, *58*, 159–172. [CrossRef]
10. Xiao, L.; Ryan, U.; Feng, Y. *Biology of Foodborne Parasites*; CRC Press: Boca Raton, FL, USA, 2015; Volume 1.
11. Dei-Cas, E.; Aliouat, C.-M.; Certad, G.; Creusy, C.; Guyot, K. Infectious Forms of Parasites in Food: Man Embedded in Ecosystems. In *Detection of Bacteria, Viruses, Parasites and Fungi*; Springer: Dordrecht, The Netherlands, 2010; pp. 299–332.
12. Hernández-Cortez, C.; Palma-Martínez, I.; Gonzalez-Avila, L.U.; Guerrero-Mandujano, A.; Solís, R.C.; Castro-Escarpulli, G. Food Poisoning Caused by Bacteria (Food Toxins). In *Poisoning—From Specific Toxic Agents to Novel Rapid and Simplified Techniques for Analysis*; IntechOpen Limited: London, UK, 2017; pp. 33–72.
13. Walsh, C.; Fanning, S. Antimicrobial resistance in foodborne pathogens-A cause for concern? *Curr. Drug Targets* **2008**, *9*, 808–815. [CrossRef]
14. Slutsker, L.; Altekruse, S.F.; Swerdlow, D.L. Foodborne diseases: Emerging pathogens and trends. *Infect. Dis. Clin.* **1998**, *12*, 199–216. [CrossRef]
15. Abd El-Baky, H.H.; El-Baroty, G.S. The Potential Use of Microalgal Carotenoids as Dietary Supplements and Natural Preservative Ingredients. *J. Aquat. Food Prod. Technol.* **2013**, *22*, 392–406. [CrossRef]
16. Msagati, T.A. *The Chemistry of Food Additives and Preservatives*; John Wiley & Sons: Hoboken, NJ, USA, 2012.
17. Switaj, T.L.; Winter, K.J.; Christensen, S.R. Diagnosis and management of foodborne illness. *Am. Fam. Physician* **2015**, *92*, 358–365.
18. Ayaz, M.; Subhan, F.; Sadiq, A.; Ullah, F.; Ahmed, J.; Sewell, R. Cellular efflux transporters and the potential role of natural products in combating efflux mediated drug resistance. *Front. Biosci. (Landmark Ed.)* **2017**, *22*, 732–756. [CrossRef]
19. Ayaz, M.; Subhan, F.; Ahmed, J.; Khan, A.-u.; Ullah, F.; Ullah, I.; Ali, G.; Hussain, S. Sertraline enhances the activity of antimicrobial agents against pathogens of clinical relevance. *J. Biol. Res. Thessalon.* **2015**, *22*, 4. [CrossRef]
20. Ayaz, M.; Subhan, F.; Ahmed, J.; Khan, A.-U.; Ullah, F.; Sadiq, A.; Syed, N.; Ullah, I.; Hussain, S. Citalopram and venlafaxine differentially augments antimicrobial properties of antibiotics. *Acta Pol. Pharm. Drug Res.* **2015**, *72*, 1269–1278.
21. Shahid, M.; Subhan, F.; Ahmad, N.; Ullah, I. A bacosides containing *Bacopa monnieri* extract alleviates allodynia and hyperalgesia in the chronic constriction injury model of neuropathic pain in rats. *BMC Complement. Altern. Med.* **2017**, *17*, 293. [CrossRef]
22. Shahid, M.; Subhan, F.; Ullah, I.; Ali, G.; Alam, J.; Shah, R. Beneficial effects of *Bacopa monnieri* extract on opioid induced toxicity. *Heliyon* **2016**, *2*, e00068. [CrossRef] [PubMed]
23. Aman, U.; Subhan, F.; Shahid, M.; Akbar, S.; Ahmad, N.; Ali, G.; Fawad, K.; Sewell, R.D. *Passiflora incarnata* attenuation of neuropathic allodynia and vulvodynia apropos GABA-ergic and opioidergic antinociceptive and behavioural mechanisms. *BMC Complement. Altern. Med.* **2016**, *16*, 77. [CrossRef]
24. Ullah, I.; Subhan, F.; Alam, J.; Shahid, M.; Ayaz, M. Suppression of cisplatin-induced vomiting by *Cannabis sativa* in pigeons: Neurochemical evidences. *Front. Pharmacol.* **2018**, *9*, 231. [CrossRef] [PubMed]
25. Ayaz, M.; Sadiq, A.; Junaid, M.; Ullah, F.; Subhan, F.; Ahmed, J. Neuroprotective and anti-aging potentials of essential oils from aromatic and medicinal plants. *Front. Aging Neurosci.* **2017**, *9*, 168. [CrossRef]
26. Ovais, M.; Ayaz, M.; Khalil, A.T.; Shah, S.A.; Jan, M.S.; Raza, A.; Shahid, M.; Shinwari, Z.K. HPLC-DAD finger printing, antioxidant, cholinesterase, and α-glucosidase inhibitory potentials of a novel plant Olax nana. *BMC Complement. Altern. Med.* **2018**, *18*, 1. [CrossRef] [PubMed]
27. Odeyemi, O.A.; Sani, N.A. Antibiotic resistance and burden of foodborne diseases in developing countries. *Future Sci.* **2016**, *2*, FSO139. [CrossRef] [PubMed]
28. Grace, D. Food safety in low and middle income countries. *Int. J. Environ. Res. Public Health* **2015**, *12*, 10490–10507. [CrossRef] [PubMed]
29. Ayaz, M.; Ullah, F.; Sadiq, A.; Ullah, F.; Ovais, M.; Ahmed, J.; Devkota, H.P. Synergistic interactions of phytochemicals with antimicrobial agents: Potential strategy to counteract drug resistance. *Chem. Biol. Interact.* **2019**, *308*, 294–303. [CrossRef]
30. Smid, E.J.; Gorris, L.G. Natural antimicrobials for food preservation. In *Handbook of Food Preservation*; CRC Press: Boca Raton, FL, USA, 2007; pp. 237–358.

31. Ehiri, J.E.; Morris, G. Food safety control strategies: A critical review of traditional approaches. *Int. J. Environ. Health Res.* **1994**, *4*, 254–263. [CrossRef]
32. Castillo, S.L.; Heredia, N.; Contreras, J.F.; Garcia, S. Extracts of edible and medicinal plants in inhibition of growth, adherence, and cytotoxin production of Campylobacter jejuni and Campylobacter coli. *J. Food Sci.* **2011**, *76*, M421–M426. [CrossRef]
33. Harris, J.C.; Plummer, S.; Turner, M.P.; Lloyd, D. The microaerophilic flagellate Giardia intestinalis: Allium sativum (garlic) is an effective antigiardial. *Microbiology* **2000**, *146*, 3119–3127. [CrossRef]
34. Silver, L.; Bostian, K. Screening of natural products for antimicrobial agents. *Eur. J. Clin. Microbiol. Infect. Dis.* **1990**, *9*, 455–461. [CrossRef]
35. Nachamkin, I.; Szymanski, C.M.; Blaser, M.J. *Campylobacter*, 3rd ed.; American Society for Microbiology Press: Washington, DC, USA, 2008.
36. Kirk, M.D.; Pires, S.M.; Black, R.E.; Caipo, M.; Crump, J.A.; Devleesschauwer, B.; Dopfer, D.; Fazil, A.; Fischer-Walker, C.L.; Hald, T.; et al. World Health Organization Estimates of the Global and Regional Disease Burden of 22 Foodborne Bacterial, Protozoal, and Viral Diseases, 2010: A Data Synthesis. *PLoS Med.* **2015**, *12*, e1001921. [CrossRef]
37. Cha, W.; Mosci, R.E.; Wengert, S.L.; Venegas Vargas, C.; Rust, S.R.; Bartlett, P.C.; Grooms, D.L.; Manning, S.D. Comparing the Genetic Diversity and Antimicrobial Resistance Profiles of *Campylobacter jejuni* Recovered from Cattle and Humans. *Front. Microbiol.* **2017**, *8*, 818. [CrossRef]
38. Szczepanska, B.; Andrzejewska, M.; Spica, D.; Klawe, J.J. Prevalence and antimicrobial resistance of *Campylobacter jejuni* and *Campylobacter coli* isolated from children and environmental sources in urban and suburban areas. *BMC Microbiol.* **2017**, *17*, 80. [CrossRef]
39. Dholvitayakhun, A.; Cushnie, T.P.; Trachoo, N. Antibacterial activity of three medicinal Thai plants against *Campylobacter jejuni* and other foodborne pathogens. *Nat. Prod. Res.* **2012**, *26*, 356–363. [CrossRef] [PubMed]
40. Singh, G.; Passsari, A.K.; Leo, V.V.; Mishra, V.K.; Subbarayan, S.; Singh, B.P.; Kumar, B.; Kumar, S.; Gupta, V.K.; Lalhlenmawia, H.; et al. Evaluation of Phenolic Content Variability along with Antioxidant, Antimicrobial, and Cytotoxic Potential of Selected Traditional Medicinal Plants from India. *Front. Plant Sci.* **2016**, *7*, 407. [CrossRef]
41. Ouahouo, B.M.; Azebaze, A.G.; Meyer, M.; Bodo, B.; Fomum, Z.T.; Nkengfack, A.E. Cytotoxic and antimicrobial coumarins from *Mammea africana*. *Ann. Trop. Med. Parasitol.* **2004**, *98*, 733–739. [CrossRef]
42. Canning, C.; Sun, S.; Ji, X.; Gupta, S.; Zhou, K. Antibacterial and cytotoxic activity of isoprenylated coumarin mammea A/AA isolated from *Mammea africana*. *J. Ethnopharmacol.* **2013**, *147*, 259–262. [CrossRef]
43. Fais, T.; Delmas, J.; Serres, A.; Bonnet, R.; Dalmasso, G. Impact of CDT Toxin on Human Diseases. *Toxins* **2016**, *8*, 220. [CrossRef]
44. Sanchez, E.; Garcia, S.; Heredia, N. Extracts of edible and medicinal plants damage membranes of *Vibrio cholerae*. *Appl. Environ. Microbiol.* **2010**, *76*, 6888–6894. [CrossRef]
45. Upadhyay, A.; Arsi, K.; Wagle, B.R.; Upadhyaya, I.; Shrestha, S.; Donoghue, A.M.; Donoghue, D.J. Trans-Cinnamaldehyde, Carvacrol, and Eugenol Reduce *Campylobacter jejuni* Colonization Factors and Expression of Virulence Genes in Vitro. *Front. Microbiol.* **2017**, *8*, 713. [CrossRef] [PubMed]
46. Kovacs, J.K.; Felso, P.; Makszin, L.; Papai, Z.; Horvath, G.; Abraham, H.; Palkovics, T.; Boszormenyi, A.; Emody, L.; Schneider, G. Antimicrobial and Virulence-Modulating Effects of Clove Essential Oil on the Foodborne Pathogen *Campylobacter jejuni*. *Appl. Environ. Microbiol.* **2016**, *82*, 6158–6166. [CrossRef] [PubMed]
47. Friedman, M.; Henika, P.R.; Mandrell, R.E. Bactericidal activities of plant essential oils and some of their isolated constituents against *Campylobacter jejuni*, *Escherichia coli*, *Listeria monocytogenes*, and *Salmonella enterica*. *J. Food Prot.* **2002**, *65*, 1545–1560. [CrossRef] [PubMed]
48. Fisher, K.; Phillips, C.A. The effect of lemon, orange and bergamot essential oils and their components on the survival of Campylobacter jejuni, Escherichia coli O157, Listeria monocytogenes, Bacillus cereus and Staphylococcus aureus in vitro and in food systems. *J. Appl. Microbiol.* **2006**, *101*, 1232–1240. [CrossRef] [PubMed]
49. Kurekci, C.; Padmanabha, J.; Bishop-Hurley, S.L.; Hassan, E.; Al Jassim, R.A.; McSweeney, C.S. Antimicrobial activity of essential oils and five terpenoid compounds against *Campylobacter jejuni* in pure and mixed culture experiments. *Int. J. Food Microbiol.* **2013**, *166*, 450–457. [CrossRef]

50. Rattanachaikunsopon, P.; Phumkhachorn, P. Potential of coriander (*Coriandrum sativum*) oil as a natural antimicrobial compound in controlling Campylobacter jejuni in raw meat. *Biosci. Biotechnol. Biochem.* **2010**, *74*, 31–35. [CrossRef]
51. Rossi, P.G.; Bao, L.; Luciani, A.; Panighi, J.; Desjobert, J.M.; Costa, J.; Casanova, J.; Bolla, J.M.; Berti, L. (E)-Methylisoeugenol and elemicin: Antibacterial components of *Daucus carota* L. essential oil against Campylobacter jejuni. *J. Agric. Food Chem.* **2007**, *55*, 7332–7336. [CrossRef]
52. Hernandez-Ochoa, L.; Aguirre-Prieto, Y.B.; Nevarez-Moorillon, G.V.; Gutierrez-Mendez, N.; Salas-Munoz, E. Use of essential oils and extracts from spices in meat protection. *J. Food Sci. Technol.* **2014**, *51*, 957–963. [CrossRef]
53. Lu, X.; Rasco, B.A.; Jabal, J.M.; Aston, D.E.; Lin, M.; Konkel, M.E. Investigating antibacterial effects of garlic (*Allium sativum*) concentrate and garlic-derived organosulfur compounds on *Campylobacter jejuni* by using Fourier transform infrared spectroscopy, Raman spectroscopy, and electron microscopy. *Appl. Environ. Microbiol.* **2011**, *77*, 5257–5269. [CrossRef] [PubMed]
54. Smith-Palmer, A.; Stewart, J.; Fyfe, L. Antimicrobial properties of plant essential oils and essences against five important food-borne pathogens. *Lett. Appl. Microbiol.* **1998**, *26*, 118–122. [CrossRef]
55. Ozogul, Y.; Kuley, E.; Ucar, Y.; Ozogul, F. Antimicrobial Impacts of Essential Oils on Food Borne-Pathogens. *Recent Pat. Food Nutr. Agric.* **2015**, *7*, 53–61. [CrossRef]
56. Sela, F.; Karapandzova, M.; Stefkov, G.; Cvetkovikj, I.; Kulevanova, S. Chemical composition and antimicrobial activity of essential oils of *Juniperus excelsa* Bieb. (Cupressaceae) grown in R. Macedonia. *Pharmacogn. Res.* **2015**, *7*, 74–80. [CrossRef]
57. Silva, O.; Duarte, A.; Pimentel, M.; Viegas, S.; Barroso, H.; Machado, J.; Pires, I.; Cabrita, J.; Gomes, E. Antimicrobial activity of *Terminalia macroptera* root. *J. Ethnopharmacol.* **1997**, *57*, 203–207. [CrossRef]
58. Samie, A.; Obi, C.L.; Lall, N.; Meyer, J.J. In-vitro cytotoxicity and antimicrobial activities, against clinical isolates of *Campylobacter* species and *Entamoeba histolytica*, of local medicinal plants from the Venda region, in South Africa. *Ann. Trop. Med. Parasitol.* **2009**, *103*, 159–170. [CrossRef] [PubMed]
59. Paulo, A.; Pimentel, M.; Viegas, S.; Pires, I.; Duarte, A.; Cabrita, J.; Gomes, E.T. *Cryptolepis sanguinolenta* activity against diarrhoeal bacteria. *J. Ethnopharmacol.* **1994**, *44*, 73–77. [CrossRef]
60. Jarriyawattanachaikul, W.; Chaveerach, P.; Chokesajjawatee, N. Antimicrobial Activity of Thai-herbal Plants against Food-borne Pathogens *E. coli*, *S. aureus* and *C. jejuni*. *Agric. Agric. Sci. Procedia* **2016**, *11*, 20–24. [CrossRef]
61. Sreeramulu, G.; Zhu, Y.; Knol, W. Kombucha fermentation and its antimicrobial activity. *J. Agric. Food Chem.* **2000**, *48*, 2589–2594. [CrossRef] [PubMed]
62. Diker, K.S.; Akan, M.; Hascelik, G.; Yurdakök, M. The bactericidal activity of tea against *Campylobacter jejuni* and *Campylobacter coli*. *Lett. Appl. Microbiol.* **1991**, *12*, 34–35. [CrossRef]
63. Aslim, B.; Yucel, N. In vitro antimicrobial activity of essential oil from endemic Origanum minutiflorum on ciprofloxacin-resistant Campylobacter spp. *Food Chem.* **2008**, *107*, 602–606. [CrossRef]
64. Kurekci, C.; Bishop-Hurley, S.L.; Vercoe, P.E.; Durmic, Z.; Al Jassim, R.A.; McSweeney, C.S. Screening of Australian plants for antimicrobial activity against *Campylobacter jejuni*. *Phytother. Res.* **2012**, *26*, 186–190. [CrossRef]
65. Welkos, S.; Schreiber, M.; Baer, H. Identification of *Salmonella* with the O-1 bacteriophage. *Appl. Environ. Microbiol.* **1974**, *28*, 618–622. [CrossRef]
66. Letellier, A.; Messier, S.; Quessy, S. Prevalence of Salmonella spp. and Yersinia enterocolitica in finishing swine at Canadian abattoirs. *J. Food Prot.* **1999**, *62*, 22–25. [CrossRef]
67. Robinson, R. Salmonella infection: Diagnosis and control. *N. Z. Vet. J.* **1970**, *18*, 259–277. [CrossRef]
68. Thorns, C. Bacterial food-borne zoonoses. *Rev. Sci. Et Tech. Off. Int. Des Epizoot.* **2000**, *19*, 226–239. [CrossRef]
69. *Salmonella—A Dangerous Foodborne Pathogen*; Mahmoud, B.S.M. (Ed.) InTechOpen Limited: London, UK, 2016.
70. Sadiq, M.B.; Tarning, J.; Aye Cho, T.Z.; Anal, A.K. Antibacterial Activities and Possible Modes of Action of *Acacia nilotica* (L.) Del. against Multidrug-Resistant Escherichia coli and Salmonella. *Molecules* **2017**, *22*, 47. [CrossRef]
71. Khan, R.; Islam, B.; Akram, M.; Shakil, S.; Ahmad, A.A.; Ali, S.M.; Siddiqui, M.; Khan, A. Antimicrobial Activity of Five Herbal Extracts Against Multi Drug Resistant (MDR) Strains of Bacteria and Fungus of Clinical Origin. *Molecules* **2009**, *14*, 586. [CrossRef] [PubMed]

72. Zhao, Y.; Chen, M.; Zhao, Z.; Yu, S. The antibiotic activity and mechanisms of sugarcane (*Saccharum officinarum* L.) bagasse extract against food-borne pathogens. *Food Chem.* **2015**, *185*, 112–118. [CrossRef] [PubMed]
73. Bisi-Johnson, M.A.; Obi, C.L.; Samuel, B.B.; Eloff, J.N.; Okoh, A.I. Antibacterial activity of crude extracts of some South African medicinal plants against multidrug resistant etiological agents of diarrhoea. *BMC Complement. Altern. Med.* **2017**, *17*, 321. [CrossRef] [PubMed]
74. Elisha, I.L.; Botha, F.S.; McGaw, L.J.; Eloff, J.N. The antibacterial activity of extracts of nine plant species with good activity against *Escherichia coli* against five other bacteria and cytotoxicity of extracts. *BMC Complement. Altern. Med.* **2017**, *17*, 133. [CrossRef] [PubMed]
75. Dzoyem, J.P.; Melong, R.; Tsamo, A.T.; Tchinda, A.T.; Kapche, D.G.; Ngadjui, B.T.; McGaw, L.J.; Eloff, J.N. Cytotoxicity, antimicrobial and antioxidant activity of eight compounds isolated from *Entada abyssinica* (Fabaceae). *BMC Res. Notes* **2017**, *10*, 118. [CrossRef]
76. Rahman, M.A.; Imran, T.B.; Islam, S. Antioxidative, antimicrobial and cytotoxic effects of the phenolics of *Leea indica* leaf extract. *Saudi J. Biol. Sci.* **2013**, *20*, 213–225. [CrossRef]
77. Razwinani, M.; Tshikalange, T.E.; Motaung, S.C. Antimicrobial and anti-inflammatory activities of *Pleurostylia capensis* Turcz (Loes) (Celastraceae). *Afr. J. Tradit Complement. Altern Med.* **2014**, *11*, 452–457. [CrossRef]
78. Tanih, N.F.; Ndip, R.N. Evaluation of the Acetone and Aqueous Extracts of Mature Stem Bark of *Sclerocarya birrea* for Antioxidant and Antimicrobial Properties. *Evid. Based Complement. Altern. Med.* **2012**, *2012*, 834156. [CrossRef]
79. Gull, I.; Sohail, M.; Aslam, M.S.; Amin Athar, M. Phytochemical, toxicological and antimicrobial evaluation of *Lawsonia inermis* extracts against clinical isolates of pathogenic bacteria. *Ann. Clin. Microbiol. Antimicrob.* **2013**, *12*, 36. [CrossRef]
80. Shrestha, S.; Subaramaihha, S.R.; Subbaiah, S.G.; Eshwarappa, R.S.; Lakkappa, D.B. Evaluating the antimicrobial activity of methonolic extract of *Rhus succedanea* leaf gall. *Bioimpacts* **2013**, *3*, 195–198. [CrossRef] [PubMed]
81. Stojanovic, G.; Radulovic, N.; Hashimoto, T.; Palic, R. In vitro antimicrobial activity of extracts of four Achillea species: The composition of *Achillea clavennae* L. (Asteraceae) extract. *J. Ethnopharmacol.* **2005**, *101*, 185–190. [CrossRef] [PubMed]
82. Ozbay, H.; Alim, A. Antimicrobial activity of some water plants from the northeastern Anatolian region of Turkey. *Molecules* **2009**, *14*, 321–328. [CrossRef] [PubMed]
83. Mbosso Teinkela, J.E.; Assob Nguedia, J.C.; Meyer, F.; Vouffo Donfack, E.; Lenta Ndjakou, B.; Ngouela, S.; Tsamo, E.; Adiogo, D.; Guy Blaise Azebaze, A.; Wintjens, R. In vitro antimicrobial and anti-proliferative activities of plant extracts from *Spathodea campanulata*, *Ficus bubu*, and *Carica papaya*. *Pharm. Biol.* **2016**, *54*, 1086–1095. [CrossRef]
84. Assob, J.C.; Kamga, H.L.; Nsagha, D.S.; Njunda, A.L.; Nde, P.F.; Asongalem, E.A.; Njouendou, A.J.; Sandjon, B.; Penlap, V.B. Antimicrobial and toxicological activities of five medicinal plant species from Cameroon traditional medicine. *BMC Complement. Altern. Med.* **2011**, *11*, 70. [CrossRef]
85. Fu, L.; Lu, W.; Zhou, X. Phenolic Compounds and In Vitro Antibacterial and Antioxidant Activities of Three Tropic Fruits: Persimmon, Guava, and Sweetsop. *BioMed Res. Int.* **2016**, *2016*, 4287461. [CrossRef] [PubMed]
86. Liu, H.; Wang, Q.; Liu, Y.; Chen, G.; Cui, J. Antimicrobial and antioxidant activities of *Cichorium intybus* root extract using orthogonal matrix design. *J. Food Sci.* **2013**, *78*, M258–M263. [CrossRef]
87. Onivogui, G.; Diaby, M.; Chen, X.; Zhang, H.; Kargbo, M.R.; Song, Y. Antibacterial and antifungal activities of various solvent extracts from the leaves and stem bark of *Anisophyllea laurina* R. Br ex Sabine used as traditional medicine in Guinea. *J. Ethnopharmacol.* **2015**, *168*, 287–290. [CrossRef]
88. Benevides Bahiense, J.; Marques, F.M.; Figueira, M.M.; Vargas, T.S.; Kondratyuk, T.P.; Endringer, D.C.; Scherer, R.; Fronza, M. Potential anti-inflammatory, antioxidant and antimicrobial activities of *Sambucus australis*. *Pharm. Biol.* **2017**, *55*, 991–997. [CrossRef]
89. Akinyemi, K.; Mendie, U.; Smith, S.; Oyefolu, A.; Coker, A. Screening of some medicinal plants used in south-west Nigerian traditional medicine for anti-*Salmonella typhi* activity. *J. Herb. Pharmacother.* **2005**, *5*, 45–60. [CrossRef] [PubMed]
90. Franklyne, J.S.; Mukherjee, A.; Chandrasekaran, N. Essential oil micro- and nanoemulsions: Promising roles in antimicrobial therapy targeting human pathogens. *Lett. Appl. Microbiol.* **2016**, *63*, 322–334. [CrossRef]
91. Raut, J.S.; Karuppayil, S.M. A status review on the medicinal properties of essential oils. *Ind. Crop. Prod.* **2014**, *62*, 250–264. [CrossRef]

92. Ovais, M.; Zia, N.; Khalil, A.T.; Ayaz, M.; Khalil, A.; Ahmad, I. Nanoantibiotics: Recent Developments and Future Prospects. *Front. Clin. Drug Res. Anti. Infect.* **2019**, *5*, 158.
93. Qasim Nasar, M.; Zohra, T.; Khalil, A.T.; Saqib, S.; Ayaz, M.; Ahmad, A.; Shinwari, Z.K. *Seripheidium quettense* mediated green synthesis of biogenic silver nanoparticles and their theranostic applications. *Green Chem. Lett. Rev.* **2019**, *12*, 310–322. [CrossRef]
94. Ovais, M.; Ahmad, I.; Khalil, A.T.; Mukherjee, S.; Javed, R.; Ayaz, M.; Raza, A.; Shinwari, Z.K. Wound healing applications of biogenic colloidal silver and gold nanoparticles: Recent trends and future prospects. *Appl. Microbiol. Biotechnol.* **2018**, *102*, 4305–4318. [CrossRef]
95. Ovais, M.; Khalil, A.T.; Islam, N.U.; Ahmad, I.; Ayaz, M.; Saravanan, M.; Shinwari, Z.K.; Mukherjee, S. Role of plant phytochemicals and microbial enzymes in biosynthesis of metallic nanoparticles. *Appl. Microbiol. Biotechnol.* **2018**, *102*, 6799–6814. [CrossRef]
96. Ayaz, M.; Ovais, M.; Ahmad, I.; Sadiq, A.; Khalil, A.T.; Ullah, F. Biosynthesized metal nanoparticles as potential Alzheimer's disease therapeutics. In *Metal Nanoparticles for Drug Delivery and Diagnostic Applications*; Elsevier: Amsterdam, The Netherlands, 2020; pp. 31–42.
97. Elemike, E.; Onwudiwe, D.; Ekennia, A.; Sonde, C.; Ehiri, R. Green Synthesis of Ag/Ag2O Nanoparticles Using Aqueous Leaf Extract of *Eupatorium odoratum* and Its Antimicrobial and Mosquito Larvicidal Activities. *Molecules* **2017**, *22*, 674. [CrossRef]
98. Elemike, E.E.; Onwudiwe, D.C.; Ekennia, A.C.; Ehiri, R.C.; Nnaji, N.J. Phytosynthesis of silver nanoparticles using aqueous leaf extracts of *Lippia citriodora*: Antimicrobial, larvicidal and photocatalytic evaluations. *Mater. Sci. Eng. C Mater. Biol. Appl.* **2017**, *75*, 980–989. [CrossRef]
99. Rashid, M.M.O.; Akhter, K.N.; Chowdhury, J.A.; Hossen, F.; Hussain, M.S.; Hossain, M.T. Characterization of phytoconstituents and evaluation of antimicrobial activity of silver-extract nanoparticles synthesized from *Momordica charantia* fruit extract. *BMC Complement. Altern. Med.* **2017**, *17*, 336. [CrossRef]
100. Zia, M.; Gul, S.; Akhtar, J.; Haq, I.U.; Abbasi, B.H.; Hussain, A.; Naz, S.; Chaudhary, M.F. Green synthesis of silver nanoparticles from grape and tomato juices and evaluation of biological activities. *IET Nanobiotechnol.* **2017**, *11*, 193–199. [CrossRef] [PubMed]
101. Balakrishnan, S.; Sivaji, I.; Kandasamy, S.; Duraisamy, S.; Kumar, N.S.; Gurusubramanian, G. Biosynthesis of silver nanoparticles using *Myristica fragrans* seed (nutmeg) extract and its antibacterial activity against multidrug-resistant (MDR) Salmonella enterica serovar Typhi isolates. *Environ. Sci. Pollut. Res. Int.* **2017**, *24*, 14758–14769. [CrossRef] [PubMed]
102. Bettelheim, K. Escherichia coli in the normal flora of humans and animals. In *Escherichia Coli: Mechanisms of Virulence*; Cambridge University Press: Cambridge, UK, 1997; pp. 85–109.
103. Meng, J.; LeJeune, J.T.; Zhao, T.; Doyle, M.P. Enterohemorrhagic *Escherichia coli*. In *Food Microbiology*; American Society of Microbiology: Washington, DC, USA, 2013; pp. 287–309.
104. Prescott, L.M.; Harley, J.P.; Klein, D.A. *Microbiology*; McGraw-Hill: Boston, MA, USA, 2002; Volume fifth.
105. Johnson, J.K.; Robinson, G.L.; Pineles, L.L.; Ajao, A.O.; Zhao, L.; Albrecht, J.S.; Harris, A.D.; Thom, K.A.; Furuno, J.P. Carbapenem MICs in *Escherichia coli* and *Klebsiella Species* Producing Extended-Spectrum beta-Lactamases in Critical Care Patients from 2001 to 2009. *Antimicrob. Agents Chemother.* **2017**, *61*. [CrossRef]
106. Lu, Z.; Dockery, C.R.; Crosby, M.; Chavarria, K.; Patterson, B.; Giedd, M. Antibacterial Activities of Wasabi against *Escherichia coli* O157:H7 and *Staphylococcus aureus*. *Front. Microbiol.* **2016**, *7*, 1403. [CrossRef]
107. Lansky, E.P.; Newman, R.A. Punica granatum (pomegranate) and its potential for prevention and treatment of inflammation and cancer. *J. Ethnopharmacol.* **2007**, *109*, 177–206. [CrossRef]
108. Rahmani, A.H.; Alsahli, M.A.; Almatroodi, S.A. Active constituents of pomegranates (*Punica granatum*) as potential candidates in the management of health through modulation of biological activities. *Pharmacogn. J.* **2017**, *9*, 689–695. [CrossRef]
109. Rahimi, H.R.; Arastoo, M.; Ostad, S.N. A Comprehensive Review of *Punica granatum* (Pomegranate) Properties in Toxicological, Pharmacological, Cellular and Molecular Biology Researches. *Iran. J. Pharm. Res. IJPR* **2012**, *11*, 385–400. [PubMed]
110. Mostafa, A.A.; Al-Askar, A.A.; Almaary, K.S.; Dawoud, T.M.; Sholkamy, E.N.; Bakri, M.M. Antimicrobial activity of some plant extracts against bacterial strains causing food poisoning diseases. *Saudi J. Biol. Sci.* **2018**, *25*, 361–366. [CrossRef]

111. Zohra, T.; Ovais, M.; Khalil, A.T.; Qasim, M.; Ayaz, M.; Shinwari, Z.K.; Ahmad, S.; Zahoor, M. Bio-guided profiling and HPLC-DAD finger printing of *Atriplex lasiantha* Boiss. *BMC Complement. Altern. Med.* **2019**, *19*, 4. [CrossRef]
112. Al-Zoreky, N.S. Antimicrobial activity of pomegranate (*Punica granatum* L.) fruit peels. *Int. J. Food Microbiol.* **2009**, *134*, 244–248. [CrossRef]
113. Mahwasane, S.; Middleton, L.; Boaduo, N. An ethnobotanical survey of indigenous knowledge on medicinal plants used by the traditional healers of the Lwamondo area, Limpopo province, South Africa. *S. Afr. J. Bot.* **2013**, *88*, 69–75. [CrossRef]
114. Mathabe, M.C.; Nikolova, R.V.; Lall, N.; Nyazema, N.Z. Antibacterial activities of medicinal plants used for the treatment of diarrhoea in Limpopo Province, South Africa. *J. Ethnopharmacol.* **2006**, *105*, 286–293. [CrossRef] [PubMed]
115. Meléndez, P.A.; Capriles, V.A. Antibacterial properties of tropical plants from Puerto Rico. *Phytomedicine* **2006**, *13*, 272–276. [CrossRef] [PubMed]
116. Yang, P.C.; Wang, C.S.; An, Z.Y. A murine model of ulcerative colitis: Induced with sinusitis-derived superantigen and food allergen. *BMC Gastroenterol.* **2005**, *5*, 6. [CrossRef]
117. Lina, G.; Cozon, G.; Ferrandiz, J.; Greenland, T.; Vandenesch, F.; Etienne, J. Detection of *Staphylococcal* superantigenic toxins by a CD69-specific cytofluorimetric assay measuring T-cell activation. *J. Clin. Microbiol.* **1998**, *36*, 1042–1045. [CrossRef]
118. Llewelyn, M.; Cohen, J. Superantigens: Microbial agents that corrupt immunity. *Lancet Infect. Dis.* **2002**, *2*, 156–162. [CrossRef]
119. Letertre, C.; Perelle, S.; Dilasser, F.; Fach, P. Identification of a new putative enterotoxin SEU encoded by the egc cluster of *Staphylococcus aureus*. *J. Appl. Microbiol.* **2003**, *95*, 38–43. [CrossRef]
120. Fueyo, J.M.; Mendoza, M.C.; Rodicio, M.R.; Muniz, J.; Alvarez, M.A.; Martin, M.C. Cytotoxin and pyrogenic toxin superantigen gene profiles of *Staphylococcus aureus* associated with subclinical mastitis in dairy cows and relationships with macrorestriction genomic profiles. *J. Clin. Microbiol.* **2005**, *43*, 1278–1284. [CrossRef]
121. Umeda, K.; Nakamura, H.; Yamamoto, K.; Nishina, N.; Yasufuku, K.; Hirai, Y.; Hirayama, T.; Goto, K.; Hase, A.; Ogasawara, J. Molecular and epidemiological characterization of staphylococcal foodborne outbreak of Staphylococcus aureus harboring seg, sei, sem, sen, seo, and selu genes without production of classical enterotoxins. *Int. J. Food Microbiol.* **2017**, *256*, 30–35. [CrossRef]
122. Naz, R.; Ayub, H.; Nawaz, S.; Islam, Z.U.; Yasmin, T.; Bano, A.; Wakeel, A.; Zia, S.; Roberts, T.H. Antimicrobial activity, toxicity and anti-inflammatory potential of methanolic extracts of four ethnomedicinal plant species from Punjab, Pakistan. *BMC Complement. Altern. Med.* **2017**, *17*, 302. [CrossRef]
123. Hoekou, Y.P.; Tchacondo, T.; Karou, S.D.; Yerbanga, R.S.; Achoribo, E.; Da, O.; Atakpama, W.; Batawila, K. Therapeutic Potentials of Ethanolic Extract of Leaves of *Holarrhena floribunda* (G. Don) Dur. and Schinz (Apocynaceae). *Afr. J. Tradit. Complement. Altern. Med.* **2017**, *14*, 227–233. [CrossRef] [PubMed]
124. Tamokou, J.D.D.; Tala, M.F.; Wabo, H.K.; Kuiate, J.R.; Tane, P. Antimicrobial activities of methanol extract and compounds from stem bark of Vismia rubescens. *J. Ethnopharmacol.* **2009**, *124*, 571–575. [CrossRef] [PubMed]
125. Kuete, V.; Nguemeving, J.R.; Beng, V.P.; Azebaze, A.G.B.; Etoa, F.-X.; Meyer, M.; Bodo, B.; Nkengfack, A.E. Antimicrobial activity of the methanolic extracts and compounds from *Vismia laurentii* De Wild (Guttiferae). *J. Ethnopharmacol.* **2007**, *109*, 372–379. [CrossRef] [PubMed]
126. Idowu, T.O.; Ogundaini, A.O.; Adesanya, S.A.; Onawunmi, G.O.; Osungunna, M.O.; Obuotor, E.M.; Abegaz, B.M. Isolation and Characterization of Chemical Constituents from *Chrysophyllum Albidum* G. Don-Holl. Stem-Bark Extracts and Their Antioxidant and Antibacterial Properties. *Afr. J. Tradit. Complement. Altern. Med.* **2016**, *13*, 182–189. [CrossRef] [PubMed]
127. Coulibaly, K.; Zirihi, G.N.; Guessennd-Kouadio, N.; Oussou, K.R.; Dosso, M. Antibacterial properties studies of trunk barks of *Terminalia ivorensis*, a commercial and medicinal species on some methicillin-resistant Staphylococci species strains. *Afr. Health Sci.* **2014**, *14*, 753–756. [CrossRef]
128. Elegami, A.; El-Nima, E.; El Tohami, M.; Muddathir, A. Antimicrobial activity of some species of the family Combretaceae. *Phytother. Res.* **2002**, *16*, 555–561. [CrossRef]
129. Tayel, A.A.; Hussein, H.; Sorour, N.M.; El-Tras, W.F. Foodborne Pathogens Prevention and Sensory Attributes Enhancement in Processed Cheese via Flavoring with Plant Extracts. *J. Food Sci.* **2015**, *80*, M2886–M2891. [CrossRef]

130. Ferhat, M.; Erol, E.; Beladjila, K.A.; Cetintas, Y.; Duru, M.E.; Ozturk, M.; Kabouche, A.; Kabouche, Z. Antioxidant, anticholinesterase and antibacterial activities of *Stachys guyoniana* and *Mentha aquatica*. *Pharm. Biol.* **2017**, *55*, 324–329. [CrossRef]
131. Zater, H.; Huet, J.; Fontaine, V.; Benayache, S.; Stevigny, C.; Duez, P.; Benayache, F. Chemical constituents, cytotoxic, antifungal and antimicrobial properties of *Centaurea diluta* Ait. subsp. *algeriensis* (Coss. & Dur.) Maire. *Asian Pac. J. Trop. Med.* **2016**, *9*, 554–561. [CrossRef]
132. Bouchouka, E.; Djilani, A.; Bekkouche, A. Antibacterial and antioxidant activities of three endemic plants from Algerian Sahara. *Acta Sci. Pol. Technol. Aliment.* **2012**, *11*, 61–65.
133. Njeru, S.N.; Obonyo, M.; Nyambati, S.; Ngari, S.; Mwakubambanya, R.; Mavura, H. Antimicrobial and cytotoxicity properties of the organic solvent fractions of *Clerodendrum myricoides* (Hochst.) R. Br. ex Vatke: Kenyan traditional medicinal plant. *J. Intercult Ethnopharmacol.* **2016**, *5*, 226–232. [CrossRef] [PubMed]
134. Wang, J.; Wang, Z.; Wu, R.; Jiang, D.; Bai, B.; Tan, D.; Yan, T.; Sun, X.; Zhang, Q.; Wu, Z. Proteomic Analysis of the Antibacterial Mechanism of Action of Juglone against *Staphylococcus aureus*. *Nat. Prod. Commun.* **2016**, *11*, 825–827. [CrossRef]
135. Lee, Y.S.; Han, S.H.; Lee, S.H.; Kim, Y.G.; Park, C.B.; Kang, O.H.; Keum, J.H.; Kim, S.B.; Mun, S.H.; Seo, Y.S.; et al. The mechanism of antibacterial activity of tetrandrine against *Staphylococcus aureus*. *Foodborne Pathog. Dis.* **2012**, *9*, 686–691. [CrossRef] [PubMed]
136. Wang, H.; Zou, D.; Xie, K.; Xie, M. Antibacterial mechanism of fraxetin against *Staphylococcus aureus*. *Mol. Med. Rep.* **2014**, *10*, 2341–2345. [CrossRef]
137. Kim, Y.S.; Kim, H.; Jung, E.; Kim, J.H.; Hwang, W.; Kang, E.J.; Lee, S.; Ha, B.J.; Lee, J.; Park, D. A novel antibacterial compound from *Siegesbeckia glabrescens*. *Molecules* **2012**, *17*, 12469–12477. [CrossRef]
138. Bajpai, V.K.; Kang, S.C. Antibacterial abietane-type diterpenoid, taxodone from *Metasequoia glyptostroboides* Miki ex Hu. *J. Biosci.* **2010**, *35*, 533–538. [CrossRef] [PubMed]
139. Lee, L.Y.; Shim, J.S.; Rukayadi, Y.; Hwang, J.K. Antibacterial activity of xanthorrhizol isolated from *Curcuma xanthorrhiza* Roxb. against foodborne pathogens. *J. Food Prot.* **2008**, *71*, 1926–1930. [CrossRef]
140. Linde, G.A.; Gazim, Z.C.; Cardoso, B.K.; Jorge, L.F.; Tesevic, V.; Glamoclija, J.; Sokovic, M.; Colauto, N.B. Antifungal and antibacterial activities of *Petroselinum crispum* essential oil. *Genet Mol. Res.* **2016**, *15*. [CrossRef]
141. Tavakoli, H.R.; Mashak, Z.; Moradi, B.; Sodagari, H.R. Antimicrobial Activities of the Combined Use of *Cuminum cyminum* L. Essential Oil, Nisin and Storage Temperature Against *Salmonella typhimurium* and *Staphylococcus aureus* In Vitro. *Jundishapur J. Microbiol.* **2015**, *8*, e24838. [CrossRef]
142. Monu, E.A.; David, J.R.; Schmidt, M.; Davidson, P.M. Effect of white mustard essential oil on the growth of foodborne pathogens and spoilage microorganisms and the effect of food components on its efficacy. *J. Food Prot.* **2014**, *77*, 2062–2068. [CrossRef] [PubMed]
143. Park, M.J.; Choi, W.S.; Kang, H.Y.; Gwak, K.S.; Lee, G.S.; Jeung, E.B.; Choi, I.G. Inhibitory effect of the essential oil from *Chamaecyparis obtusa* on the growth of food-borne pathogens. *J. Microbiol.* **2010**, *48*, 496–501. [CrossRef]
144. Hale, T.L. Genetic basis of virulence in Shigella species. *Microbiol. Mol. Biol. Rev.* **1991**, *55*, 206–224. [CrossRef]
145. Surawicz, C.M. Mechanisms of diarrhea. *Curr. Gastroenterol. Rep.* **2010**, *12*, 236–241. [CrossRef]
146. Mattock, E.; Blocker, A.J. How Do the Virulence Factors of Shigella Work Together to Cause Disease? *Front. Cell. Infect. Microbiol.* **2017**, *7*, 64. [CrossRef] [PubMed]
147. Mahboubi, A.; Asgarpanah, J.; Sadaghiyani, P.N.; Faizi, M. Total phenolic and flavonoid content and antibacterial activity of Punica granatum L. var. pleniflora flowers (Golnar) against bacterial strains causing foodborne diseases. *BMC Complement. Altern. Med.* **2015**, *15*, 366. [CrossRef]
148. Mahboubi, A.; Kamalinejad, M.; Ayatollahi, A.M.; Babaeian, M. Total Phenolic Content and Antibacterial Activity of Five Plants of Labiatae against Four Foodborne and Some Other Bacteria. *Iran. J. Pharm. Res. IJPR* **2014**, *13*, 559–566.
149. van Vuuren, S.F.; Nkwanyana, M.N.; de Wet, H. Antimicrobial evaluation of plants used for the treatment of diarrhoea in a rural community in northern Maputaland, KwaZulu-Natal, South Africa. *BMC Complement. Altern. Med.* **2015**, *15*, 53. [CrossRef]

150. Nasir, M.; Tafess, K.; Abate, D. Antimicrobial potential of the Ethiopian *Thymus schimperi* essential oil in comparison with others against certain fungal and bacterial species. *BMC Complement. Altern. Med.* **2015**, *15*, 260. [CrossRef]
151. Srivastava, U.; Ojha, S.; Tripathi, N.N.; Singh, P. In vitro antibacterial, antioxidant activity and total phenolic content of some essential oils. *J. Environ. Biol.* **2015**, *36*, 1329–1336.
152. Hamon, M.; Bierne, H.; Cossart, P. Listeria monocytogenes: A multifaceted model. *Nat. Rev. Microbiol.* **2006**, *4*, 423–434. [CrossRef]
153. Portnoy, D.A.; Chakraborty, T.; Goebel, W.; Cossart, P. Molecular determinants of *Listeria monocytogenes* pathogenesis. *Infection and immunity.* **1992**, *60*, 1263. [CrossRef]
154. Gray, M.L.; Killinger, A. *Listeria monocytogenes* and listeric infections. *Bacteriol. Rev.* **1966**, *30*, 309. [CrossRef]
155. Farber, J.M.; Peterkin, P.I. *Listeria monocytogenes*, a food-borne pathogen. *Microbiol. Rev.* **1991**, *55*, 476–511. [CrossRef] [PubMed]
156. Yoon, Y.; Choi, K.H. Antimicrobial activities of therapeutic herbal plants against Listeria monocytogenes and the herbal plant cytotoxicity on Caco-2 cell. *Lett. Appl. Microbiol.* **2012**, *55*, 47–55. [CrossRef] [PubMed]
157. Upadhyay, A.; Johny, A.K.; Amalaradjou, M.A.; Ananda Baskaran, S.; Kim, K.S.; Venkitanarayanan, K. Plant-derived antimicrobials reduce *Listeria monocytogenes* virulence factors in vitro, and down-regulate expression of virulence genes. *Int. J. Food Microbiol.* **2012**, *157*, 88–94. [CrossRef]
158. Xu, Y.; Li, G.; Zhang, B.; Wu, Q.; Wang, X.; Xia, X. Tannin-rich pomegranate rind extracts reduce adhesion to and invasion of Caco-2 cells by *Listeria monocytogenes* and decrease its expression of virulence genes. *J. Food Prot.* **2015**, *78*, 128–133. [CrossRef]
159. Raeisi, M.; Tajik, H.; Razavi Rohani, S.M.; Tepe, B.; Kiani, H.; Khoshbakht, R.; Shirzad Aski, H.; Tadrisi, H. Inhibitory effect of *Zataria multiflora* Boiss. essential oil, alone and in combination with monolaurin, on Listeria monocytogenes. *Vet. Res. Forum.* **2016**, *7*, 7–11.
160. Rabiey, S.; Hosseini, H.; Rezaei, M. Use Carum copticum essential oil for controlling the *Listeria monocytogenes* growth in fish model system. *Braz. J. Microbiol.* **2014**, *45*, 89–96. [CrossRef]
161. El Abed, N.; Kaabi, B.; Smaali, M.I.; Chabbouh, M.; Habibi, K.; Mejri, M.; Marzouki, M.N.; Ben Hadj Ahmed, S. Chemical Composition, Antioxidant and Antimicrobial Activities of *Thymus capitata* Essential Oil with Its Preservative Effect against *Listeria monocytogenes* Inoculated in Minced Beef Meat. *Evid. Based Complement. Altern. Med.* **2014**, *2014*, 152487. [CrossRef]
162. Leite, C.J.; de Sousa, J.P.; Medeiros, J.A.; da Conceicao, M.L.; dos Santos Falcao-Silva, V.; de Souza, E.L. Inactivation of *Escherichia coli*, *Listeria monocytogenes*, and *Salmonella enteritidis* by *Cymbopogon citratus* D.C. Stapf. Essential Oil in Pineapple Juice. *J. Food Prot.* **2016**, *79*, 213–219. [CrossRef]
163. Ngang, J.J.; Nyegue, M.A.; Ndoye, F.C.; Tchuenchieu Kamgain, A.D.; Sado Kamdem, S.L.; Lanciotti, R.; Gardini, F.; Etoa, F.X. Characterization of Mexican coriander (*Eryngium foetidum*) essential oil and its inactivation of Listeria monocytogenes in vitro and during mild thermal pasteurization of pineapple juice. *J. Food Prot.* **2014**, *77*, 435–443. [CrossRef] [PubMed]
164. Poxton, I.R. Other *Clostridium* spp. In *Principles and Practice of Clinical Bacteriology*, 2nd ed.; John Wiley & Sons Ltd.: West Sussex, UK, 2006; pp. 567–574.
165. Sugiyama, H. Clostridium botulinum neurotoxin. *Microbiol. Rev.* **1980**, *44*, 419. [CrossRef] [PubMed]
166. Sakaguchi, G. Clostridium botulinum toxins. *Pharmacol. Ther.* **1982**, *19*, 165–194. [CrossRef]
167. Doyle, M.P.; Buchanan, R.L. *Food Microbiology: Fundamentals and Frontiers*; American Society for Microbiology Press: Washington, DC, USA, 2012.
168. Shukla, H.D.; Sharma, S.K. *Clostridium botulinum*: A bug with beauty and weapon. *Crit. Rev. Microbiol.* **2005**, *31*, 11–18. [CrossRef]
169. Nakai, Y.; Pellett, S.; Tepp, W.H.; Johnson, E.A.; Janda, K.D. Toosendanin: Synthesis of the AB-ring and investigations of its anti-botulinum properties (Part II). *Bioorganic Med. Chem.* **2010**, *18*, 1280–1287. [CrossRef]
170. Uzal, F.A.; Freedman, J.C.; Shrestha, A.; Theoret, J.R.; Garcia, J.; Awad, M.M.; Adams, V.; Moore, R.J.; Rood, J.I.; McClane, B.A. Towards an understanding of the role of *Clostridium perfringens* toxins in human and animal disease. *Future Microbiol.* **2014**, *9*, 361–377. [CrossRef]
171. Garcia, S.; Araiza, M.; Gomez, M.; Heredia, N. Inhibition of growth, enterotoxin production, and spore formation of *Clostridium perfringens* by extracts of medicinal plants. *J. Food Prot.* **2002**, *65*, 1667–1669. [CrossRef]

172. De Oliveira, T.L.C.; de Araújo Soares, R.; Ramos, E.M.; das Graças Cardoso, M.; Alves, E.; Piccoli, R.H. Antimicrobial activity of *Satureja montana* L. essential oil against *Clostridium perfringens* type A inoculated in mortadella-type sausages formulated with different levels of sodium nitrite. *Int. J. Food Microbiol.* **2011**, *144*, 546–555. [CrossRef] [PubMed]
173. David, X.Y.; Zhiyong, H.; Wenyue, W.; Colin, P.; Zhi-cheng, X. The Effects of Berberine on *Clostridium perfringens* Induced Necrotic Enteritis in Broiler Chickens. *Arch. Clin. Microbiol.* **2017**, *8*. [CrossRef]
174. Ahn, Y.; Kwon, J.; Chae, S.; Park, J.; Yoo, J. Growth-inhibitory responses of human intestinal bacteria to extracts of oriental medicinal plants. *Microb. Ecol. Health Dis.* **1994**, *7*, 257–261.
175. Bottone, E.J. *Bacillus cereus*, a volatile human pathogen. *Clin. Microbiol. Rev.* **2010**, *23*, 382–398. [CrossRef] [PubMed]
176. Jun, H.; Kim, J.; Bang, J.; Kim, H.; Beuchat, L.R.; Ryu, J.-H. Combined effects of plant extracts in inhibiting the growth of *Bacillus cereus* in reconstituted infant rice cereal. *Int. J. Food Microbiol.* **2013**, *160*, 260–266. [CrossRef] [PubMed]
177. Hamdan, M.; Al-Ismail, K.; Al-Delaimy, K. The antibacterial activity of selected edible plant extracts against *Bacillus cereus*. *Jordan J. Agric. Sci.* **2007**, *3*, 148–155.
178. Silva, A.J.; Benitez, J.A. *Vibrio cholerae* biofilms and cholera pathogenesis. *PLoS Negl. Trop. Dis.* **2016**, *10*, e0004330. [CrossRef] [PubMed]
179. Faruque, S.M.; Albert, M.J.; Mekalanos, J.J. Epidemiology, Genetics, and Ecology of Toxigenic *Vibrio cholerae*. *Microbiol. Mol. Biol. Rev.* **1998**, *62*, 1301–1314. [CrossRef]
180. Sánchez, E.; Heredia, N.; del Camacho-Corona, M.R.; García, S. Isolation, characterization and mode of antimicrobial action against *Vibrio cholerae* of methyl gallate isolated from *Acacia farnesiana*. *J. Appl. Microbiol.* **2013**, *115*, 1307–1316. [CrossRef]
181. Yamasaki, S.; Asakura, M.; Neogi, S.B.; Hinenoya, A.; Iwaoka, E.; Aoki, S. Inhibition of virulence potential of *Vibrio cholerae* by natural compounds. *Indian J. Med Res.* **2011**, *133*, 232.
182. García, S.; Alarcón, G.; Rodríguez, C.; Heredia, N. Extracts of *Acacia farnesiana* and *Artemisia ludoviciana* inhibit growth, enterotoxin production and adhesion of Vibrio cholerae. *World J. Microbiol. Biotechnol.* **2006**, *22*, 669–674. [CrossRef]
183. Acharyya, S.; Patra, A.; Bag, P.K. Evaluation of the antimicrobial activity of some medicinal plants against enteric bacteria with particular reference to multi-drug resistant *Vibrio cholerae*. *Trop. J. Pharm. Res.* **2009**, *8*, 231–237. [CrossRef]
184. Lopman, B.A.; Reacher, M.; Gallimore, C.; Adak, G.K.; Gray, J.J.; Brown, D.W. A summertime peak of" winter vomiting disease": Surveillance of noroviruses in England and Wales, 1995 to 2002. *BMC Public Health* **2003**, *3*, 13. [CrossRef]
185. Chan, C.M.V.; Chan, C.W.D.; Ma, C,k.; Chan, H.B. Norovirus as cause of benign convulsion associated with gastro-enteritis. *J. Paediatr. Child Health* **2011**, *47*, 373–377. [CrossRef] [PubMed]
186. Glass, R.I.; Parashar, U.D.; Estes, M.K. Norovirus Gastroenteritis. *N. Engl. J. Med.* **2009**, *361*, 1776–1785. [CrossRef] [PubMed]
187. Choudhuri, B.S.; Bhakta, S.; Barik, R.; Basu, J.; Kundu, M.; Chakrabati, P. Overexpression and functional characterization of an ABC (ATP-binding cassette) transporter encoded by the genes drrA and drrB of *Mycobacterium tuberculosis*. *J. Bacteriol.* **2002**, *367*, 279–285. [CrossRef] [PubMed]
188. Zhang, X.-F.; Dai, Y.-C.; Zhong, W.; Tan, M.; Lv, Z.-P.; Zhou, Y.-C.; Jiang, X. Tannic acid inhibited norovirus binding to HBGA receptors, a study of 50 Chinese medicinal herbs. *Bioorganic Med. Chem.* **2012**, *20*, 1616–1623. [CrossRef] [PubMed]
189. Su, X.; D'Souza, D.H. Grape seed extract for control of human enteric viruses. *Appl. Environ. Microbiol.* **2011**, *77*, 3982–3987. [CrossRef]
190. Gilling, D.H.; Kitajima, M.; Torrey, J.R.; Bright, K.R. Mechanisms of antiviral action of plant antimicrobials against murine norovirus. *Appl. Environ. Microbiol.* **2014**, *80*, 4898–4910. [CrossRef]
191. Cortez, V.; Meliopoulos, V.A.; Karlsson, E.A.; Hargest, V.; Johnson, C.; Schultz-Cherry, S. Astrovirus biology and pathogenesis. *Annu. Rev. Virol.* **2017**, *4*, 327–348. [CrossRef]
192. Téllez, M.; Téllez, A.; Vélez, F.; Ulloa, J. In vitro antiviral activity against rotavirus and astrovirus infection exerted by substances obtained from *Achyrocline bogotensis* (Kunth) DC.(Compositae). *BMC Complement. Altern. Med.* **2015**, *15*, 428.

193. El-Baz, F.; El-Senousy, W.; El-Sayed, A.; Kamel, M. In vitro antiviral and antimicrobial activities of *Spirulina platensis* extract. *J. Appl. Pharm. Sci.* **2013**, *3*, 52–56.
194. Kudi, A.; Myint, S. Antiviral activity of some Nigerian medicinal plant extracts. *J. Ethnopharmacol.* **1999**, *68*, 289–294. [CrossRef]
195. Cuthbert, J.A. Hepatitis A: Old and new. *Clin. Microbiol. Rev.* **2001**, *14*, 38–58. [CrossRef] [PubMed]
196. Seo, D.J.; Lee, M.; Jeon, S.B.; Park, H.; Jeong, S.; Lee, B.-H.; Choi, C. Antiviral activity of herbal extracts against the hepatitis A virus. *Food Control* **2017**, *72*, 9–13. [CrossRef]
197. Abd-Elshafy, D.N. Effect of methanolic-extracted green tea on hepatitis A virus and its usage in clearing the virus from drinking Water. *J. Virol. Sci.* **2018**, *3*, 58–67.
198. Ogilvie, I.; Khoury, H.; El Khoury, A.C.; Goetghebeur, M.M. Burden of rotavirus gastroenteritis in the pediatric population in Central and Eastern Europe: Serotype distribution and burden of illness. *Hum. Vaccines* **2011**, *7*, 523–533. [CrossRef]
199. Grimwood, K.; Lambert, S.B.; Milne, R.J. Rotavirus infections and vaccines. *Pediatr. Drugs* **2010**, *12*, 235–256. [CrossRef]
200. Cecílio, A.B.; de Faria, D.B.; de Carvalho Oliveira, P.; Caldas, S.; de Oliveira, D.A.; Sobral, M.E.G.; Duarte, M.G.R.; de Souza Moreira, C.P.; Silva, C.G.; de Almeida, V.L. Screening of Brazilian medicinal plants for antiviral activity against rotavirus. *J. Ethnopharmacol.* **2012**, *141*, 975–981. [CrossRef]
201. Knipping, K.; Garssen, J.; van't Land, B. An evaluation of the inhibitory effects against rotavirus infection of edible plant extracts. *Virol. J.* **2012**, *9*, 137. [CrossRef]
202. Sun, Y.; Gong, X.; Tan, J.Y.; Kang, L.; Li, D.; Yang, J.; Du, G. In vitro Antiviral Activity of *Rubia cordifolia* Aerial Part Extract against Rotavirus. *Front. Pharmacol.* **2016**, *7*, 308. [CrossRef]
203. Mohamed, S.; Mamdouh, E.; Adel, M.; Samy, M.; Nagwa, E. Antiviral activity of *Bauhinia variegata* extracts against rotavirus in vitro. *Curr. Sci. Int.* **2014**, *3*, 172–178.
204. Shaheen, M.; Mostafa, S.; El-Esnawy, N. Anti-Rotaviral Effects of *Calliandra haematocephala* Leaf Extracts In-vitro and In-vivo. *J. Virol. Antivir. Res.* **2015**, *4*, 1–7. [CrossRef]
205. Kawahara, T.; Tomono, T.; Hamauzu, Y.; Tanaka, K.; Yasui, H. Inhibitory effect of a hot-water extract of leaves of Japanese big-leaf magnolia (*Magnolia obovata*) on rotavirus-induced diarrhea in mouse pups. *Evid. Based Complement. Altern. Med.* **2014**, *2014*, 365831. [CrossRef] [PubMed]
206. Farthing, M.J. Giardiasis. *Gastroenterol. Clin.* **1996**, *25*, 493–515. [CrossRef]
207. Derda, M.; Hadaś, E. The use of phytotherapy in diseases caused by parasitic protozoa. *Acta Parasitol.* **2015**, *60*, 1–8. [CrossRef]
208. Hawrelak, J. Giardiasis: Pathophysiology and management. *Altern. Med. Rev.* **2003**, *8*, 129–142.
209. Phillipson, J.D.; Wright, C.W.; Kirby, G.C.; Warhurst, D.C. Tropical plants as sources of antiprotozoal agents. In *Phytochemical Potential of Tropical Plants*; Springer: New York, NY, USA, 1993; pp. 1–40.
210. Ross, I. *Medicinal Plants of the World: Chemical Constituents, Traditional and Modern Medicinal Uses*; Humana Press: Totowa, NJ, USA, 2002; pp. 25–63.
211. Soffar, S.; Mokhtar, G. Evaluation of the antiparasitic effect of aqueous garlic (*Allium sativum*) extract in hymenolepiasis nana and giardiasis. *J. Egypt. Soc. Parasitol.* **1991**, *21*, 497–502.
212. Ankri, S.; Mirelman, D. Antimicrobial properties of allicin from garlic. *Microbes Infect.* **1999**, *1*, 125–129. [CrossRef]
213. Jiménez, J.; Uzcanga, G.; Zambrano, A.; Di Prisco, M.; Lynch, N. Identification and partial characterization of excretory/secretory products with proteolytic activity in Giardia intestinalis. *J. Parasitol.* **2000**, *86*, 859–862. [CrossRef]
214. Frawley, D.; Lad, V. *The Yoga of Herbs: An Ayurvedic Guide to Herbal Medicine*; Lotus Press: Twin Lakeswi, Kenosha County, WI, USA, 1986; pp. 180–182.
215. Tripathi, D.; Gupta, N.; Lakshmi, V.; Saxena, K.; Agrawal, A. Antigiardial and immunostimulatory effect of *Piper longum* on giardiasis due to *Giardia lamblia*. *Phytother. Res.* **1999**, *13*, 561–565. [CrossRef]
216. Agarwal, A.; Singh, M.; Gupta, N.; Saxena, R.; Puri, A.; Verma, A.; Saxena, R.; Dubey, C.; Saxena, K. Management of giardiasis by an immuno-modulatory herbal drug Pippali Rasayana. *J. Ethnopharmacol.* **1994**, *44*, 143–146. [CrossRef]
217. Agrawal, A.; Tripathi, D.; Sahai, R.; Gupta, N.; Saxena, R.; Puri, A.; Singh, M.; Misra, R.; Dubey, C.; Saxena, K. Management of Giardiasis by a herbal drug 'Pippali Rasayana': A clinical study. *J. Ethnopharmacol.* **1997**, *56*, 233–236. [CrossRef]

218. Miyares, C.; Hollands, I.; Castaneda, C.; Gonzalez, T.; Fragoso, T.; Curras, R.; Soria, C. Clinical trial with a preparation based on propolis"propolisina" in human giardiasis. *Acta Gastroenterol. Latinoam.* **1987**, *18*, 195–201.
219. Snow, J.M. *Hydrastis canadensis* L. (Ranunculaceae). *Protoc. J. Bot. Med.* **1997**, *2*, 25–30.
220. Willard, T. *The Wild Rose Scientific Herbal*; Wild Rose College of Natural Healing: Calgary, AB, Canada, 1991; pp. 24–29.
221. Kaneda, Y.; Torii, M.; Tanaka, T.; Aikawa, M. In vitro effects of berberine sulphate on the growth and structure of Entamoeba histolytica, Giardia lamblia and *Trichomonas vaginalis*. *Ann. Trop. Med. Parasitol.* **1991**, *85*, 417–425. [CrossRef] [PubMed]
222. Choudhry, V.; Sabir, M.; Bhide, V. Berberine in giardiasis. *Indian Pediatr.* **1972**, *9*, 143. [PubMed]
223. Gupte, S. Use of berberine in treatment of giardiasis. *Am. J. Dis. Child.* **1975**, *129*, 866. [CrossRef]
224. Kaneda, Y.; Tanaka, T.; Saw, T. Effects of berberine, a plant alkaloid, on the growth of anaerobic protozoa in axenic culture. *Tokai J. Exp. Clin. Med.* **1990**, *15*, 417–423.
225. Calzada, F.; Meckes, M.; Cedillo-Rivera, R. Antiamoebic and antigiardial activity of plant flavonoids. *Planta Med.* **1999**, *65*, 78–80. [CrossRef]
226. Cai, Y.; Evans, F.; Roberts, M.; Phillipson, J.; Zenk, M.; Gleba, Y. Polyphenolic compounds from *Croton lechleri*. *Phytochemistry* **1991**, *30*, 2033–2040. [CrossRef]
227. Blumenthal, M.; Goldberg, A.; Brinckmann, J. *Herbal Medicine: Expanded Commission E Monographs*; Integrative Medicine Communications: Austintx, TX, USA, 2000; pp. 413–417.
228. Ponce-Macotela, M.; Navarro-Alegria, I.; Martinez-Gordillo, M.; Alvarez-Chacon, R. In vitro effect against Giardia of 14 plant extracts. *Rev. Investig. Clin. Organo Hosp. Enferm. Nutr.* **1993**, *46*, 343–347.
229. Barbosa, E.; Calzada, F.; Campos, R. In vivo antigiardial activity of three flavonoids isolated of some medicinal plants used in Mexican traditional medicine for the treatment of diarrhea. *J. Ethnopharmacol.* **2007**, *109*, 552–554. [CrossRef]
230. Orozco, E.; Pérez, D.; Gómez, M.; Ayala, P. Multidrug resistance in *Entamoeba histolytica*. *Parasitol. Today* **1995**, *11*, 473–475. [CrossRef]
231. Bruckner, D.A. Amebiasis. *Clin. Microbiol. Rev.* **1992**, *5*, 356–369. [CrossRef] [PubMed]
232. Tengku, S.; Norhayati, M. Review Paper Public health and clinical importance of amoebiasis in Malaysia: A review. *Trop. Biomed.* **2011**, *28*, 194–222.
233. Kammanadiminti, S.J. *Early Interactions between* Entamoeba histolytica *and Mucosal Cells*; McGill University Libraries: Montreal, QC, Canada, 2006.
234. Otshudi, A.L.; Vercruysse, A.; Foriers, A. Contribution to the ethnobotanical, phytochemical and pharmacological studies of traditionally used medicinal plants in the treatment of dysentery and diarrhoea in Lomela area, Democratic Republic of Congo (DRC). *J. Ethnopharmacol.* **2000**, *71*, 411–423. [CrossRef]
235. Taylor, M.; Pillai, G.; Kvalsvig, J. Targeted chemotherapy for parasite infestations in rural black preschool children. *S. Afr. Med. J.* **1995**, *85*, 870–874.
236. Swetman, S.C. Martindale. In: The Complete Drug Reference 33th ed. *Pharm. Presslondon* **2002**, 594.
237. Kapoor, K.; Chandra, M.; Nag, D.; Paliwal, J.; Gupta, R.; Saxena, R. Evaluation of metronidazole toxicity: A prospective study. *Int. J. Clin. Pharmacol. Res.* **1998**, *19*, 83–88.
238. Azam, A.; Agarwal, S. Targeting Amoebiasis: Status and developments. *Curr. Bioact. Compd.* **2007**, *3*, 121–133. [CrossRef]
239. Ayaz, M.; Junaid, M.; Ullah, F.; Sadiq, A.; Ovais, M.; Ahmad, W.; Zeb, A. Chemical profiling, antimicrobial and insecticidal evaluations of *Polygonum hydropiper* L. *BMC Complement. Altern. Med.* **2016**, *16*, 502. [CrossRef]
240. Ahmad, S.; Ullah, F.; Ayaz, M.; Sadiq, A.; Imran, M. Antioxidant and anticholinesterase investigations of *Rumex hastatus* D. Don: Potential effectiveness in oxidative stress and neurological disorders. *Biol. Res.* **2015**, *48*, 1–8. [CrossRef]
241. Ayaz, M.; Junaid, M.; Ullah, F.; Sadiq, A.; Subhan, F.; Khan, M.A.; Ahmad, W.; Ali, G.; Imran, M.; Ahmad, S. Molecularly characterized solvent extracts and saponins from *Polygonum hydropiper* L show high anti-angiogenic, anti-tumor, brine shrimp and fibroblast NIH/3T3 cell line cytotoxicity. *Front. Pharmacol.* **2016**, *7*, 74. [CrossRef]
242. Zeb, A.; Ahmad, S.; Ullah, F.; Ayaz, M.; Sadiq, A. Anti-nociceptive activity of ethnomedicinally important analgesic plant *Isodon rugosus* Wall. ex Benth: Mechanistic study and identifications of bioactive compounds. *Front. Pharmacol.* **2016**, *7*, 200. [CrossRef]

243. Gillin, F.; Reiner, D.; Suffness, M. Bruceantin, a potent amoebicide from a plant, *Brucea antidysenterica*. *Antimicrob. Agents Chemother.* **1982**, *22*, 342–345. [CrossRef]
244. Sharma, G.; Bhutani, K. Plant based amoebicidal activity of parthenin isolated from *Parthenium hysterophorus*. *Planta Med.* **1987**, *2*, 120–122.
245. Wright, C.; O'neill, M.; Phillipson, J.; Warhurst, D. Use of microdilution to assess in vitro antiamoebic activities of *Brucea javanica* fruits, *Simarouba amara* stem, and a number of quassinoids. *Antimicrob. Agents Chemother.* **1988**, *32*, 1725–1729. [CrossRef]
246. Wright, C.; Allen, D.; Cai, Y.; Phillipson, J.; Said, I.; Kirby, G.; Warhurst, D. In vitro antiamoebic and antiplasmodial activities of alkaloids isolated from *Alstonia angustifolia* roots. *Phytother. Res.* **1992**, *6*, 121–124. [CrossRef]
247. Cimanga, R.; Kambu, K.; Tona, L.; Hermans, N.; Apers, S.; Totte, J.; Pieters, L.; Vlietinck, A. Cytotoxicity and in vitro susceptibility of *Entamoeba histolytica* to *Morinda morindoides* leaf extracts and its isolated constituents. *J. Ethnopharmacol.* **2006**, *107*, 83–90. [CrossRef]
248. Tona, L.; Kambu, K.; Ngimbi, N.; Cimanga, K.; Vlietinck, A. Antiamoebic and phytochemical screening of some Congolese medicinal plants. *J. Ethnopharmacol.* **1998**, *61*, 57–65. [CrossRef]
249. Sohni, Y.R.; Kaimal, P.; Bhatt, R.M. The antiamoebic effect of a crude drug formulation of herbal extracts against *Entamoeba histolytica* in vitro and in vivo. *J. Ethnopharmacol.* **1995**, *45*, 43–52. [CrossRef]
250. Calzada, F.; Yepez-Mulia, L.; Tapia-Contreras, A.; Bautista, E.; Maldonado, E.; Ortega, A. Evaluation of the antiprotozoal activity of neo-clerodane type diterpenes from Salvia polystachya against *Entamoeba histolytica* and *Giardia lamblia*. *Phytother. Res.* **2010**, *24*, 662–665.
251. Calzada, F.; Yépez-Mulia, L.; Aguilar, A. In vitro susceptibility of *Entamoeba histolytica* and *Giardia lamblia* to plants used in Mexican traditional medicine for the treatment of gastrointestinal disorders. *J. Ethnopharmacol.* **2006**, *108*, 367–370. [CrossRef]
252. Calzada, F.; Cervantes-Martínez, J.A.; Yépez-Mulia, L. In vitro antiprotozoal activity from the roots of *Geranium mexicanum* and its constituents on *Entamoeba histolytica* and *Giardia lamblia*. *J. Ethnopharmacol.* **2005**, *98*, 191–193. [CrossRef]
253. Alanís, A.D.; Calzada, F.; Cedillo-Rivera, R.; Meckes, M. Antiprotozoal activity of the constituents of *Rubus coriifolius*. *Phytother. Res.* **2003**, *17*, 681–682. [CrossRef]
254. Kijlstra, A.; Jongert, E. Control of the risk of human toxoplasmosis transmitted by meat. *Int. J. Parasitol.* **2008**, *38*, 1359–1370. [CrossRef]
255. Jones, J.L.; Dubey, J. Foodborne toxoplasmosis. *Clin. Infect. Dis.* **2012**, *55*, 845–851. [CrossRef]
256. Choi, W.-Y.; Nam, H.-W.; Kwak, N.-H.; Huh, W.; Kim, Y.-R.; Kang, M.-W.; Cho, S.-Y.; Dubey, J. Foodborne outbreaks of human toxoplasmosis. *J. Infect. Dis.* **1997**, *175*, 1280–1282. [CrossRef]
257. Jones, J.L.; Hanson, D.L.; Dworkin, M.S.; Alderton, D.L.; Fleming, P.L.; Kaplan, J.E.; Ward, J. Surveillance for AIDS-defining opportunistic illnesses, 1992–1997. *Arch. Dermatol.* **1999**, *135*, 897–902. [CrossRef]
258. Gkogka, E.; Reij, M.W.; Havelaar, A.H.; Zwietering, M.H.; Gorris, L.G. Risk-based estimate of effect of foodborne diseases on public health, Greece. *Emerg. Infect. Dis.* **2011**, *17*, 1581. [CrossRef]
259. Youn, H.; Lakritz, J.; Kim, D.; Rottinghaus, G.; Marsh, A. Anti-protozoal efficacy of medicinal herb extracts against *Toxoplasma gondii* and *Neospora caninum*. *Vet. Parasitol.* **2003**, *116*, 7–14. [CrossRef]
260. Wright, C.W.; Anderson, M.M.; Allen, D.; Phillipson, J.D.; Kirby, G.C.; Warhurst, D.C.; Chang, H.R. Quassinoids exhibit greater selectivity against Plasmodium falciparum than against *Entamoeba histolytica*, *Giardia intestinalis* or *Toxoplasma gondii* in vitro. *J. Eukaryot. Microbiol.* **1993**, *40*, 244–246. [CrossRef] [PubMed]
261. Choi, K.-M.; Gang, J.; Yun, J. Anti-Toxoplasma gondii RH strain activity of herbal extracts used in traditional medicine. *Int. J. Antimicrob. Agents* **2008**, *32*, 360–362. [CrossRef]
262. Vanathy, K.; Parija, S.C.; Mandal, J.; Hamide, A.; Krishnamurthy, S. Cryptosporidiosis: A mini review. *Trop. Parasitol.* **2017**, *7*, 72–80.
263. Checkley, W.; White, A.C., Jr.; Jaganath, D.; Arrowood, M.J.; Chalmers, R.M.; Chen, X.-M.; Fayer, R.; Griffiths, J.K.; Guerrant, R.L.; Hedstrom, L. A review of the global burden, novel diagnostics, therapeutics, and vaccine targets for cryptosporidium. *Lancet Infect. Dis.* **2015**, *15*, 85–94. [CrossRef]
264. Teichmann, K.; Kuliberda, M.; Schatzmayr, G.; Pacher, T.; Zitterl-Eglseer, K.; Joachim, A.; Hadacek, F. In vitro inhibitory effects of plant-derived by-products against *Cryptosporidium parvum*. *Parasite* **2016**, *23*, 41. [CrossRef]

265. Al-Jboori, A.H.; Al-Alousi, T.I.; Obiad, H.M. The in vivo effect of some medicinal plant extracts on *Cryptosporidium* parasite. *J. Univ. Anbar Pure Sci.* **2012**, *6*, 15–26.
266. Almoradie, A.M.; Angeles, R.J.; Beltran, E.V.; Ugali, M.; Valles, N.S.; Los Banos, Z.D.; Mahboob, T.; Barusrux, S.; Nissapatorn, V. Cryptosporicidal Activity of Plant Extracts against *Cryptosporidium parvum* and *Cryptosporidium hominis*. *Asian J. Pharmacogn.* **2018**, *2*, 22–31.
267. Khater, M.M.; El-Sayed, S.H.; Yousof, H.-A.S.; Mahmoud, S.S.; El-Dib, N.; El-Badry, A.A. Anti-*Cryptosporidium* efficacy of *Olea europaea* and *Actinidia deliciosa* in a neonatal mouse model. *Kasr Al Ainy Med J.* **2017**, *23*, 32–37. [CrossRef]
268. Saritha, K.; Rajesh, A.; Manjulatha, K.; Setty, O.H.; Yenugu, S. Mechanism of antibacterial action of the alcoholic extracts of *Hemidesmus indicus* (L.) R. Br. ex Schult, *Leucas aspera* (Wild.), *Plumbago zeylanica* L., and *Tridax procumbens* (L.) R. Br. ex Schult. *Front. Microbiol.* **2015**, *6*, 577. [CrossRef]
269. Yadav, A.K.; Saraswat, S.; Sirohi, P.; Rani, M.; Srivastava, S.; Singh, M.P.; Singh, N.K. Antimicrobial action of methanolic seed extracts of *Syzygium cumini* Linn. on *Bacillus subtilis*. *AMB Express* **2017**, *7*, 196. [CrossRef]
270. Chandar, B.; Poovitha, S.; Ilango, K.; MohanKumar, R.; Parani, M. Inhibition of New Delhi Metallo-β-Lactamase 1 (NDM-1) producing *Escherichia coli* IR-6 by selected plant extracts and their synergistic actions with antibiotics. *Front. Microbiol.* **2017**, *8*, 1580. [CrossRef]
271. Ono, K.; Nakane, H.; Fukushima, M.; Chermann, J.-C.; Barré-Sinoussi, F. Inhibition of reverse transcriptase activity by a flavonoid compound, 5,6,7-trihydroxyflavone. *Biochem. Biophys. Res. Commun.* **1989**, *160*, 982–987. [CrossRef]
272. Brinkworth, R.I.; Stoermer, M.J.; Fairlie, D.P. Flavones are inhibitors of HIV-1 proteinase. *Biochem. Biophys. Res. Commun.* **1992**, *188*, 631–637. [CrossRef]
273. Gonelimali, F.D.; Lin, J.; Miao, W.; Xuan, J.; Charles, F.; Chen, M.; Hatab, S.R. Antimicrobial properties and mechanism of action of some plant extracts against food pathogens and spoilage microorganisms. *Front. Microbiol.* **2018**, *9*, 1639. [CrossRef]
274. Trombetta, D.; Castelli, F.; Sarpietro, M.G.; Venuti, V.; Cristani, M.; Daniele, C.; Saija, A.; Mazzanti, G.; Bisignano, G. Mechanisms of antibacterial action of three monoterpenes. *Antimicrob. Agents Chemother.* **2005**, *49*, 2474–2478. [CrossRef]
275. Alexopoulos, A.; Plessas, S.; Kimbaris, A.; Varvatou, M.; Mantzourani, I.; Fournomiti, M. Mode of antimicrobial action of Origanum vulgare essential oil against clinical pathogens. *Curr. Res. Nutr. Food Sci. J.* **2017**, *5*, 109–115. [CrossRef]
276. Faleiro, M. The mode of antibacterial action of essential oils. *Sci. Against Microb. Pathog. Commun. Curr. Res. Technol. Adv.* **2011**, *2*, 1143–1156.
277. Sledz, W.; Los, E.; Paczek, A.; Rischka, J.; Motyka, A.; Zoledowska, S.; Piosik, J.; Lojkowska, E. Antibacterial activity of caffeine against plant pathogenic bacteria. *Acta Biochim. Pol.* **2015**, *62*, 605–612. [CrossRef]
278. Saad, N.Y.; Muller, C.D.; Lobstein, A. Major bioactivities and mechanism of action of essential oils and their components. *Flavour Fragr. J.* **2013**, *28*, 269–279. [CrossRef]
279. Cushnie, T.T.; Cushnie, B.; Lamb, A.J. Alkaloids: An overview of their antibacterial, antibiotic-enhancing and antivirulence activities. *Int. J. Antimicrob. Agents* **2014**, *44*, 377–386. [CrossRef]
280. Awasthi, L.; Verma, H.; Kluge, S. A Possible mechanism of action for the inhibition of plant viruses by an antiviral glycoprotein isolated from *Boerhaavia diffusa* roots. *Virol. Antivir. Res.* **2016**, *2016*. [CrossRef]
281. Ngan, L.T.M.; Jang, M.J.; Kwon, M.J.; Ahn, Y.J. Antiviral activity and possible mechanism of action of constituents identified in *Paeonia lactiflora* root toward human rhinoviruses. *PLoS ONE* **2015**, *10*, e0121629. [CrossRef] [PubMed]
282. Idriss, M.T.; Suliman, M.M.; Khongwichit, S.; Tongluan, N.; Smith, D.R.; Abdurahman, N.; Elnima, A.I. Antiviral activity and possible mechanisms of action of Aristolochia bracteolate against influenza A virus. *Microbiol. Curr. Res.* **2017**, *1*, 22.
283. Lecoin, M.O.P. Mechanism of action of antiviral compounds isolated from plants: HIV virus as a model. *Univ. Tor. Repos.* **2008**, va07012.
284. Aziz, Q.; Doré, J.; Emmanuel, A.; Guarner, F.; Quigley, E. Gut microbiota and gastrointestinal health: Current concepts and future directions. *Neurogastroenterol. Motil.* **2013**, *25*, 4–15. [CrossRef] [PubMed]
285. Robinson, C.J.; Young, V.B. Antibiotic administration alters the community structure of the gastrointestinal microbiota. *Gut Microbes* **2010**, *1*, 279–284. [CrossRef] [PubMed]

286. Zweifel, C.; Stephan, R. Spices and herbs as source of *Salmonella*-related foodborne diseases. *Food Res. Int.* **2012**, *45*, 765–769. [CrossRef]
287. Kim, M.; Zahn, M.; Reporter, R.; Askar, Z.; Green, N.; Needham, M.; Terashita, D. Outbreak of foodborne botulism associated with prepackaged pouches of liquid herbal tea. *Open Forum. Infect. Dis.* **2019**, *6*. [CrossRef]
288. Farkas, J. Irradiation as a method for decontaminating food: A review. *Int. J. Food Microbiol.* **1998**, *44*, 189–204. [CrossRef]
289. Pelaez, F. The historical delivery of antibiotics from microbial natural products—Can history repeat? *Biochem. Pharmacol.* **2006**, *71*, 981–990. [CrossRef]
290. Cowan, M.M. Plant products as antimicrobial agents. *Clin. Microbiol. Rev.* **1999**, *12*, 564–582. [CrossRef]
291. Ulrich-Merzenich, G.S. Combination screening of synthetic drugs and plant derived natural products—Potential and challenges for drug development. *Synergy* **2014**, *1*, 59–69. [CrossRef]

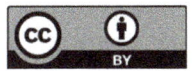

© 2020 by the authors. Licensee MDPI, Basel, Switzerland. This article is an open access article distributed under the terms and conditions of the Creative Commons Attribution (CC BY) license (http://creativecommons.org/licenses/by/4.0/).

Review

Vaccinium Species (Ericaceae): From Chemical Composition to Bio-Functional Activities

Rosa Tundis [1,*], Maria C. Tenuta [1,2], Monica R. Loizzo [1], Marco Bonesi [1], Federica Finetti [3], Lorenza Trabalzini [3] and Brigitte Deguin [2]

1. Department of Pharmacy, Health and Nutritional Sciences, University of Calabria, 87036 Rende, Italy; mary.tn2006@hotmail.it (M.C.T.); monica_rosa.loizzo@unical.it (M.R.L.); marco.bonesi@unical.it (M.B.)
2. Université de Paris, UFR de Pharmacie de Paris, U.M.R. n°8038, -CiTCoM- (CNRS, Université de Paris), F-75006 Paris, France; brigitte.deguin@parisdescartes.fr
3. Department of Biotechnology, Chemistry and Pharmacy, University of Siena, 53100 Siena, Italy; finetti2@unisi.it (F.F.); lorenza.trabalzini@unisi.it (L.T.)
* Correspondence: rosa.tundis@unical.it

Abstract: The genus *Vaccinium* L. (Ericaceae) includes more than 450 species, which mainly grow in cooler areas of the northern hemisphere. *Vaccinium* species have been used in traditional medicine of different cultures and the berries are widely consumed as food. Indeed, *Vaccinium* supplement-based herbal medicine and functional food, mainly from *V. myrtillus* and *V. macrocarpon*, are used in Europe and North America. Biological studies support traditional uses since, for many *Vaccinium* components, important biological functions have been described, including antioxidant, antitumor, anti-inflammatory, antidiabetic and endothelium protective activities. *Vaccinium* components, such as polyphenols, anthocyanins and flavonoids, are widely recognized as modulators of cellular pathways involved in pathological conditions, thus indicating that *Vaccinium* may be an important source of bioactive molecules. This review aims to better describe the bioactivity of *Vaccinium* species, focusing on anti-inflammatory and endothelial protective cellular pathways, modulated by their components, to better understand their importance for public health.

Keywords: *Vaccinium* species; phytochemicals; berry; leaf; anti-inflammatory pathways; endothelial dysfunction

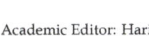

Citation: Tundis, R.; Tenuta, M.C.; Loizzo, M.R.; Bonesi, M.; Finetti, F.; Trabalzini, L.; Deguin, B. *Vaccinium* Species (Ericaceae): From Chemical Composition to Bio-Functional Activities. *Appl. Sci.* **2021**, *11*, 5655. https://doi.org/10.3390/app11125655

Academic Editor: Hari Prasad Devkota

Received: 30 May 2021
Accepted: 16 June 2021
Published: 18 June 2021

Publisher's Note: MDPI stays neutral with regard to jurisdictional claims in published maps and institutional affiliations.

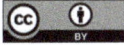

Copyright: © 2021 by the authors. Licensee MDPI, Basel, Switzerland. This article is an open access article distributed under the terms and conditions of the Creative Commons Attribution (CC BY) license (https:// creativecommons.org/licenses/by/ 4.0/).

1. Introduction

In recent years, *Vaccinium* species, mainly their fruits, have gained great attention for their potential health benefits. *Vaccinium* L. (Ericaceae) is a morphologically various genus of terrestrial or epiphytic shrubs and sub-shrubs, comprising approximately 450 species across Europe, North and Central America, South East and Central Africa, and Asia [1]. Deciduous or evergreen dwarf shrubs, shrubs or small trees characterize the genus, and the fruits of each variety are edible. The European flora comprises *V. corymbosum* (blueberry), *V. oxycoccos* (cranberry), *V. microcarpum*, *V. macrocarpon*, *V. vitis-idaea*, *V. uliginosum*, *V. myrtillus*, *V. arctostaphylos*, and *V. cylindraceum*. *V. corymbosum* was imported by North America, and now is cultivated in Europe for its big edible fruits [2]. *V. myrtillus* (bilberry) is a woody dwarf shrub, present in the forests of the Northern Hemisphere. It needs acid and well-drained soils for its growth, and it is considered to be an indicator of the biodiversity of forests due to its abundance.

Fruits of several *Vaccinium* species have been extensively investigated for their chemical profile. They are described as being a rich source of polyphenols and carotenoids. Nevertheless, especially due to their high content of anthocyanins, these fruits are recognized for their bioactive properties, such as prevention or treatment of cardiovascular diseases, diabetes, obesity, cancer, urinary tract infections, and aging diseases [3,4].

Polyphenols are the subject of increasing interest because of their potential beneficial effects on human health [5–9]. In fact, several epidemiological studies suggested that long term consumption of foods rich in polyphenols offered protection against the development of cardiovascular diseases, diabetes, cancers, and neurodegenerative diseases [5,6]. Polyphenols have been recognized due to their potent antioxidant activity and ability to modulate key signalling pathways of several inflammatory cytokines and enzymes [5]. Therefore, beyond these modulatory roles, their antioxidant activity related to the capacity to scavenge reactive oxygen species (ROS), or to activate cellular endogenous antioxidant systems, may be of importance in countering the oxidative stress in inflammatory diseases [5,6].

The antioxidant and anti-inflammatory activities of *Vaccinum* species are also reflected in a protective role for vascular endothelium against cardiovascular diseases linked to endothelial dysfunction [10,11].

The present review is designed to report the current knowledge on the plant species that belong to the *Vaccinium* genus, their phytochemicals, and their potential biological properties, with particular emphasis on their cardiovascular protective effects. Attention is focused on the ability of *Vaccinium* species to revert endothelial dysfunction promoted by increased oxidative stress and inflammatory status. All collected data have been obtained from different databases such as PubMed, Scopus, Sci Finder, Web of Science, Science Direct, NCBI, and Google Scholar.

2. Traditional Uses of *Vaccinium* Species

Vaccinium species are extensively used in traditional medicine. As reported in Table 1, the fruits of *V. myrtillus* are used in Europe for the treatment of stomatitis, renal stones, intestinal and liver disorders, as a remedy for fevers and coughs, and for their astringent, tonic, and antiseptic properties [12,13]. The decoction and infusion of leaves are used in south-eastern Europe to treat diabetes [14].

Table 1. Traditional uses of *Vaccinium* species.

Vaccinium	Traditional Uses	Part Used	References
V. myrtillus	Fevers and coughs	Fruits	[12]
	Antidiabetic and anti-inflammatory diabetic	Leaves	[13,14]
	Respiratory inflammations	Leaves and fruits	[15]
	Stomatitis	Fruits	[12]
	Eye inflammation	Fruits	[15]
	Intestinal and liver disorders	Fruits	[12]
	Hepatitis	Fruits	[15]
	Digestive and urinary tract disorders	Fruits	[15]
	Renal stones	Leaves and fruits	[12,15]
	Antiseptic, astringent, tonic	Fruits	[13]
	Anti-anemic	Leaves and fruits	[15]
V. vitis idaea	Antipyretic	Leaves and fruits	[15]
	Sore eyes, abscesses, toothache, thrush and snow blindness	Fruits	[16]
	Colds, coughs and sore throats	Fruits	[17]
	Anti-inflammatory properties in urinary tract	Leaves	[15]
	Respiratory system infections	Stems and leaves	[18]
	Frequent urination	Fruits	[16]
	Urinary tract infection properties	Fruits	[15]
	Kidney stones	Fruits	[15]
	Anti-inflammatory	Stems and leaves	[18]
	Wound healing, anti-rheumatic, anti-convulsant, diuretic and anti-diabetic	Leaves and fruits	[15]
V. arctostaphylos	Anti-hypertensive and anti-diabetic	Leaves and fruits	[19]
V. corymbosum	Anti-diabetic, antioxidant, and anti-inflammatory	Fruits	[20,21]
	Gastrointestinal disorders	Fruits	[22]

In Macedonia and Kosovo, the juice of *V. myrtillus* fruits are employed as anti-anemic agents, and to treat digestive and urinary tract infections, eye inflammations and hepatitis, while the infusions of leaves and fruits are used as lithontriptic and anti-anemic treatments, and for respiratory inflammations [15]. *V. vitis idaea* berries are effective in the traditional medicine of Cree Nation (Quebec) to treat frequent urination, sore eyes, abscesses, toothache, thrush and snow blindness [16]. Among the Alaska Natives, berries are also used to treat colds, coughs and sore throats [17]. From ancient times, stems and leaves have shown anti-inflammatory properties and are known for treating respiratory system infections in Chinese Traditional Medicine [18].

In Macedonia and Kosovo, an infusion of the leaves was used for their anti-rheumatic properties, as well as anti-inflammatory effects in the urinary tract, while the fruit infusion was useful for treating urinary tract infections and the presence of kidney stones. Fruits and leaves are also used as diuretic, anti-rheumatic, antipyretic, anti-diabetic and anti-convulsant medicines, as well as for wound healing [15]. *V. arctostaphylos* leaves and fruits have been utilized as anti-hypertensive and anti-diabetic agents in Iranian folk medicine [19]. In Quebec, *V. corymbosum* fruits have mainly been used to treat diabetes [20–22].

3. Phytochemicals of *Vaccinium* Fruits

Anthocyanins are present in the outer layer of fruits, together with polyphenolic compounds, and a small content was found also in pulp and seeds. Environmental factors can affect the content and composition of secondary metabolites in berries.

Growing conditions also affect the content of anthocyanins and other phenolic compounds in the berries of wild and cultivated species [23]. Prior to berry ripening, proanthocyanidins, flavonols and hydroxycinnamic acids are the major phenolic compounds. During the ripening process, flavonoid profiles vary, and anthocyanins accumulate in the skin. High levels—and a wide variety—of anthocyanins provide the red, blue, and purple colours that characterize berries of this genus.

Vaccinium berries have a well-deserved reputation as potential healthy products and functional foods, supported by many studies, which have identified and quantified various bioactive phytochemicals with known benefits for human health.

Many studies have demonstrated the benefits of anthocyanin-rich extracts of *Vaccinium* species in the prevention of several diseases [24]. Nonetheless, it is important to note that their efficacy is subject to their bioavailability. Once ingested, anthocyanins are metabolized into various conjugates, which are metabolized into phenolic acid degradation products. Accumulated evidence suggests synergistic effects between all possible metabolites to explain their health-promoting properties.

An inter-individual and intra-individual variability in anthocyanins absorption, metabolism, distribution, and excretion is also evident.

Six anthocyanidins (cyanidin, delphinidin, malvidin, pelargonidin, petunidin, and peonidin), which are also the most common anthocyanidin skeletons in higher plants, have been isolated from *Vaccinium* species [25]. To date, more than 35 anthocyanin glycosides have been isolated from the genus *Vaccinium*.

In *Vaccinium* berries, mono, di, or trisaccharide derivatives of delphinidin, cyanidin, peonidin, petunidin, and malvidin are common (Figure 1) [25]. The principal sugars are glucose, galactose, xylose, rhamnose, and arabinose.

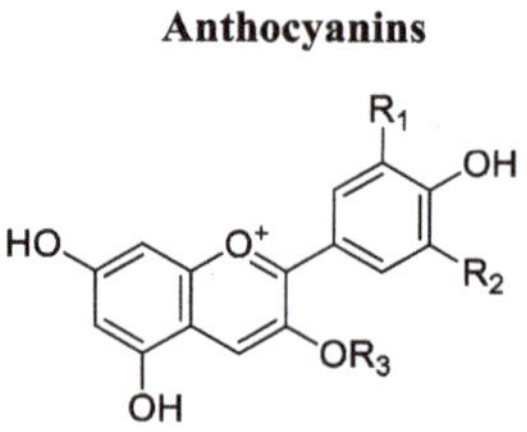

Anthocyanins

	R₁	R₂	R₃
Cyanidin 3-O-arabinoside	OH	H	Ara
Cyanidin 3-O-galactoside	OH	H	Gal
Cyanidin 3-O-glucoside	OH	H	Glc
Cyanidin 3-O-glucuronide	OH	H	Glc A
Cyanidin 3-O-sambubioside	OH	H	Xyl(1→2)Glc
Delphinidin 3-O-arabinoside	OH	OH	Ara
Delphinidin 3-O-glucoside	OH	OH	Glc
Delphinidin 3-O-galactoside	OH	OH	Gal
Delphinidin 3-O-sambubioside	OH	OH	Xyl(1→2)Glc
Delphinidin 3-O-xyloside	OH	OH	Xyl
Malvidin 3-O-arabinoside	OCH₃	OCH₃	Ara
Malvidin 3-O-galactoside	OCH₃	OCH₃	Gal
Malvidin 3-O-glucoside	OCH₃	OCH₃	Glc
Malvidin 3-O-xyloside	OCH₃	OCH₃	Xyl
Peonidin 3-O-arabinoside	OCH₃	H	Ara
Peonidin 3-O-galactoside	OCH₃	H	Gal
Peonidin 3-O-glucoside	OCH₃	H	Glc
Petunidin 3-O-arabinoside	OH	OCH₃	Ara
Petunidin 3-O-galactoside	OH	OCH₃	Gal
Petunidin 3-O-glucoside	OH	OCH₃	Glc
Petunidin 3-O-xyloside	OH	OCH₃	Xyl

Figure 1. Anthocyanins from *Vaccinium* species [25–36].

The fruits of *V. myrtillus* are characterized by the presence of different types of anthocyanins. In particular, cyanidin 3-O-galactoside, cyanidin 3-O-glucoside, cyanidin 3-O-arabinoside, delphinidin 3-O-galactoside, delphinidin 3-O-arabinoside, delphinidin 3-O-glucoside, malvidin 3-O-galactoside, malvidin 3-O-arabinoside, malvidin 3-O-glucoside, petunidin 3-O-galactoside, petunidin 3-O-arabinoside, petunidin 3-O-acetylglucoside, peonidin 3-O-galactoside, and peonidin 3-O-arabinoside were identified [26–31].

In *V. myrtillus*, cyanidin 3-O-xyloside, cyanidin 5-O-glucoside, cyanidin 3,5-O-diglucoside, cyanidin 3-O-(6″-O-2-rhamnopyranpsyl-2″-O-β-xylopranosyl-β-glucopyranoside), cyanidin 3-O-sambubioside, delphinidin 3-O-sambuobiside, and peonidin-3-glycoside have also been identified [31–34].

Malvidin and delphinidin derivatives represent about 75% of the total anthocyanins content of *V. corymbosum* fruits [35,36]. Cho et al. [29] reported percentages of 27–40% for delphinidin, 22–33% for malvidin, 19–26% for petunidin, 6–14% for cyanidin, and 1–5% for peonidin. Petunidin 3-O-glucoside has been also identified in *V. corymbosum* and *V. myrtillus* [27,31]. The 3-O-galactosides and 3-O-arabinosides of cyanidin and peonidin are the most abundant recognised anthocyanins in the fruits of *V. oxycoccos* [27,37,38].

Twelve anthocyanins, namely cyanidin 3-O-glucoside, delphinidin 3-O-glucoside cyanidin 3-O-arabinoside, peonidin 3-O-arabinoside, peonidin 3-O-glucoside, peonidin 3-O-galactoside, delphinidin 3-O-arabinoside, delphinidin 3-O-galactoside, petunidin 3-O-galactoside, petunidin 2-O-glucoside, malvidin 3-O-galactoside, and malvidin 3-O-glucoside, were isolated from the extract of the edible berries of *V. vitis-idaea* by a combination of chromatography techniques [39–44].

Delphinidin-3-*O*-xyloside, delphinidin-3-*O*-glucoside, malvidin-3-*O*-galactoside, malvidin-3-*O*-glucoside petunidin-3-*O*-galactoside, petunidin-2-*O*-glucoside, malvidin-3-*O*-xyloside, and petunidin-3-*O*-xyloside were isolated from *V. arctostaphylos* [45,46].

Except anthocyanins, to date, more than 50 other flavonoids (mainly flavanols and proanthocyanidins) have been isolated and identified from the genus *Vaccinium* (Figure 2) [25,28–31,40–44].

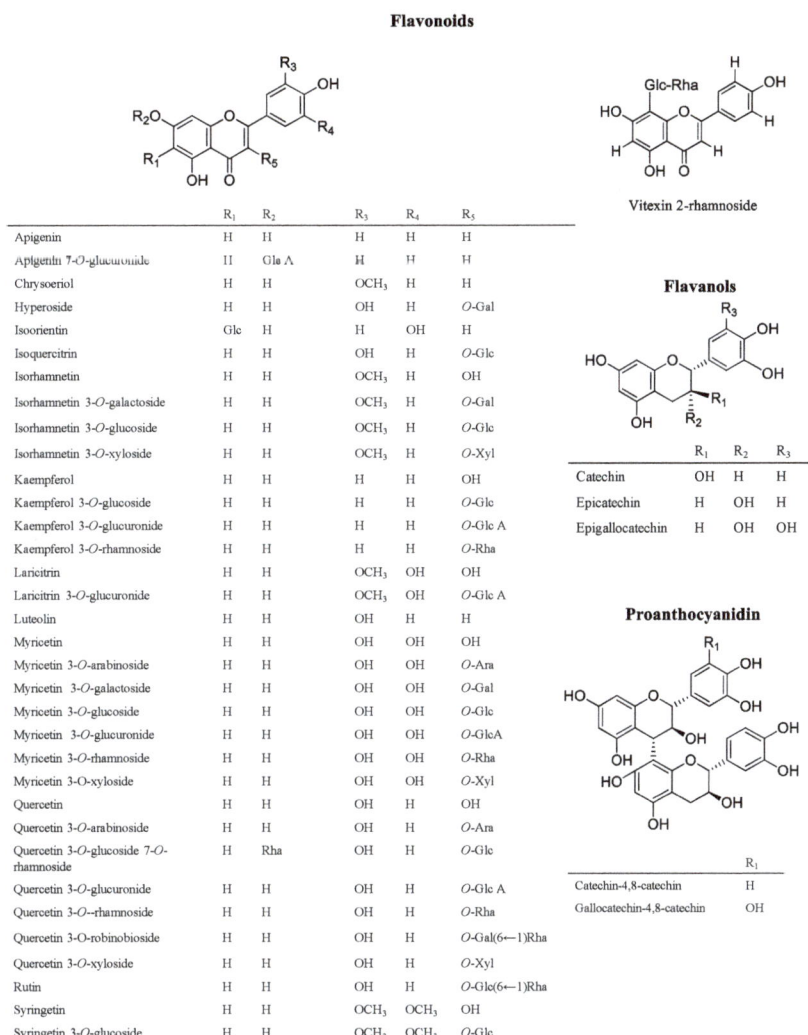

	R_1	R_2	R_3	R_4	R_5
Apigenin	H	H	H	H	H
Apigenin 7-*O*-glucuronide	H	Glc A	H	H	H
Chrysoeriol	H	H	OCH$_3$	H	H
Hyperoside	H	H	OH	H	*O*-Gal
Isoorientin	Glc	H	H	OH	H
Isoquercitrin	H	H	OH	H	*O*-Glc
Isorhamnetin	H	H	OCH$_3$	OH	
Isorhamnetin 3-*O*-galactoside	H	H	OCH$_3$	H	*O*-Gal
Isorhamnetin 3-*O*-glucoside	H	H	OCH$_3$	H	*O*-Glc
Isorhamnetin 3-*O*-xyloside	H	H	OCH$_3$	H	*O*-Xyl
Kaempferol	H	H	H	H	OH
Kaempferol 3-*O*-glucoside	H	H	H	H	*O*-Glc
Kaempferol 3-*O*-glucuronide	H	H	H	H	*O*-Glc A
Kaempferol 3-*O*-rhamnoside	H	H	H	H	*O*-Rha
Laricitrin	H	H	OCH$_3$	OH	OH
Laricitrin 3-*O*-glucuronide	H	H	OCH$_3$	OH	*O*-Glc A
Luteolin	H	H	OH	H	H
Myricetin	H	H	OH	OH	OH
Myricetin 3-*O*-arabinoside	H	H	OH	OH	*O*-Ara
Myricetin 3-*O*-galactoside	H	H	OH	OH	*O*-Gal
Myricetin 3-*O*-glucoside	H	H	OH	OH	*O*-Glc
Myricetin 3-*O*-glucuronide	H	H	OH	OH	*O*-GlcA
Myricetin 3-*O*-rhamnoside	H	H	OH	OH	*O*-Rha
Myricetin 3-*O*-xyloside	H	H	OH	OH	*O*-Xyl
Quercetin	H	H	OH	H	OH
Quercetin 3-*O*-arabinoside	H	H	OH	H	*O*-Ara
Quercetin 3-*O*-glucoside 7-*O*-rhamnoside	H	Rha	OH	H	*O*-Glc
Quercetin 3-*O*-glucuronide	H	H	OH	H	*O*-Glc A
Quercetin 3-*O*-rhamnoside	H	H	OH	H	*O*-Rha
Quercetin 3-*O*-robinobioside	H	H	OH	H	*O*-Gal(6←1)Rha
Quercetin 3-*O*-xyloside	H	H	OH	H	*O*-Xyl
Rutin	H	H	OH	H	*O*-Glc(6←1)Rha
Syringetin	H	H	OCH$_3$	OCH$_3$	OH
Syringetin 3-*O*-glucoside	H	H	OCH$_3$	OCH$_3$	*O*-Glc

Flavanols

	R_1	R_2	R_3
Catechin	OH	H	H
Epicatechin	H	OH	H
Epigallocatechin	H	OH	OH

Proanthocyanidin

	R_1
Catechin-4,8-catechin	H
Gallocatechin-4,8-catechin	OH

Figure 2. The main flavonoids identified in *Vaccinium* species [25,28–31,41].

Glycosides are usually *O*-glycosides, with the sugar moiety bound to the hydroxyl group at the C-3 or C-7 position. The most common sugar moieties include D-glucose, L-rhamnose, D-xylose, D-galactose, and L-arabinose [25].

Quercetin is the most common flavonoid isolated from *Vaccinium* species [25]. It was found in high quantities in *V. uliginosum* and *V. myrtillus* [29]; however, the richest source of quercetin is *V. oxycoccos* with 20–40 mg/100 g fresh weight [38].

Several glycosides of myricetin and quercetin were identified in *V. myrtillus*. Different studies reported the presence of myricetin 3-glucoside, myricetin 3-arabinoside, myricetin 3-*O*-rhamnoside, quercetin 3-*O*-arabinoside, quercetin 3-*O*-rhamnoside, quercetin 3-*O*-galactoside, quercetin 3-*O*-glucoside, and quercetin 3-*O*-rutinoside [28–31]. Apigenin, chrysoeriol, myricetin, myricetin-3-xyloside, quercetin 3-*O*-glucuronide, quercetin 3-*O*-xyloside, isorhamnetin 3-*O*-glucoside [41], luteolin are other flavonoids described in *V. myrtillus* [47]. Kaempferol, isorhamnetin, laricitrin, syringetin, isorhamnetin 3-*O*-galactoside, myricetin 3-*O*-glucuronide, laricitrin 3-*O*-glucoside, syringetin 3-*O*-glucoside [35,41,48], kaempferol 3-*O*-glucoside, myricetin 3-*O*-galactoside, and isorhamnetin 3-*O*-xyloside are also described [48].

The flavonoids identified in *V. oxycoccos* are mainly glycosides of quercetin and myricetin, and to a lesser extent, of kaempferol [49]. Quercetin 3-*O*-galactoside is the dominant compound, but at least 11 other glycosides are present in lower concentrations [38].

Epicatechin is the dominant constitutive unit of *V. oxycoccos*, whereas catechin and (epi)gallocatechins are present only in trace amounts [24,40].

The major flavonoids described in *V. vitis idaea* are kaempferol [41], quercetin [41,50], myricetin, myricetin 3-*O*-glucoside [44], quercetin derivatives (bond to glucose, galactose, glucuronide, rhamnose, arabinose, and xylose), kaempferol 3-*O*-rhamnoside, isorhamnetin 3-*O*-galactoside [40,51], isorhamnetin 3-*O*-glucoside, syringetin-3-*O*-glucoside, kaempferol 3-*O*-glucoside, and rutin [51].

The fruits of *V. uliginosum* are characterized by the presence of kaempferol, laricitrin [50], quercetin [50,52–54], myricetin [54], syringetin, quercetin 3-*O*-glucoside, quercetin 3-*O*-galactoside, quercetin 3-*O*-glucuronide, isorhamnetin 3-*O*-galactoside, isorhamnetin 3-*O*-glucoside, syringetin 3-*O*-glucoside, myricetin 3-*O*-galactoside, rutin [50,52], and myricetin 3-*O*-glucuronide [48].

Sellappan et al. [55] described, in *V. corymbosum*, the presence of catechin, myricetin, quercetin and kaempferol, but not the presence of epicatechin.

Seventeen phenolic acids were identified in some varieties of *V. myrtillus* (Figure 3) [56]. Sellappan et al. [55] found gallic, *p*-coumaric, ferulic, ellagic and caffeic acids as phenolic acids in *V. corymbosum* produced in the state of Georgia (US). These results were confirmed by Taruscio et al. [30] who analysed the phenolic acids composition of *V. corymbosum* and *V. oxycoccos*. The two species have different compositions. In fact, *V. corymbosum* was characterised by the presence of chlorogenic acid as a major phenolic acid, followed by caffeic, ferulic, *p*-coumaric and traces of *p*-hydroxybenzoic acids, while *p*-coumaric acid was the principal phenolic acid of *V. oxycoccos*, followed by ferulic, chlorogenic, caffeic and *p*-hydroxybenzoic acids.

Other studies have reported *p*-coumaric, sinapic, caffeic, and ferulic acids as the main hydroxycinnamic acids identified in *V. oxycoccos* [57–59]. Ellagic acid and ellagitannins have not been detected in significant amounts [24].

Thirteen phenolic acids (gallic, protocatechuic, *p*-hydroxybenzoic, *m*-hydroxybenzoic, gentisic, chlorogenic, *p*-coumaric, caffeic, ferulic, syringic, sinapic, salicylic, and *trans*-cinnamic acids) were identified in *V. arctostaphylos*.

The dominant phenolic acids were caffeic and *p*-coumaric acids. The phenolic acid concentrations are mostly lower in *V. arctostaphylos* in comparison to the other berries of the *Vaccinium* genus [60].

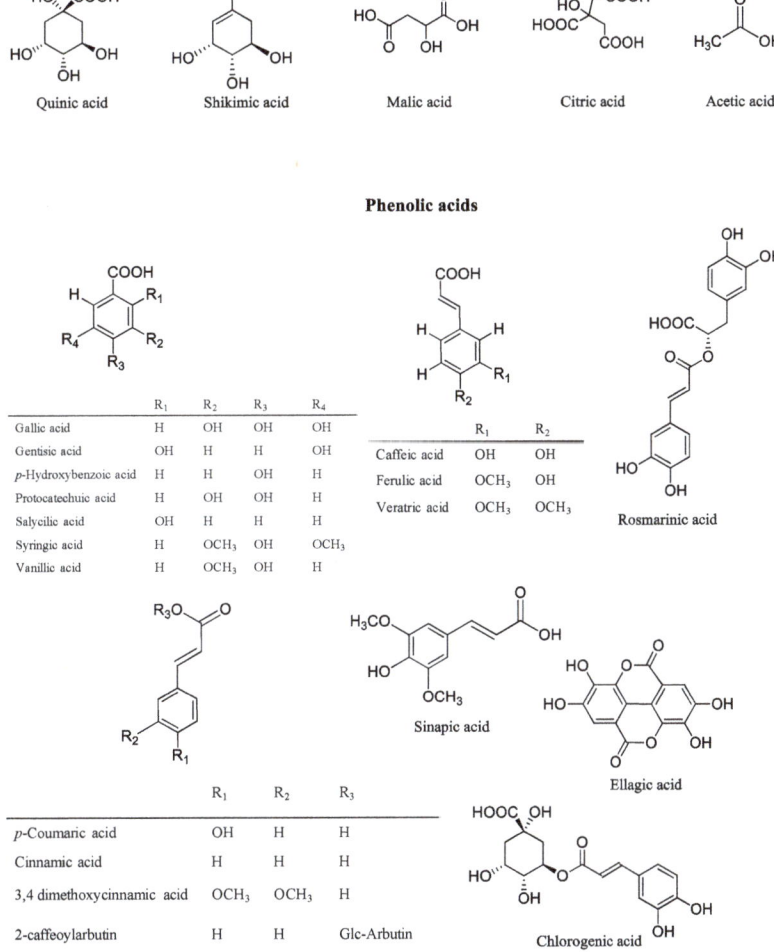

Figure 3. Main acids and phenolic acids in the *Vaccinium* genus [56–60].

Iridoids are a widespread group of monoterpenoids comprising a generally glycosylated cyclopentan[c]pyran skeleton. They are specifically produced by several botanical families and are a class of secondary metabolites that is characteristic of the Ericaceae. Iridoids from the *Vaccinium* genus have been less studied than anthocyanins and other phenolic compounds. However, iridoids have known human health benefits including anti-inflammatory, anticancer, antimicrobial, antioxidant, antispasmodic, cardioprotective, choleretic, hepatoprotective, hypoglycaemic, hypolipidemic, neuroprotective, and purgative activities [61–63].

The Figure 4 shows the main iridoids identified in *Vaccinium* species. These compounds have often been identified in mixtures and have not always been isolated. The stereochemistry of the asymmetric carbons of some of them has not been elucidated. Asperuloside, scandoside, and monotropein, and their derivatives, seem to be representative of the genus [64,65].

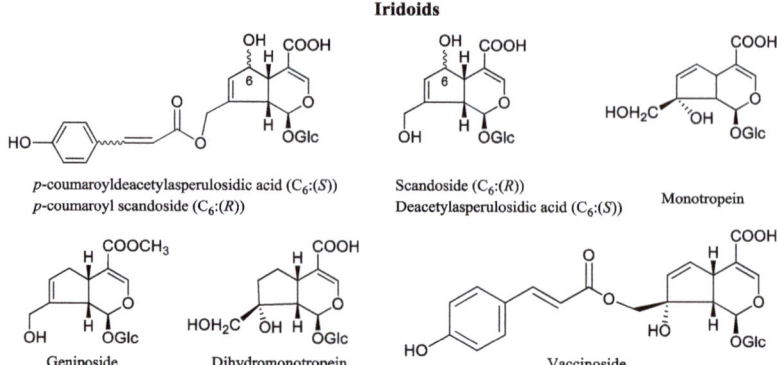

Figure 4. The chemical structures of the main iridoids isolated from *Vaccinium* species [64,65].

Heffels et al. [64] have tentatively identified, in *V. uliginosum* and *V. myrtillus*, 14 iridoid glucosides, including vaccinoside, monotropein, *p*-coumaroyl-scandoside, deacetylasperulosidic acid (C_6: (S)), scandoside (C_6: (R)), *p*-coumaroyl-deacetylasperulosidic acid, *p*-coumaroyl-monotropein, and *p*-coumaroyldihydromonotropein (C_6-C_7 hydrogenated). *V. oxycoccos* juice showed the presence of two new coumaroyl iridoid glycosides, namely 10-*p*-trans- and 10-*p*-cis-coumaroyl-1S-dihydromonotropein [66].

Detection and isolation of iridoids from fruits is not straightforward. Surprisingly, iridoid glycosides have not been identified in *V. corymbosum* [64,67,68], whereas scandoside, geniposide, vaccinoside, and dihydromonotropein have recently been identified in *V. corymbosum* extracts [65].

Ursolic acid, which showed to possess strong anti-inflammatory effects, is abundant in *V. oxycoccos*, which also contains two rare derivatives of ursolic acid: *cis*-3-*O*-*p*-hydroxycinnamoyl ursolic acid and *trans*-3-*O*-*p*-hydroxycinnamoyl ursolic acid [69].

Triterpenoids are the most predominant components in the cuticular wax of blueberry fruits, together with the triterpene alcohols α-amyrin, β-amyrin, and lupeol [70].

Ursolic acid was the dominant triterpene in *V. corymbosum* (southern highbush blueberry) cultivars, whereas oleanolic acid was the most abundant in northern highbush blueberry cultivars. Hentriacontan-10,12-dione was detected for the first time in *V. corymbosum* [70].

Malic, citric, and quinic acids are the non-volatile acids identified and quantified in *V. arctostaphylos* and *V. myrtillus* species. It is interesting to note that the level of malic acid in both berries increases gradually during maturation. In contrast, the level of citric and quinic acids, as well as the total acid level, decreases towards ripening in both species [71]. Citric and malic acids are the main organic acids in *V. oxycoccos* [72]. In *V. corymbosum*, the major acids (organic and phenolic) present are citric, malic, quinic, and chlorogenic acids. The minor acids, acetic and shikimic acid are present and their contribution to the total acid equivalents is 3.0% [73].

4. The Chemical Profile of *Vaccinium* Leaves

A body of scientific research studies proved the contribution of berries' consumption to the main targets of functional foods, such as health maintenance and reduced risk of some chronic diseases. However, in addition to fruits, the leaves of the *Vaccinium* species have also been used in traditional remedies (Table 1).

Leaves are considered to be by-products of berries' cultivation. Their traditional use against several diseases, such as inflammation, diabetes, and ocular dysfunction, has been almost forgotten in recent times. The scientific interest regarding the leaves' composition and beneficial properties has grown, demonstrating that leaves may be considered to be an alternative source of bioactive compounds. Analytical studies reveal that the chemical composition of leaves is similar to that of the fruits or even higher, indicating that they may be used as an alternative source of bioactive compounds for the development of functional foods, nutraceuticals, and/or food supplements.

Riihinen et al. [74] showed that red leaves of *Vaccinium* genus contain anthocyanins, which are absent in green leaves. Both green and red leaves contain proanthocyanidins, especially procyanidin. Teleszko and Wojdyło [75] analysed the phytochemical composition of fruits and leaves of several *Vaccinium* species; among them, *V. myrtillus* leaves were the first source of phenolic compounds, followed by *V. oxycoccos* leaves. The major polyphenolic group was proanthocyanidins, followed by flavonols. Proanthocyanidins, flavan-3-ols, phenolic acids and flavonols were in higher concentration than the respective fruits [76].

Proanthocyanidins were detected in small quantities in the leaves of *V. vitis-idaea* [41]. Ferlemi et al. [76,77] have detected proanthocyanidin B1/B2 and cinchonain in the leaves of *V. corymbosum*. In the same year, Wang et al. [78] identified the presence of cyanidin 3-*O*-glucoside, cyanidin 3-*O*-glucuronide, and cyanidin 3-*O*-arabinoside in the methanolic leaf extract of *V. corymbosum*, confirming that *V. corymbosum* leaves possess a higher total anthocyanins content compared to *V. virgatum* and *V. formosum* leaves.

After proanthocyanidins, flavonoids are the most important classes of constituents of *Vaccinium* leaves. Quercetin-3-*O*-glucuronide is the most abundant flavonoid (70–93% of total flavonoids) [79]. Other identified flavonoids in the leaves are quercetin-3-*O*-galactoside, quercetin-3-*O*-(4″-3-hydroxy-3-methylglutaroyl)-α-rhamnoside, quercetin-3-*O*-arabinoside, quercetin-3-*O*-glucoside, quercitrin, and quercetin, as well as three kaempferol glycosides [41,79]. In addition, Hokkanen et al. [41] have detected several other bioactive compounds in the leaves, such as flavan-3-ols, six different isomers of cinchonain, three proanthocyanidins, and two coumaroyl iridoids.

Sidorova et al. [80] investigated the flavonoids present in *V. myrtillus*, and found flavonoid C-glycosides and *O*-derivatives of apigenin and luteolin; the main ones are apigenin-7-glucuronide, vitexin-2-*O*-rhamnoside, and isoorientin. Flavonoid glycosides are represented mainly in quercetin derivatives, particularly rutin and quercetin-3-glucoside-7-rhamnoside. Isorhamnetin-3-glucoside and kaempferol-3-glucuronide were also found in the extract. Additionally, free aglycones were also present (myricetin, quercetin, luteolin and kaempferol).

The main flavonols detected in the *V. oxycoccos* leaves were hyperoside and quercetin-3-*O*-rhamnoside, together with quercetin-3-*O*-xyloside, quercetin-3-*O*-arabinoside and procyanidin A2 [66].

The green leaves of *V. vitis-idaea* have similar phytochemical profiles to those of *V. myrtillus* [41,79]. Ieri et al. [79] and Hokkanen et al. [41] have quantified the phenolic compounds in methanolic and hydroalcoholic leaf extracts of *V. vitis-idaea*. In general, hydroxycinnamic acids and flavonoids were the most abundant compounds. In the methanolic extract, the content of flavonoids was higher than that of hydroxycinnamic acids, but in the hydroalcoholic extract, the opposite was observed. In both extracts, the main acid was 2-*O*-caffeoylarbutin, which is not present in other *Vaccinium* leaves.

Other phenolic acids detected in the methanolic extract were chlorogenic, caffeic, *p*-coumaric and caffeoyl-shikimic acids, together with the coumaroyl quinic acid isomers [41]. Moreover, *V. vitis-idaea* leaves were characterised by coumaroyl- and caffeoyl-hexose hydroxyphenols.

The most abundant flavonoid was quercetin-3-*O*-(4″-3-hydroxy-3-methylglutaroyl)-α-rhamnoside, which represents 5–6% of total phenols in the hydroalcoholic extract and 32% of the methanolic extract.

Rutin, hyperoside, and quercitrin were also detected in significant amounts in the methanolic extract, while traces of four quercetin glycosides and kaempferol glycosides were also found. Proanthocyanidins and coumaroyl iridoids were also identified [41].

Quercetin-3-*O*-glucoside, quercetin-3-*O*-rutinoside, kaempferol-3-*O*-glucoside, and kaempferol-3-*O*-rhamnoside were identified in the leaves of *V. arctostaphylos* [45,81].

The main flavonoids detected in the leaves of *V. corymbosum* were hyperoside, isoquercetin and rutin. Other flavonoids found were: myricetin [54], quercetin-3-*O*-glucoside, quercetine-3-*O*-galactoside, quercetine-3-*O*-arabinoside [82], quercetin-3-*O*-rhamnoside [35,82,83], myricetin-3-*O*-glucoside, quercetin-3-*O*-rutinoside [83], syringetin-3-*O*-glucoside, and kaempferol-3-*O*-glucoside [35,83].

Several studies have demonstrated the role of collection time of *Vaccinium* leaves in influencing their phenolic content [79]. In fact, contrary to the fruits, the flavonoid content increases during the development of the leaves, while hydroxycinnamic acid content strongly decreases [84]. Previously, Riihinen et al. [74] have indicated that the red leaves of *V. corymbosum* have higher quantities of quercetin and kaempferol, as well as of ferulic, caffeic and *p*-coumaric acid, than green leaves. The main bioactive compounds of *V. myrtillus* leaves are hydroxycinnamic acids, especially chlorogenic acid [41,79]; its concentration ranges from 59 to 74% of the total hydroxycinnamic acids [79]. Sidorova et al. [80] also reported the presence of rosmarinic acid, caffeoylquinic acid, *p*-coumaric and ferulic acid. Hokkanen et al. [41] analysed the methanolic extract of *V. myrtillus* leaves and identified thirty-five compounds. Other than the abundant chlorogenic acid and its isomers, caffeoyl-shikimic acid, feruloylquinic acid isomer, and traces of caffeic acid were found.

In addition, Neto et al. [85] have performed an HPLC-MS analysis of the phenolic profile of *V. oxycoccos* leaves; the phenolic acids are mainly chlorogenic and neo-chlorogenic acid, as well as 3-*O*- and 5-*O*-coumaroylquinic acids. Mzhavanadze et al. [86] reported the isolation of caffeic, chlorogenic, neochlorogenic, 3- and 5-*p*-coumaroylquinic acids, and 3,5-dicaffeoylquinic acid from the leaves of *V. arctostaphylos*.

Continuing the investigation of the qualitative composition of the leaves, they have isolated six phenolic substances: cryptochlorogenic (4-caffeoyl-quinic) acid, arbutin, rosmarinic acid, caffeoylarbutin, 1-*p*-coumaroylgalactoglucose, and *p*-coumaroylarbutin.

Twenty different compounds, mainly phenolic acids and flavonols, were identified in the red dried leaves of *V. corymbosum* by Liquid Chromatography Electrospray Ionization Tandem Mass Spectrometry (LC/ESI-MS/MS) and High-Performance Liquid Chromatography-Diode-Array Detection (HPLC-DAD) [76,77]. Interestingly, these two groups were in almost equal concentration in the crude extract (chlorogenic acid and quercetin-3-*O*-galactoside); as in *V. myrtillus* leaves, the most abundant compound was chlorogenic acid. LC-MS analysis showed the presence of quinic and caffeic acid.

Even though the triperpenes in the leaves comprised only the 4–6% of those in the respective fruits, several compounds were identified in the diethyl ether leaf extract. The principal compound was β-amyrin, followed by oleanane- and ursane-type triterpenes. The triterpene oleanolic and ursolic acids were also identified [87].

Two coumaroyl iridoid isomers (*trans*- and *cis*- form) previously documented in *V. oxycoccos* fruits were also reported in the leaves [66]. In *V. vitis ideae* coumaroyl, iridoids were quantified in small concentrations [41]. The three iridoids found in the leaf extracts of *V. corymbosum* are identical to those found in the fruit. However, it should be noted that a fourth iridoid, vaccinoside (monotropein-10-trans-*p*-coumarate), was detected in fresh leaves but not in dried leaves [65].

5. Biological Properties of *Vaccinium* Species

Many biological properties have been reported for extracts and derivatives of different *Vaccinium* species, and the anti-inflammatory, antioxidant, anti-carcinogenic, cardiovascular and neurodegenerative protective effects have been extensively described [11,88–90]. High antioxidant activity has been demonstrated for *V. corymbosum* [76,91], *V. oxycoccos* [92], *V. myrtillus* [93], and many others. This activity appears to be linked to cultivar, genotype, growing site, cultivation techniques and conditions, processing, and storage.

Similarly, in different anti-inflammatory tests, *Vaccinium* exhibited high anti-inflammatory activity [11]. High concentrations of anthocyanins (such as cyanidin, delphinidin and malvidin) and flavonoids (such as astragalin, hyperoside, isoquercitrin, and quercitrin) appear to be related to the anti-inflammatory and antioxidant activities ascribed to these berries [94,95]. Considering that berries of *Vaccinium* are edible, their consumption may be helpful for the treatment of inflammatory illnesses.

In this review, we will focus on the activity of *Vaccinium* extracts and derivatives in cardiovascular diseases, closely associated with the inflammation processes and oxidative stress. The vascular endothelium occupies a catalogue of functions that contribute to the homeostasis of the cardiovascular system. Endothelial cells (ECs) play a variety of roles, including the control of tone regulation, blood coagulation and vascular permeability, and local regulation of coagulative, immune and inflammatory stimuli [96].

Indeed, many cardiovascular diseases are either a direct or indirect result of a dysfunction of the endothelium that fails to maintain body homeostasis [97,98]. Endothelial dysfunction (ED) is considered as a predictor of cardiovascular events, and it is characterized by alterations in vascular tone and endothelial production of procoagulant and prothrombotic factors [97,98].

Several risk factors including smoking, obesity, insulin resistance, diabetes, hypercholesterolemia, and physical inactivity have been described for ED. In addition, ED occurs with aging, as a consequence of senescence processes [99,100]. *Vaccinium* extracts have long been used in traditional medicine and appear to be promising nutraceuticals to prevent endothelial dysfunction and cardiovascular diseases.

5.1. Vaccinium and Diabetes

Several reports indicate a potential role of *Vaccinium* in the control of diabetes, and it has been used in traditional medicine for centuries to ameliorate its symptoms [101–103]. Approximately 90% of the diabetic patients have type 2 diabetes that is characterized by peripheral insulin resistance and by a reduction in the number and the activity of pancreatic β-cells [104]. Anthocyanins from *Vaccinium* have potential in terms of lowering the risk of developing various chronic diseases due to their ability to regulate energy metabolism as well as through their anti-inflammatory and anti-oxidative effects [11]. Furthermore, anthocyanins inhibit the activities of α-glucosidase and pancreatic α-amylase, important targets for some antidiabetic drugs [105–107]. Phenolic compounds affect key pathways of carbohydrate metabolism and hepatic glucose homeostasis including glycolysis, glycogenesis, and gluconeogenesis, which are usually impaired in diabetes.

In addition, *Vaccinium* extracts and derivatives protect pancreatic β-cells from glucose-induced oxidative stress, increase insulin secretion, possess glucose-lowering effects, restore glutathione concentration, inhibit DPP-4, enhance insulin response, and attenuate the secretion of glucose-dependent insulinotropic polypeptide and GLP-1 [80,106,108,109]. Blueberry metabolites reduce the expression of inflammatory markers and restore the glycosaminoglycan levels increased by high glucose in in vitro models of diabetic ECs [110]. Moreover, malvidin, a major anthocyanin present in blueberries, decreases reactive oxygen species levels, increases the enzyme activity of catalase and superoxide dismutase, and downregulates NADPH oxidase 4 (NOX4) expression in ECs exposed to high glucose levels [111], indicating a protective role against diabetes-induced oxidative stress. In similar models, this compound also reduces vascular endothelial growth factor (VEGF) up-regulation, ICAM-1 expression, and NF-κB (p65) levels [112]. In addition, malvidin has been shown to be able to restore PI3K and Akt levels, which are reduced by high glucose [113].

These observations are also confirmed in the retina of diabetic rats, where blueberry anthocyanins reduce oxidative stress, vascular endothelial growth factor (VEGF) and interleukin 1β (IL-1β) expression, and activate the Nrf2-related/heme oxygenase 1 (Nrf2/HO-1) signalling pathway [114], suggesting that *Vaccinium* anthocyanin may be helpful in inhibiting diabetes-induced retinal abnormalities and preventing the development of diabetic retinopathy.

5.2. Vaccinium and Atherosclerosis

Atherosclerosis is one of the major causes of cardiovascular diseases and is characterized by the accumulation of lipids and fibrous plaques in the large arteries, which may lead to heart attacks, strokes, and peripheral vascular diseases [115].

Cignarella et al. [116] tested a dried hydroalcoholic extract of *V. myrtillus* leaves showing a lipid-lowering activity with decrease of 39% of the triglycerides in the blood of dyslipidemic animals. Similarly, *V. corymbosum* berries decreased blood cholesterol levels, thus reducing cardiovascular risk and promoting atherosclerosis prevention [117,118]. In addition, consumption of cranberry anthocyanins improved lipid profiles, increasing HDL and decreasing LDL in rats, hamsters fed a high-fat diet and hypercholesterolemic swine [119–121]. Wu et al. [122] showed that blueberries induce a regression of atherosclerotic plaques in arteries. In this manuscript, the apolipoprotein-E deficient (apoE−/−) mice were fed either a control diet or an enriched diet supplemented with 1% freeze-dried wild blueberries for 20 weeks. The plaques, measured at two sites, were 39 and 58% smaller in the mice fed blueberries compared to those fed the control diet, and these effects were associated with the reduction in biomarkers of lipid peroxidation in the liver, such as F2-isoprostane [122]. Similarly, Matziouridou et al. [123] showed that in Apoe−/− mice fed either a low-fat diet or high-fat diet, with or without lingonberries, the size of the atherosclerotic plaques, the total, HDL and LDL-VLDL blood cholesterol, and triglycerides, as well as the hepatic gene expression of bile acid synthesis genes (cholesterol 7 α-hydroxylase (Cyp7a1), sterol 12α-hydroxylase (Cyp8b1)) were reduced.

Although published animal studies primarily focused on the specific cardiovascular disease risk factors or biomarkers, and the antioxidant and anti-inflammatory effects, of *Vaccinium* and its derivatives, clinical data have also been published [10]. Indeed, good results were also observed with cranberry juice in obese men, and hyper-triglyceridemic or diabetic patients [24].

The molecular mechanisms of atheroprotective effects of *Vaccinium* are not completely understood and are often associated with antioxidant and anti-inflammatory activities. In fact, the protective activity in atherosclerosis development have been associated with the reduction in oxidative stress, inhibition of inflammation, and regulation of cholesterol accumulation and trafficking [10].

In apoE−/− mice, the treatment with 1% wild blueberries for 20 weeks modulated gene expression and protein levels of scavenger receptors CD36 and SR-A, the principal receptors responsible for the binding and uptake of modified LDL in macrophages [124].

CD36 and SR-A were found to be lower in peritoneal macrophages of blueberry-fed mice, and fewer ox-LDL-induced foam cells were formed, probably through a mechanism involving PPARγ [124]. In addition, Xie et al. [125] demonstrated that blueberry consumption increased the levels of the cholesterol transporter ABCA1, indicating that blueberries may facilitate cholesterol efflux and lowering cholesterol accumulation. Overall, it has been shown that blueberry consumption increased PPARα, PPARγ, ABCA1 and fatty acid synthase expression, while reducing SREBP-1 levels [10].

Although several sources of experimental evidence support the atheroprotective effects of *Vaccinium*, further and more in-depth studies are needed to completely elucidate the molecular mechanisms underlying this activity.

5.3. Vaccinium and Endothelial Dysfunction

Endothelial dysfunction is an early predictor of cardiovascular diseases, and it is well known that oxidative stress and low grade of inflammation contributes to endothelial cell activation, priming it for adhesion, infiltration, and immune cell activation [126].

In this context, data from the literature indicate that *Vaccinium* extracts and derivatives may prevent or delay cardiovascular diseases due to their capability to revert endothelial dysfunction. Very recently, Curtis et al. [127] showed that one cup of blueberries/day, for six months, promotes 12–15% reductions in cardiovascular disease risk, demonstrating that higher intakes of blueberries improve markers of vascular function and ameliorate lipid status. Similarly, the intake of blueberry acutely improved peripheral arterial dysfunction in smoker and in non-smoker subjects [128,129], improved endothelial function over six weeks in subjects with metabolic syndrome [130], and improved endothelium-dependent vasodilation in hypercholesterolemic individuals through the induction of the NO-cGMP signaling pathway [131].

In animal models, blueberry anthocyanin-enriched extracts were shown to be able to increase Bcl-2 protein expression, as well as to decrease interleukin 6, malondialdehyde, endothelin 1, and angiotensin II levels and to reduce Bax protein expression after rat exposure to fine particulate matter [132]. Blueberry consumption was also able to protect endothelial function in obese Zucker rats, through the attenuation of local inflammation in perivascular adipose tissue (PVAT) [133]. In diabetic rats, the *Vaccinium* treatment decreased markers of diabetic retinopathy, such as retinal VEGF expression and degradation of zonula occludens-1, occludin and claudin-5 [134]. Finally, in experiments of hypoperfusion-reperfusion in rats, the administration of the extract of *Vaccinium myrtillus* protected pial microcirculation by preventing vasoconstriction, microvascular permeability, and leukocyte adhesion [135].

The endothelium protective role of *Vaccinium* has also been reported in in vitro experimental models. Human aortic endothelial cell (HAECs) treated with palmitate exhibited elevated ROS levels, and increased expression of several markers of endothelial dysfunction including NOX4, chemokines, adhesion molecules, and IκBα.

The effects of palmitate were ameliorated in HAECs previously treated with blueberry metabolites [136]. In human umbilical vein endothelial cells (HUVEC), pterostilbene, an active constituent of blueberries, is able to induce a concentration-dependent nitric oxide release via endothelial nitric oxide synthase (eNOS) phosphorylation, mediated by activation of the PI3K/Akt signaling pathway [137]. Similarly, blueberry anthocyanins protect endothelial cells from oxidative deterioration by decreasing the levels of ROS and Xanthine Oxidase -1 (XO-1) and increasing the levels of superoxide dismutase and HO-1 [138].

6. Conclusions and Future Perspectives

The fruits and leaves of different *Vaccinium* species have been used for a long time in the traditional medicine of different cultures to treat several diseases including renal, gastrointestinal and liver disorders, respiratory system infections, cough, fever, diabetes, and convulsions. Biological studies support traditional uses since many *Vaccinium* components exhibit important biological properties, including antioxidant, antitumor, anti-inflammatory, antidiabetic and endothelium protective activities. In particular, the high antioxidant and anti-inflammatory activity of *Vaccinium* has been related to the high content in polyphenols, anthocyanins, and flavonoids.

In addition, *Vaccinium* extracts appear to be safe and mostly lacking in side effects, with the exception of a few case reports, without statistical significance, describing an aspirin-like effect (increased bleeding) [139,140].

Herein, we reported the chemical composition of fruits and leaves of *Vaccinium* species and provided an overview of their biological properties, focusing on the activity of *Vaccinium* extracts and derivatives in cardiovascular diseases and endothelial dysfunctions, closely associated with inflammation processes and oxidative stress.

Many studies indicate that *Vaccinium* is an important source of bioactive molecules that appear to satisfy all the requirements to develop drugs and nutraceuticals against endothelial dysfunction, thus preventing cardiovascular disease onset and progression. Well-designed and specific clinical trials are necessary in order to explore the intriguing potential of *Vaccinium* in the treatment of metabolic syndrome and in cardiovascular protection.

In conclusion, as fruits and leaves of *Vaccinium* species represent a rich source of phenolic compounds with a high biological potential, they can serve as commercial sources of specific compounds or fractions for pharmaceutics, cosmetics and natural product markets. However, because of the wide variety of constituents that characterizes the chemical profile of *Vaccinium* species, their possible interactions with other constituents, and the complexity of their metabolism, further and more in-depth studies will be necessary to better define and characterize the contribution of each single active component, possible synergisms between the different compounds, and the molecular mechanisms underlying their biological effects.

Author Contributions: Conceptualization, R.T. and F.F.; writing—original draft preparation, investigation, resources, data curation, M.C.T., F.F., M.B., R.T., M.R.L., L.T. and B.D.; writing—review and editing, R.T., M.R.L., F.F., L.T. and B.D.; supervision, B.D., R.T. and L.T. All authors have read and agreed to the published version of the manuscript.

Funding: This work was supported by MIUR (Progetto Dipartimento di Eccellenza 2018–2022) to L.T. and F.F.

Institutional Review Board Statement: Not applicable.

Informed Consent Statement: Not applicable.

Data Availability Statement: All data related to the review manuscript are presented in the manuscript in the form of tables and figures.

Conflicts of Interest: The authors declare no conflict of interest.

References

1. Kloet, V.E. Manual of the flowering plants of Hawaii. *Bishop Museum Spec. Publ.* **1990**, *83*, 591–595.
2. Tutin, T.G.; Heywood, V.H.; Burges, N.A.; Valentine, D.H.; Walters, S.M.; Webb, D.A. *Flora Europea*; Cambridge University Press: Cambridge, UK, 1972; Volume 3, pp. 12–13.
3. Colak, N.; Primetta, A.K.; Riihinen, K.R.; Jaakola, L.; Jiři Grúz, J.; Strnad, M.; Torun, H.; Ayaz, F.A. Phenolic compounds and antioxidant capacity in different-colored and non-pigmented berries of bilberry (*Vaccinium myrtillus* L.). *Food Biosci.* **2017**, *20*, 67–78. [CrossRef]
4. Abreu, O.A.; Barreto, G.; Prieto, S. *Vaccinium* (*Ericaceae*): Ethnobotany and pharmacological potentials. *Emir. J. Food A* **2014**, *26*, 577–591. [CrossRef]
5. Esposito, D.; Chen, A.; Grace, M.H.; Komarnytsky, S.; Lila, M.A. Inhibitory effects of wild blueberry anthocyanins and other flavonoids on biomarkers of acute and chronic inflammation in vitro. *J. Agric. Food Chem.* **2014**, *62*, 7022–7028. [CrossRef]
6. Donnini, S.; Finetti, F.; Lusini, L.; Morbidelli, L.; Cheynier, V.; Barron, D.; Williamson, G.; Waltenberger, J.; Ziche, M. Divergent effects of quercetin conjugates on angiogenesis. *Br. J. Nutr.* **2006**, *95*, 1016–1023. [CrossRef]
7. Tenuta, M.C.; Deguin, B.; Loizzo, M.R.; Dugay, A.; Acquaviva, R.; Malfa, G.A.; Bonesi, M.; Bouzidi, C.; Tundis, R. Contribution of flavonoids and iridoids to the hypoglycaemic, antioxidant, and nitric oxide (NO) inhibitory activities of *Arbutus unedo* L. *Antioxidants* **2020**, *9*, 184. [CrossRef] [PubMed]
8. Brindisi, M.; Bouzidi, C.; Frattaruolo, L.; Loizzo, M.R.; Tundis, R.; Dugay, A.; Deguin, B.; Cappello, A.R.; Cappello, M.S. Chemical profile, antioxidant, anti-inflammatory, and anti-cancer effects of Italian *Salvia rosmarinus* spenn. methanol leaves extracts. *Antioxidants* **2020**, *9*, 826. [CrossRef]
9. Brindisi, M.; Bouzidi, C.; Frattaruolo, L.; Loizzo, M.R.; Cappello, M.S.; Dugay, A.; Deguin, B.; Lauria, G.; Cappello, A.R.; Tundis, R. New Insights into the antioxidant and anti-inflammatory effects of Italian *Salvia officinalis* leaf and flower extracts in lipopolysaccharide and tumor-mediated inflammation models. *Antioxidants* **2021**, *10*, 311. [CrossRef]
10. Wu, X.; Wang, T.T.Y.; Prior, R.L.; Pehrsson, P.R. Prevention of atherosclerosis by berries: The case of blueberries. *J. Agric. Food Chem.* **2018**, *66*, 9172–9188. [CrossRef]
11. Kalt, W.; Cassidy, A.; Howard, L.R.; Krikorian, R.; Stull, A.J.; Tremblay, F.; Zamora-Ros, R. Recent research on the health benefits of blueberries and their anthocyanins. *Adv. Nutr.* **2020**, *11*, 224–236. [CrossRef]
12. Kemper, K.J. Bilberry (Vaccinium myrtillus). *Longwood Herb. Task Force* **1999**, *20115386*, 55–71.
13. Morazzoni, P.; Bombardelli, E. *Vaccinium myrtillus* L. *Fitoterapia* **1996**, *68*, 3–29.
14. Frohne, D. *Heidelbeerblätter*; Teedrogen., M.W., Ed.; Wissenschaftliche Verlagsgesell: Stuttgart, Germany, 1990; pp. 217–219.
15. Mustafa, B.; Hajdari, A.; Pieroni, A.; Pulaj, B.; Koro, X.; Quave, C.L. A cross-cultural comparison of folk plant uses among Albanians, Bosniaks, Gorani and Turks living in south Kosovo. *J. Ethnobiol. Ethnomed.* **2015**, *12*, 11–39. [CrossRef]
16. Leduc, C.; Coonishish, J.; Haddad, P.; Cuerrier, A. Plants used by the Cree Nation of Eeyou Istchee (Quebec, Canada) for the treatment of diabetes: A novel approach in quantitative ethnobotany. *J. Ethnopharmacol.* **2006**, *105*, 55–63. [CrossRef] [PubMed]
17. Kari, P.R. *Upper Tanana Ethnobotany*; Alaska Historical Commission: Anchorage, Alaska, 1985.
18. *Standard for the Plant Drug of Heilongjiang Province*; Heilongjiang Provincial Drug Administration: Harbin, China, 2001; p. 198.
19. Mozaffarian, V. Identification of medicinal and aromatic plants of Iran. *Farhang Moaser Tehran* **2013**, 391–392.
20. Pervin, M.; Hasnat, M.A.; Lim, B.O. Antibacterial and antioxidant activities of *Vaccinium corymbosum* L. leaf extract. *Asian Pac. J. Trop. Dis.* **2013**, *3*, 444–453. [CrossRef]

21. Pervin, M.; Hasnat, M.A.; Lim, J.H.; Lee, Y.M.; Kim, E.O.; Um, B.H.; Lim, B.O. Preventive and therapeutic effects of blueberry (*Vaccinium corymbosum*) extract against DSS-induced ulcerative colitis by regulation of antioxidant and inflammatory mediators. *J. Nutr. Biochem.* **2016**, *28*, 103–113. [CrossRef] [PubMed]
22. Branning, C.; Hakansson, A.; Ahrne, S.; Jeppsson, B.; Molin, G.; Nyman, M. Blueberry husks and multi-strain probiotics affect colonic fermentation in rats. *Br. J. Nutr.* **2009**, *101*, 859–870. [CrossRef]
23. Karppinen, K.; Zoratti, L.; Nguyenquynh, N.; Häggman, H.; Jaakola, L. Molecular and metabolic mechanisms associated with fleshy fruit quality. *Front. Plant Sci.* **2016**, *7*, 657.
24. Blumberg, J.B.; Camesano, T.A.; Cassidy, A.; Kris-Etherton, P.; Howell, A.; Manach, C.; Ostertag, L.M.; Sies, H.; Skulas-Ray, A.; Vita, J.A. Cranberries and their bioactive constituents in human health. *Adv. Nutr.* **2013**, *4*, 618–632. [CrossRef]
25. Su, Z. Anthocyanins and flavonoids of *Vaccinium*, L. *Pharm. Crops* **2012**, *3*, 7–37. [CrossRef]
26. Gao, L.; Mazza, G. Quantitation and distribution of simple and acylated anthocyanins and other phenolics in blueberries. *J. Food Sci.* **1994**, *59*, 1057–1059. [CrossRef]
27. Beattie, J.; Crozier, A.; Duthie, G.G. Potential health benefits of berries. *Curr. Nutr. Food Sci.* **2005**, *1*, 71–86. [CrossRef]
28. Borges, G.; Degeneve, A.; Mullen, W.; Crozier, A. Identification of flavonoid and phenolic antioxidants in black currants, blueberries, raspberries, red currants, and cranberries. *J. Agric. Food Chem.* **2010**, *58*, 3901–3909. [CrossRef] [PubMed]
29. Cho, M.J.; Howard, L.R.; Prior, R.L.; Clark, J.R. Flavonoid glycosides and antioxidant capacity of various blackberry, blueberry, and red grape genotypes determined by high-performance liquid chromatography/mass spectrometry. *J. Sci. Food Agric.* **2004**, *84*, 1771–1782. [CrossRef]
30. Taruscio, T.G.; Barney, D.L.; Exon, J. Content and profile of flavanoid and phenolic acid compounds in conjunction with the antioxidant capacity for a variety of northwest *Vaccinium* berries. *J. Agric. Food Chem.* **2004**, *52*, 3169–3176. [CrossRef] [PubMed]
31. Zheng, W.; Wang, S.Y. Oxygen radical absorbing capacity of phenolics in blueberries, cranberries, chokeberries, and lingonberries. *J. Agric. Food Chem.* **2003**, *51*, 502–509. [CrossRef]
32. Suomalainen, H.; Keranen, A.J.A. The first anthocyanins appearing during the ripening of blueberries. *Nature* **1961**, *191*, 498–499. [CrossRef]
33. Cabrita, L.; Froystein, N.A.; Andersen, O.M. Anthocyanin trisaccharides in blueberries of *Vaccinium padifolium*. *Food Chem.* **2000**, *69*, 33–36. [CrossRef]
34. Du, Q.; Jerz, G.; Winterhalter, P. Isolation of two anthocyanin sambubiosides from bilberry (*Vaccinium myrtillus*) by high-speed counter-current chromatography. *J. Chromatogr. A* **2004**, *1045*, 59–63. [CrossRef]
35. Spela, M.; Tomaz, P.; Lea, G.; Darinka, K.; Andreja, V.; Natasa, P.U.; Veronika, A. Phenolics in Slovenian bilberries (*Vaccinium myrtillus* L.) and blueberries (*Vaccinium corymbosum* L.). *J. Agric. Food Chem.* **2011**, *59*, 6998–7004.
36. Scibisz, I.; Mitek, M. Influence of freezing process and frozen storage on anthocyanin contents of highbush blueberries. *Food Sci. Technol. Qual.* **2007**, *5*, 231–238.
37. Wu, X.; Prior, R.L. Systematic identification and characterization of anthocyanins by HPLC-ESI-MS/MS in common foods in the United States: Fruits and berries. *J. Agric. Food Chem.* **2005**, *53*, 2589–2599. [CrossRef] [PubMed]
38. Pappas, E.; Schaich, K.M. Phytochemicals of cranberries and cranberry products: Characterization, potential health effects, and processing stability. *Crit. Rev. Food Sci. Nutr.* **2009**, *49*, 741–781. [CrossRef]
39. Andersen, O.M. Chromatographic separation of anthocyanins in cowberry (lingonberry) *Vaccinium vites-idaea* L. *J. Food Sci.* **1985**, *50*, 1230–1232. [CrossRef]
40. Ek, S.; Kartimo, H.; Mattila, S.; Tolonen, A. Characterization of phenolic compounds from lingonberry (*Vaccinium vitis-idaea* L.). *J. Agric. Food. Chem.* **2006**, *54*, 9834–9842. [CrossRef] [PubMed]
41. Hokkanen, J.; Mattila, S.; Jaakola, L.; Pirttila, A.M.; Tolonen, A. Identification of phenolic compounds from lingonberry (*Vaccinium vitis-idaea* L.), bilberry (*Vaccinium myrtillus* L.) and hybrid bilberry (*Vaccinium x intermedium* Ruthe, L.) leaves. *J. Agric. Food Chem.* **2009**, *57*, 9437–9447. [CrossRef] [PubMed]
42. Laetti, A.K.; Riihinen, K.R.; Jaakola, L. Phenolic compounds in berries and flowers of a natural hybrid between bilberry and lingonberry (*Vaccinium intermedium* Ruthe). *Phytochemistry* **2011**, *72*, 810–815. [CrossRef]
43. Madhavi, D.L.; Bomser, J.; Smith, M.A.L.; Singleton, K. Isolation of bioactive constituents of *Vaccinium myrtillus* (bilberry) fruits and cell cultures. *Plant Sci.* **1998**, *131*, 95–103. [CrossRef]
44. Pan, Y.F.; Qu, W.J.; Li, J.G.; Gu, Y.B. Qualitative and quantitative analysis of flavonoid aglycones from fruit residue of *Vaccinium vitis-idaea* L. by HPLC. *Nat. Prod. Res. Develop.* **2005**, *17*, 641–644.
45. Latti, A.K.; Kainulainen, P.S.; Hayirlioglu-Ayaz, S.; Ayaz, F.A.; Riihinen, K.R. Characterization of anthocyanins in Caucasian blueberries (*Vaccinium arctostaphylos* L.) native to Turkey. *J. Agric. Food Chem.* **2009**, *57*, 5244–5249. [CrossRef] [PubMed]
46. Nickavar, B.; Amin, G.; Salehi-Sormagi, M.H. Anthocyanins from *Vaccinium arctostaphylos* berries. *Pharm. Biol.* **2004**, *42*, 289–291. [CrossRef]
47. Witzell, J.; Gref, R.; Näsholm, T. Plant-part specific and temporal variation in phenolic compounds of boreal bilberry (*Vaccinium myrtillus*) plants. *Biochem. Syst. Ecol.* **2003**, *31*, 115–127. [CrossRef]
48. Laaksonen, O.; Sandell, M.; Kallio, H. Chemical factors contributing to orosensory profiles of bilberry (*Vaccinium myrtillus*) fractions. *Eur. Food Res. Technol.* **2010**, *231*, 271–285. [CrossRef]

49. Cesoniene, L.; Daubaras, R.; Jasutiene, I.; Vencloviene, J.; Miliauskiene, I. Evaluation of the biochemical components and chromatic properties of the juice of *Vaccinium macrocarpon* Aiton and *Vaccinium oxycoccos* L. *Plant Food Hum. Nutr.* **2011**, *66*, 238–244. [CrossRef]
50. Cui, Z.H.; Yuan, C.S. Flavones of *Vaccinium uliginosum* fruits. *Fitoterapia* **1992**, *63*, 283.
51. Lehtonen, H.M.; Lehtinen, O.; Suomela, J.P.; Viitanen, M.; Kallio, H. Flavonol glycosides of sea buckthorn (*Hippophae rhamnoides* ssp. sinensis) and lingonberry (*Vaccinium vitis-idaea*) are bioavailable in humans and monoglucuronidated for excretion. *J. Agric. Food Chem.* **2010**, *58*, 620–627. [CrossRef]
52. Latti, A.K.; Jaakola, L.; Riihinen, K.R.; Kainulainen, P.S. Anthocyanin and flavonol variation in bog bilberries (*Vaccinium uliginosum* L.) in Finlan. *J. Agric. Food Chem.* **2009**, *58*, 427–433. [CrossRef] [PubMed]
53. Li, R.; Wang, P.; Guo, P.; Wang, Z.Y. Anthocyanin composition and content of the *Vaccinium uliginosum* berry. *Food Chem.* **2011**, *125*, 116–120. [CrossRef]
54. Yang, G.X.; Fan, H.L.; Zheng, Y.N.; Li, Y.D. Separation and identification of the flavonoids in the fruit of *Vaccinium uliginosum* L. blueberry. *J. Jilin. Agric. Univ.* **2005**, *27*, 643–644.
55. Sellappan, S.; Akoh, C.C.; Krewer, G. Phenolic compounds and antioxidant capacity of Georgia-grown blueberries and blackberries. *J. Agric. Food Chem.* **2002**, *50*, 2432–2438. [CrossRef] [PubMed]
56. Zadernowski, R.; Naczk, M.; Nesterowicz, J. Phenolic acid profiles in some small berries. *J. Agric. Food Chem.* **2005**, *53*, 2118–2124. [CrossRef]
57. Wang, C.; Zuo, Y. Ultrasound-assisted hydrolysis and gas chromatography-mass spectrometric determination of phenolic compounds in cranberry products. *Food Chem.* **2011**, *128*, 562–568. [CrossRef] [PubMed]
58. Zhang, K.; Zuo, Y. GC-MS determination of flavonoids and phenolic and benzoic acids in human plasma after consumption of cranberry juice. *J. Agric. Food Chem.* **2004**, *52*, 222–227. [CrossRef] [PubMed]
59. Zuo, Y.; Wang, C.; Zhan, J. Separation, characterization, and quantitation of benzoic and phenolic antioxidants in American cranberry fruit by GC-MS. *J. Agric. Food Chem.* **2002**, *50*, 3789–3794. [CrossRef]
60. Ayaz, F.A.; Hayirlioglu-Ayaz, S.; Gruz, J.; Novak, O.; Strnad, M. Separation, characterization, and quantitation of phenolic acids in a little-known blueberry (*Vaccinium arctostaphylos* L.) fruit by HPLC-MS. *J. Agric. Food Chem.* **2005**, *53*, 8116–8122. [CrossRef] [PubMed]
61. Dinda, B.; Debnath, S.; Harigaya, Y. Naturally occurring iridoids. A review, part 1. *Chem. Pharm. Bull.* **2007**, *55*, 159–222. [CrossRef] [PubMed]
62. Tundis, R.; Loizzo, M.R.; Menichini, F.; Statti, G.A.; Menichini, F. Biological and pharmacological activities of iridoids: Recent developments. *Mini Rev. Med. Chem.* **2008**, *8*, 399–420. [CrossRef]
63. Wang, C.; Gong, X.; Bo, A.; Zhang, L.; Zhang, M.; Zang, E.; Zhang, C.; Li, M. Iridoids: Research advances in their phytochemistry, biological activities, and pharmacokinetics. *Molecules* **2020**, *25*, 287. [CrossRef]
64. Heffels, P.; Müller, L.; Schieber, A.; Weber, F. Profiling of iridoid glycosides in *Vaccinium* species by UHPLC-MS. *Food Res. Int.* **2017**, *100*, 462–468. [CrossRef]
65. Tenuta, M.C.; Malfa, G.A.; Marco, B.; Rosaria, A.; Loizzo, M.R.; Dugay, A.; Bouzidi, C.; Tomasello, B.; Tundis, A.; Deguin, B. LC-ESI-QTOF-MS profiling, protective effects on oxidative damage, and inhibitory activity of enzymes linked to type 2 diabetes and nitric oxide production of *Vaccinium corymbosum* L. (Ericaceae) extracts. *J. Berry Res.* **2020**, *10*, 603–622. [CrossRef]
66. Turner, A.; Chen, S.N.; Nikolic, D.; van Breemen, R.; Farnsworth, N.R.; Pauli, G.F. Coumaroyl iridoids and a depside from cranberry (*Vaccinium macrocarpon*). *J. Nat. Prod.* **2007**, *70*, 253–258. [CrossRef]
67. Leisner, C.P.; Kamileen, M.O.; Conway, M.E.; O'Connor, S.E.; Buell, C.R. Differential iridoid production as revealed by a diversity panel of 84 cultivated and wild blueberry species. *PLoS ONE* **2017**, *12*, e0179417.
68. Ma, C.; Dastmalchi, K.; Flores, G.; Wu, S.B.; Pedraza-Peñalosa, P.; Long, C.; Kennelly, E.J. Antioxidant and metabolite profiling of North American and neotropical blueberries using LC-TOF-MS and multivariate analyses. *J. Agric. Food Chem.* **2013**, *61*, 3548–3559. [CrossRef]
69. Kondo, M.; MacKinnon, S.L.; Craft, C.C.; Matchett, M.D.; Hurta, R.A.; Neto, C.C. Ursolic acid and its esters: Occurrence in cranberries and other *Vaccinium* fruit and effects on matrix metalloproteinase activity in DU145 prostate tumor cells. *J. Sci. Food Agric.* **2011**, *91*, 789–796. [CrossRef]
70. Chu, W.; Gao, H.; Cao, S.; Fang, X.; Chen, H.; Xiao, S. Composition and morphology of cuticular wax in blueberry (*Vaccinium* spp.) fruits. *Food Chem.* **2017**, *219*, 436–442. [CrossRef]
71. Ayaz, F.A.; Kadioglu, A.; Bertoft, E.; Acar, C.; Turna, I. Effect of fruit maturation on sugar and organic acid composition in two blueberries (*Vaccinium arctostaphylos* and *V. myrtillus*) native to Turkey. *New Zealand. J. Crop Hort. Sci.* **2001**, *29*, 137–141. [CrossRef]
72. Huopalahti, R.; Järvenpää, E.P.; Katina, K. A novel solid-phase extraction-hplc method for the analysis of anthocyanin and organic acid composition of finish cranberry. *J. Liquid Chrom. Related Technol.* **2000**, *23*, 2695–2701. [CrossRef]
73. Kalt, W.; McDonald, J.E. Chemical composition of lowbush blueberry cultivars. *J. Am. Soc. Hort. Sci.* **1996**, *121*, 142–146. [CrossRef]
74. Riihinen, K.; Jaakola, L.; Karenlampi, S.; Hohtola, A. Organ-specific distribution of phenolic compounds in bilberry (*Vaccinium myrtillus*) and "northblue" blueberry (*Vaccinium corymbosum* × *V. angustifolium*). *Food Chem.* **2008**, *110*, 156–160. [CrossRef]

75. Teleszko, M.; Wojdyło, A. Comparison of phenolic compounds and antioxidant potential between selected edible fruits and their leaves. *J. Funct. Foods* **2015**, *14*, 736–746. [CrossRef]
76. Ferlemi, A.V.; Mermigki, P.G.; Makri, O.E.; Anagnostopoulos, D.; Koulakiotis, N.S.; Margarity, M.; Tsarbopoulos, A.; Georgakopoulos, C.D.; Lamari, F.N. Cerebral area differential redox response of neonatal rats to selenite-induced oxidative stress and to concurrent administration of highbush blueberry leaf polyphenols. *Neurochem. Res.* **2015**, *40*, 2280–2292. [CrossRef]
77. Ferlemi, A.V.; Lamari, F.N. Berry leaves: An alternative source of bioactive natural products of nutritional and medicinal value. *Antioxidants* **2016**, *5*, 17. [CrossRef]
78. Wang, L.J.; Wu, J.; Wang, H.X.; Li, S.S.; Zheng, X.C.; Du, H.; Xu, Y.J.; Wang, L.S. Composition of phenolic compounds and antioxidant activity in the leaves of blueberry cultivars. *J. Funct. Foods* **2015**, *16*, 295–304. [CrossRef]
79. Ieri, F.; Martini, S.; Innocenti, M.; Mulinacci, N. Phenolic distribution in liquid preparations of *Vaccinium myrtillus* L. and *Vaccinium vitis idaea* L. *Phytochem. Anal.* **2013**, *24*, 467–475. [CrossRef] [PubMed]
80. Sidorova, Y.; Shipelin, V.; Mazo, V.; Zorin, S.; Petrov, N.; Kochetkova, A. Hypoglycemic and hypolipidemic effect of *Vaccinium myrtillus* L. leaf and *Phaseolus vulgaris* L. seed coat extracts in diabetic rats. *Nutrition* **2017**, *41*, 107–112. [CrossRef] [PubMed]
81. Mzhavanadze, V.V. Kaempferol glycosides from the leaves of the Cancasian bilberry, *Vaccinium arctostaphylos*. *Soobshch Akad Nauk Gruz SSR* **1971**, *62*, 445–447.
82. Kader, F.; Rovel, B.; Girardin, M.; Metche, M. Fractionation and identification of the phenolic compounds of highbush blueberries (*Vaccinium corymbosum* L.). *Food Chem.* **1996**, *55*, 35–40. [CrossRef]
83. Scibisz, I.; Mitek, M. Antioxidant activity and phenolic compound content in dried highbush blueberries (*Vaccinium corymbosum* L.). *Zywnosc* **2006**, *13*, 68–76.
84. Martz, F.; Jaakola, L.; Julkunen-Tiitto, R.; Stark, S. Phenolic composition and antioxidant capacity of bilberry (*Vaccinium myrtillus*) leaves in Northern Europe following foliar development and along environmental gradients. *J. Chem. Ecol.* **2010**, *36*, 1017–1028. [CrossRef]
85. Neto, C.C.; Salvas, M.R.; Autio, W.R.; van den Heuvel, J.E. Variation in concentration of phenolic acid derivatives and quercetin glycosides in foliage of cranberry that may play a role in pest deterrence. *J. Am. Soc. Hortic. Sci.* **2010**, *135*, 494–500. [CrossRef]
86. Mzhavanadze, V.V.; Targamadze, I.L.; Dranik, L.I. Phenolic compounds of the leaves of *Vaccinium arctostaphylos*. *Chem. Nat. Comp.* **2004**, *8*, 125–126. [CrossRef]
87. Szakiel, A.; Paczkowski, C.; Huttunen, S. Triterpenoid content of berries and leaves of bilberry *Vaccinium myrtillus* from Finland and Poland. *J. Agric. Food Chem.* **2012**, *60*, 11839–11849. [CrossRef]
88. Ramassamy, C. Emerging role of polyphenolic compounds in the treatment of neurodegenerative diseases: A review of their intracellular targets. *Eur. J. Pharmacol.* **2006**, *545*, 51–64. [CrossRef]
89. Miller, K.; Feucht, W.; Schmid, M. Bioactive compounds of strawberry and blueberry and their potential health effects based on human intervention studies: A brief overview. *Nutrients* **2019**, *11*, 1510. [CrossRef] [PubMed]
90. Mantzorou, M.; Zarros, A.; Vasios, G.; Theocharis, S.; Pavlidou, E.; Giaginis, C. Cranberry: A promising natural source of potential nutraceuticals with anticancer activity. *Anticancer Agents Med. Chem.* **2019**, *19*, 1672–1686. [CrossRef] [PubMed]
91. Del Bó, C.; Riso, P.; Campolo, J.; Møller, P.; Loft, S.; Klimis-Zacas, D.; Brambilla, A.; Rizzolo, A.; Porrini, M. A single portion of blueberry (*Vaccinium corymbosum* L.) improves protection against DNA damage but not vascular function in healthy male volunteers. *Nutr. Res.* **2013**, *33*, 220–227. [CrossRef]
92. Vinson, J.A.; Bose, P.; Proch, J.; Al Kharrat, H.; Samman, N. Cranberries and cranberry products: Powerful in vitro, ex vivo, and in vivo sources of antioxidants. *J. Agric. Food Chem.* **2008**, *56*, 5884–5891. [CrossRef] [PubMed]
93. Yao, Y.; Vieira, A. Protective activities of *Vaccinium* antioxidants with potential relevance to mitochondrial dysfunction and neurotoxicity. *Neurotoxicology* **2007**, *28*, 93–100. [CrossRef] [PubMed]
94. Torri, E.; Lemos, M.; Caliari, V.A.L.; Kassuya, C.; Bastos, J.K.; Andrade, S.F. Anti-inflammatory and antinociceptive properties of blueberry extract (*Vaccinium corymbosum*). *J. Pharm. Pharmacol.* **2007**, *59*, 591–596. [CrossRef] [PubMed]
95. Pereira, S.R.; Pereira, R.; Figueiredo, I.; Freitas, V.; Dinis, T.C.; Almeida, L.M. Comparison of anti-inflammatory activities of an anthocyanin-rich fraction from Portuguese blueberries (*Vaccinium corymbosum* L.) and 5-aminosalicylic acid in a TNBS-induced colitis rat model. *PLoS ONE* **2017**, *12*, e0174116. [CrossRef] [PubMed]
96. Marziano, C.; Genet, G.; Hirschi, K.K. Vascular endothelial cell specification in health and disease. *Angiogenesis* **2021**. [CrossRef]
97. Matsuzawa, Y.; Lerman, A. Endothelial dysfunction and coronary artery disease: Assessment, prognosis, and treatment. *Coron. Artery Dis.* **2014**, *25*, 713–724. [CrossRef] [PubMed]
98. Daiber, A.; Steven, S.; Weber, A.; Shuvaev, V.V.; Muzykantov, V.R.; Laher, I.; Li, H.; Lamas, S.; Münzel, T. Targeting vascular (endothelial) dysfunction. *Br. J. Pharmacol.* **2017**, *174*, 1591–1619. [CrossRef]
99. Alfaras, I.; Di Germanio, C.; Bernier, M.; Csiszar, A.; Ungvari, Z.; Lakatta, E.G.; de Cabo, R. Pharmacological strategies to retard cardiovascular aging. *Circ. Res.* **2016**, *118*, 1626–1642. [CrossRef]
100. Mensah, G.A.; Wei, G.S.; Sorlie, P.D.; Fine, L.J.; Rosenberg, Y.; Kaufmann, P.G.; Mussolino, M.E.; Hsu, L.L.; Addou, E.; Engelgau, M.M.; et al. Decline in cardiovascular mortality: Possible causes and implications. *Circ. Res.* **2017**, *120*, 366–380. [CrossRef]
101. Cravotto, G.; Boffa, L.; Genzini, L.; Garella, D. Phytotherapeutics: An evaluation of the potential of 1000 plants. *J. Clin. Pharm. Ther.* **2010**, *35*, 11–48. [CrossRef] [PubMed]

102. Martineau, L.C.; Couture, A.; Spoor, D.; Benhaddou-Andaloussi, A.; Harris, C.; Meddah, B.; Leduc, C.; Burt, A.; Vuong, T.; Mai Le, P.; et al. Anti-diabetic properties of the Canadian lowbush blueberry *Vaccinium angustifolium* Ait. *Phytomedicine* **2006**, *13*, 612–623. [CrossRef]
103. Chan, S.W.; Chu, T.T.W.; Choi, S.W.; Benzie, I.F.F.; Tomlinson, B. Impact of short-term bilberry supplementation on glycemic control, cardiovascular disease risk factors, and antioxidant status in Chinese patients with type 2 diabetes. *Phytother. Res.* **2021**. [CrossRef]
104. Shahcheraghi, S.H.; Aljabali, A.A.A.; Al Zoubi, M.S.; Mishra, V.; Charbe, N.B.; Haggag, Y.A.; Shrivastava, G.; Almutary, A.G.; Alnuqaydan, A.M.; Barh, D.; et al. Overview of key molecular and pharmacological targets for diabetes and associated diseases. *Life Sci.* **2021**, *278*, 119632. [CrossRef]
105. McDougall, G.J.; Shpiro, F.; Dobson, P.; Smith, P.; Blake, A.; Stewart, D. Different polyphenolic components of soft fruits inhibit alpha-amylase and alpha-glucosidase. *J. Agric. Food Chem.* **2005**, *53*, 2760–2766. [CrossRef]
106. Bljajić, K.; Petlevski, R.; Vujić, L.; Čačić, A.; Šoštarić, N.; Jablan, J.; Saraiva de Carvalho, S.; Zovko Končić, M. Chemical composition, antioxidant and α-glucosidase-inhibiting activities of the aqueous and hydroethanolic extracts of *Vaccinium myrtillus* leaves. *Molecules* **2017**, *22*, 703. [CrossRef]
107. Karcheva-Bahchevanska, D.P.; Lukova, P.K.; Nikolova, M.M.; Mladenov, R.D.; Iliev, I.N. Effect of extracts of bilberries (*Vaccinium myrtillus* L.) on amyloglucosidase and α-glucosidase activity. *Folia Med.* **2017**, *59*, 197–202. [CrossRef]
108. Li, H.; Park, H.M.; Ji, H.S.; Han, J.; Kim, S.K.; Park, H.Y.; Jeong, T.S. Phenolic-enriched blueberry-leaf extract attenuates glucose homeostasis, pancreatic beta-cell function, and insulin sensitivity in high-fat diet-induced diabetic mice. *Nutr. Res.* **2020**, *73*, 83–96. [CrossRef] [PubMed]
109. Cásedas, G.; Les, F.; Gómez-Serranillos, M.P.; Smith, C.; López, V. Anthocyanin profile, antioxidant activity and enzyme inhibiting properties of blueberry and cranberry juices: A comparative study. *Food Funct.* **2017**, *8*, 4187–4193. [CrossRef]
110. Cutler, B.R.; Gholami, S.; Chua, J.S.; Kuberan, B.; Anandh Babu, P.V. Blueberry metabolites restore cell surface glycosaminoglycans and attenuate endothelial inflammation in diabetic human aortic endothelial cells. *Int. J. Cardiol.* **2018**, *261*, 155–158. [CrossRef]
111. Huang, W.; Yao, L.; He, X.; Wang, L.; Li, M.; Yang, Y.; Wan, C. Hypoglycemic activity and constituents analysis of blueberry (*Vaccinium corymbosum*) fruit extracts. *Diabetes Metab. Syndr. Obes.* **2018**, *11*, 357–366. [CrossRef]
112. Huang, W.; Yan, Z.; Li, D.; Ma, Y.; Zhou, J.; Sui, Z. Antioxidant and anti-inflammatory effects of blueberry anthocyanins on high glucose-induced human retinal capillary endothelial cells. *Oxidative Med. Cell Longev.* **2018**, *2018*, 1862462. [CrossRef] [PubMed]
113. Huang, W.; Hutabarat, R.P.; Chai, Z.; Zheng, T.; Zhang, W.; Li, D. Antioxidant blueberry anthocyanins induce vasodilation via PI3K/Akt signaling pathway in high-glucose-induced human umbilical vein endothelial cells. *Int. J. Mol. Sci.* **2020**, *21*, 1575. [CrossRef]
114. Song, Y.; Huang, L.; Yu, J. Effects of blueberry anthocyanins on retinal oxidative stress and inflammation in diabetes through Nrf2/HO-1 signaling. *J. Neuroimmunol.* **2016**, *301*, 1–6. [CrossRef] [PubMed]
115. Jafarizade, M.; Kahe, F.; Sharfaei, S.; Momenzadeh, K.; Pitliya, A.; Tajrishi, F.Z.; Singh, P.; Chi, G. The role of interleukin-27 in atherosclerosis: A contemporary review. *Cardiology* **2021**, *19*, 1–13. [CrossRef]
116. Cignarella, A.; Nastasi, M.; Cavalli, E.; Puglisi, L. Novel lipid-lowering properties of *Vaccinium myrtillus* L. leaves, a traditional antidiabetic treatment, in several models of rat dyslipidaemia: A comparison with ciprofibrate. *Thromb. Res.* **1996**, *84*, 311–322. [CrossRef]
117. Basu, A.; Lyons, T.J. Strawberries, blueberries, and cranberries in the metabolic syndrome: Clinical perspectives. *J. Agric. Food Chem.* **2012**, *60*, 5687–5692. [CrossRef]
118. Prior, R.L.; Wu, X.; Gu, L.; Hager, T.; Hager, A.; Wilkes, S.; Howard, L. Purified berry anthocyanins but not whole berries normalize lipid parameters in mice fed an obesogenic high fat diet. *Mol. Nutr. Food Res.* **2009**, *53*, 1406–1418. [CrossRef] [PubMed]
119. Kalt, W.; Foote, K.; Fillmore, S.A.; Lyon, M.; Van Lunen, T.A.; McRae, K.B. Effect of blueberry feeding on plasma lipids in pigs. *Br. J. Nutr.* **2008**, *100*, 70–78. [CrossRef]
120. Zagayko, A.L.; Kolisnyk, T.Y.; Chumak, O.I.; Ruban, O.A.; Koshovyi, O.M. Evaluation of anti-obesity and lipid-lowering properties of *Vaccinium myrtillus* leaves powder extract in a hamster model. *J. Basic Clin. Physiol. Pharmacol.* **2018**, *29*, 697–703. [CrossRef] [PubMed]
121. Peixoto, T.C.; Moura, E.G.; de Oliveira, E.; Soares, P.N.; Guarda, D.S.; Bernardino, D.N.; Ai, X.X.; Rodrigues, V.D.S.T.; de Souza, G.R.; da Silva, A.J.R.; et al. Cranberry (*Vaccinium macrocarpon*) extract treatment improves triglyceridemia, liver cholesterol, liver steatosis, oxidative damage and corticosteronemia in rats rendered obese by high fat diet. *Eur. J. Nutr.* **2018**, *57*, 1829–1844. [CrossRef]
122. Wu, X.; Kang, J.; Xie, C.; Burris, R.; Ferguson, M.E.; Badger, T.M.; Nagarajan, S. Dietary blueberries attenuate atherosclerosis in apolipoprotein E-deficient mice by upregulating antioxidant enzyme expression. *J. Nutr.* **2010**, *140*, 1628–1632. [CrossRef]
123. Matziouridou, C.; Marungruang, N.; Nguyen, T.D.; Nyman, M.; Fåk, F. Lingonberries reduce atherosclerosis in *Apoe*$^{-/-}$ mice in association with altered gut microbiota composition and improved lipid profile. *Mol. Nutr. Food Res.* **2016**, *60*, 1150–1160. [CrossRef]
124. Xie, C.; Kang, J.; Chen, J.R.; Lazarenko, O.P.; Ferguson, M.E.; Badger, T.M.; Nagarajan, S.; Wu, X. Lowbush blueberries inhibit scavenger receptors CD36 and SR-A expression and attenuate foam cell formation in ApoE-deficient mice. *Food Funct.* **2011**, *2*, 588–594. [CrossRef]

125. Xie, C.; Kang, J.; Chen, J.R.; Nagarajan, S.; Badger, T.M.; Wu, X. Phenolic acids are in vivo atheroprotective compounds appearing in the serum of rats after blueberry consumption. *J. Agric. Food Chem.* **2011**, *59*, 10381–10387. [CrossRef]
126. Heitzer, T.; Schlinzig, T.; Krohn, K.; Meinertz, T.; Münzel, T. Endothelial dysfunction, oxidative stress, and risk of cardiovascular events in patients with coronary artery disease. *Circulation* **2001**, *104*, 2673–2678. [CrossRef]
127. Curtis, P.J.; van der Velpen, V.; Berends, L.; Jennings, A.; Feelisch, M.; Umpleby, A.M.; Evans, M.; Fernandez, B.O.; Meiss, M.S.; Minnion, M.; et al. Blueberries improve biomarkers of cardiometabolic function in participants with metabolic syndrome-results from a 6-month, double-blind, randomized controlled trial. *Am. J. Clin. Nutr.* **2019**, *109*, 1535–1545. [CrossRef] [PubMed]
128. Del Bo', C.; Porrini, M.; Fracassetti, D.; Campolo, J.; Klimis-Zacas, D.; Riso, P. A single serving of blueberry (*V. corymbosum*) modulates peripheral arterial dysfunction induced by acute cigarette smoking in young volunteers: A randomized-controlled trial. *Food Funct.* **2014**, *5*, 3107–3116. [CrossRef]
129. Del Bo', C.; Deon, V.; Campolo, J.; Lanti, C.; Parolini, M.; Porrini, M.; Klimis-Zacas, D.; Riso, P. A serving of blueberry (*V. corymbosum*) acutely improves peripheral arterial dysfunction in young smokers and non-smokers: Two randomized, controlled, crossover pilot studies. *Food Funct.* **2017**, *8*, 4108–4117. [CrossRef]
130. Stull, A.J.; Cash, K.C.; Champagne, C.M.; Gupta, A.K.; Boston, R.; Beyl, R.A.; Johnson, W.D.; Cefalu, W.T. Blueberries improve endothelial function, but not blood pressure, in adults with metabolic syndrome: A randomized, double-blind, placebo-controlled clinical trial. *Nutrients* **2015**, *7*, 4107–4123. [CrossRef] [PubMed]
131. Zhu, Y.; Xia, M.; Yang, Y.; Liu, F.; Li, Z.; Hao, Y.; Mi, M.; Jin, T.; Ling, W. Purified anthocyanin supplementation improves endothelial function via NO-cGMP activation in hypercholesterolemic individuals. *Clin. Chem.* **2011**, *57*, 1524–1533. [CrossRef] [PubMed]
132. Wang, Z.; Pang, W.; He, C.; Li, Y.; Jiang, Y.; Guo, C. Blueberry anthocyanin-enriched extracts attenuate fine particulate matter (PM 2.5)-induced cardiovascular dysfunction. *J. Agric. Food Chem.* **2017**, *65*, 87–94. [CrossRef] [PubMed]
133. Vendrame, S.; Tsakiroglou, P.; Kristo, A.S.; Schuschke, D.A.; Klimis-Zacas, D. Wild blueberry consumption attenuates local inflammation in the perivascular adipose tissue of obese Zucker rats. *Appl. Physiol. Nutr. Metab.* **2016**, *41*, 1045–1051. [CrossRef] [PubMed]
134. Kim, J.; Kim, C.S.; Lee, Y.M.; Sohn, E.; Jo, K.; Kim, J.S. *Vaccinium myrtillus* extract prevents or delays the onset of diabetes-induced blood-retinal barrier breakdown. *Int. J. Food Sci. Nutr.* **2015**, *66*, 236–242. [CrossRef] [PubMed]
135. Mastantuono, T.; Starita, N.; Sapio, D.; D'Avanzo, S.A.; Di Maro, M.; Muscariello, E.; Paterni, M.; Colantuoni, A.; Lapi, D. The Effects of *Vaccinium myrtillus* extract on hamster pial microcirculation during hypoperfusion-reperfusion injury. *PLoS ONE* **2016**, *11*, e0150659. [CrossRef] [PubMed]
136. Bharat, D.; Cavalcanti, R.R.M.; Petersen, C.; Begaye, N.; Cutler, B.R.; Assis Costa, M.M.; Gomes Ramos, R.; Ferreira, M.R.; Li, Y.; Bharath, L.P.; et al. Blueberry metabolites attenuate lipotoxicity-induced endothelial dysfunction. *Mol. Nutr. Food Res.* **2018**, *62*, 1–17. [CrossRef]
137. Park, S.H.; Jeong, S.; Chung, H.T.; Pae Pterostilbene, H.E. An active constituent of blueberries, stimulates Nitric Oxide production via activation of endothelial nitric oxide synthase in human umbilical vein endothelial cells. *Plant Foods Hum. Nutr.* **2015**, *70*, 263–268. [CrossRef] [PubMed]
138. Huang, W.; Zhu, Y.; Li, C.; Sui, Z.; Min, W. Effect of blueberry anthocyanins malvidin and glycosides on the antioxidant properties in endothelial cells. *Oxidative Med. Cell. Longev.* **2016**, *2016*, 1591803. [CrossRef]
139. Morgan, K.M.; Loloi, J.; Songdej, N. Cranberry supplementation as a cause of major intraoperative bleeding during vascular surgery due to aspirin-like platelet inhibition. *Blood Coagul. Fibrinolysis* **2020**, *31*, 402–404.
140. Izzo, A.A.; Hoon-Kim, S.; Radhakrishnan, R.; Williamson, E.M. A critical approach to evaluating clinical efficacy, adverse events and drug interactions of herbal remedies. *Phytother. Res.* **2016**, *30*, 691–700. [CrossRef] [PubMed]

MDPI
St. Alban-Anlage 66
4052 Basel
Switzerland
Tel. +41 61 683 77 34
Fax +41 61 302 89 18
www.mdpi.com

Applied Sciences Editorial Office
E-mail: applsci@mdpi.com
www.mdpi.com/journal/applsci

www.ingramcontent.com/pod-product-compliance
Lightning Source LLC
LaVergne TN
LVHW070635100526
838202LV00012B/812